# *Human*
# PARASITOLOGY

BURTON J. BOGITSH
Vanderbilt University

THOMAS C. CHENG
Medical University of South Carolina

Saunders College Publishing

Philadelphia   New York   Chicago
San Francisco   Montreal   Toronto
London   Sydney   Tokyo

Cover: False-color transmission electron micrograph of a single cell infected with the apicomplexan *Toxoplasma* sp. *Toxoplasma* appears as the roughly spherical pink bodies filling the entire cell. *T. gondii* infects a variety of mammals, including humans, sometimes provoking an acute illness, toxoplasmosis (see page 134). CNRI/Science Photo Library/Photo Researchers, Inc.

Biological drawings by Cécile Duray-Bito.

Maps by Fiona King.

Additional illustration and photo credits appear on pages 421–424, which constitute a continuation of the copyright page.

Printed in the United States of America
HUMAN PARASITOLOGY
0-03-046203-7
Library of Congress Catalog Card Number: 89-84690
9012 039 987654321

To Glenn and Libby,
who left us too soon.

# PREFACE

Several years ago, the authors began to consider writing a
textbook of human parasitology designed for premedical,
medical technology, and biology students in need of basic
knowledge of the biology of parasitism. While emphasizing
the medical aspects, the book would include sufficient functional morphology, physiology, biochemistry, and immunology to foster greater appreciation of the diverse implications
of parasitism. In addition, it would explore the means by
which certain parasites cause morbidity and mortality and
would present, where known, the modes of action of certain
modern chemotherapeutic agents. Through considerable
discussion and several revisions of the manuscript, this volume evolved. The authors believe that *Human Parasitology*
serves as an intermediate between textbooks devoted almost
exclusively to the "classical" clinical parasitology approach
and more advanced treatises that provide in-depth treatments of parasite taxonomy, physiology, biochemistry, and
immunology.

In this age of radiation therapy, immunosuppressive
drugs, and AIDS (Acquired Immune Deficiency Syndrome)—all of which serve to reduce immunocompetence in
the human host—the importance of parasites once considered inconsequential has mushroomed. Toxoplasmosis,
pneumocystosis, and other parasitic infections have become
diseases of major consequence. For this reason and others,
including marked increases in world travel and immigration,
it has become imperative that students preparing for careers
in the allied health sciences, medicine, and public health acquire some knowledge of parasitic diseases of humans. This
book has been written with such students in mind.

Classification of parasites is an integral part of the discipline. This book has been organized by placing the classification schemes most widely favored in current usage at the end of the first chapter in each part. This leaves the level of emphasis to the discretion of the instructor. References that are recommended as ancillary reading are also included at the end of each chapter.

It must be recognized that the field of chemotherapy is advancing at such a rapid pace that new drugs become available constantly. Consequently, current information about drugs of choice will become obsolete more rapidly than will information presented in other sections of the book. Nevertheless, at the end of the book is an appendix listing the specific, currently prescribed chemotherapeutic regimens that may prove useful to prospective medical students.

Newly discovered organisms that can and do parasitize humans, as well as adaptations among normally nonpathogenic parasites, continue to be documented. For instance, during the past three decades there have been fascinating discoveries that free-living amoebae such as *Naegleria fowleri* and Acanthamoeba species can become highly lethal pathogens as a result of facultative parasitism. Furthermore, it has been established that a number of essentially benign protozoans can become highly pathogenic in immunologically compromised hosts. The authors have not attempted to identify and discuss all parasites that have been reported from humans but only those considered to be of major significance.

This volume is designed for a one-semester or one-quarter course and, as such, presents the material in a less detailed format.

An Instructor's Manual is available containing suggested course syllabuses, course objectives, instructional strategies, review questions, and a selected bibliography.

## ACKNOWLEDGMENTS

Numerous friends and associates have been kind enough to review and criticize several versions of this book during manuscript preparation. Among these we want to thank especially Dr. Frank J. Etges of the University of Cincinnati; Dr. Grover C. Miller of North Carolina State University; Dr. Stuart A. Krassner of the University of California, Irvine; and Dr. John Mackiewicz of the State University of New York, Albany. We also thank Dr. Laverne Buldhaupt, University of Wisconsin—La Crosse; Dr. Albert Canaris, University of Texas at El Paso; Dr. Gerald Coles, University of Massachusetts at Amherst; Dr. Paul Nollen, Western Illinois University; Dr. Leslie Uhazy, University of Missouri at Columbia; Dr. Steven Zam, University of Florida; Dr. William Chobotar, Andrews University; Dr. Brent Nickol, University of Nebraska at Lincoln; and Dr. Peter Castro, California Polytechnic State University at Pomona.

# CONTENTS

# CHAPTER ONE

# SYMBIOSIS AND PARASITISM

Parasitology, the study of parasites and their relationships to their hosts, is one of the most fascinating areas of biology. The study of parasitism is interdisciplinary, encompassing aspects of systematics and phylogeny, ecology, morphology, embryology, physiology, biochemistry, immunology, pharmacology, and nutrition, among others. Newly developed techniques in biochemistry and cellular and molecular biology have also opened significant new avenues for research on parasites.

Not only does parasitology touch upon many disciplines, but the varied nature of parasites renders their study multifaceted. While it is entirely proper to classify many bacteria and fungi and all viruses as parasites, parasitology has traditionally been limited to parasitic protozoa, helminths, arthropods, and those species of arthropods that serve as vectors for parasites. It follows, then, that parasitology encompasses elements of protozoology, helminthology, entomology, and acarology. The World Health Organization has proclaimed that, of the six major unconquered human tropical diseases, five—schistosomiasis, malaria, filariasis, African trypanosomiasis, and leishmaniasis—are parasitic in the traditional sense. Leprosy, the sixth major disease, is caused by a bacterium.

## DEFINITIONS

The complexity of the host–parasite relationship has often led to misunderstandings of the precise nature of parasitism. In order to avoid such misperceptions, researchers have devised the following concepts to distinguish among the several types of associations involving heterospecific organisms.

Any organism that spends a portion or all of its life intimately associated with another living organism of a different species is known as a **symbiont** (or symbiote), and the relationship is designated as **symbiosis.** The term *symbiosis,* as used here, does not imply mutual or unilateral physiologic dependency; rather, it is used in its original sense (living together) without any reference to "benefit" or "damage" to the symbionts.

Although the lines of demarcation between them are indistinct, at least four categories of symbiosis are commonly recognized: commensalism, phoresis, parasitism, and mutualism. The scope of this text is limited to relationships of medical importance, and, since parasitism is the major type of symbiosis meeting this criterion, definitions of the other forms are included for clarification only.

**Commensalism.** Commensalism does not involve physiologic interaction or dependency between the two partners, the **host** and the **commensal.** Literally, the term means "eating at the same table." In other words, commensalism is a type of symbiosis in which spatial proximity allows the commensal to feed on substances captured or ingested by the host. The two partners can survive independently. Although at times certain nonpathogenic organisms (e.g., protozoa) are referred to as commensals, this interpretation is incorrect since they are physiologically dependent on the host and are, therefore, parasites. An example of commensalism is the association of hermit crabs and the sea anemones they carry on their borrowed shells.

**Phoresis.** The term *phoresis* is derived from the Greek word meaning "to carry." In this type of symbiotic relationship, the **phoront,** usually the smaller organism, is mechanically carried by the other, usually larger, organism, the host. Phoresis is a form of symbiosis in which no physiologic interaction or dependency is involved. Both commensalism and phoresis can be considered spatial, rather than physiologic, relationships. Examples of phoresis are the numerous sedentary protozoans, algae, and fungi that attach to the bodies of aquatic arthropods, turtles, etc.

**Parasitism.** Parasitism is another type of symbiotic relationship between two organisms: a **parasite,** usually the smaller of the two, and a host, upon which it is physiologically dependent. The relationship may be permanent, as in the case of tapeworms found in the vertebrate intestine, or temporary, as with female mosquitoes, some leeches, and ticks, which feed intermittently on host blood. Such parasites are considered **obligatory parasites** because they are physiologically dependent upon their hosts and usually cannot survive if kept isolated from them. **Facultative parasites,** on the other hand, are essentially free-living organisms that are capable of becoming parasitic if placed in a situation conducive to such a mode. An example of a facultative parasite is the amoeba *Naegleria*.

The physiologic requirements of most parasites are only partly known and understood, but there is sufficient information to indicate certain categories of dependence, such as nutritional. Unlike commensals, parasites derive essential nutrients directly from the host, usually from such nutritive substances as blood, lymph, cytoplasm, tissue fluids, and host-digested food.

The intimate relationship between parasite and host generally exposes the host to antigenic substances of parasite origin. Sometimes these antigens consist of the molecules that make up the surface of the parasite (**somatic antigens**), or they may be molecules secreted or excreted by the parasite (**metabolic antigens**). In either case, the host typically responds to the presence of such antigens by synthesizing antibodies. Thus, unlike phoresis and commensalism, parasitism usually involves, in addition to the physiologic dependency of the parasite, immunological responses by the host. The effect upon the host is usually the result of host reaction to the presence of the parasite. One of the more important consequences of such reaction—which may be localized at the site of attachment or deposition or may be more generalized, perhaps throughout the entire host body—is the limitation of the populations of the parasite. It is axiomatic in helminthology that "all species of worms are harmful when present in massive numbers" (Fig. 1–1); therefore, internal defense responses by the host help to reduce pathological effects of the parasite.

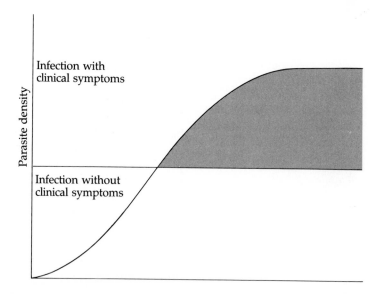

**Figure 1–1**
**Graph showing the correlation of disease with clinical symptoms and greater parasite density.**

While there are numerous systems for classifying host–parasite relationships, the one used here distinguishes between two major types of parasites, **endoparasites** and **ectoparasites,** according to location. Endoparasites live within the body of the host at sites such as the alimentary tract, liver, lungs, and urinary bladder; ectoparasites are attached to the outer surface of the host or are superficially embedded in the body surface.

According to its role, the host may be classified as (1) a **definitive host,** if the parasite attains sexual maturity therein; (2) an **intermediate host,** if it serves as a temporary, but essential, environment for the development of the parasite and/or its metamorphosis short of sexual maturity; and (3) a **transfer** or **paratenic host,** if it is not necessary for the completion of the parasite's life cycle but is utilized as a temporary refuge and a vehicle for reaching an obligatory, usually the definitive, host in the cycle.

Generally, an arthropod or some other invertebrate that serves as a host as well as a carrier for a parasite is referred to as a **vector.** Unlike the transfer host, the vector is essential for completion of the life cycle. In this text, the term is used to designate an organism, usually an arthropod, that transmits a parasite to the **human** or **vertebrate host;** for example, various species of anopheline mosquitoes serve as vectors for the malaria-producing protozoan parasites, *Plasmodium* spp., and transmit the organisms to humans, who serve as vertebrate hosts. From an evolutionary perspective, some intermediate hosts, or vectors as in the case of the *Plasmodium*–mosquito relationship, may once have been definitive hosts, while others may have been transfer or paratenic hosts.

Infected animals that serve as sources of infective organisms for humans are known as **reservoir hosts.** A wild animal in this role is called a **sylvatic reservoir host;** a domestic animal, a **domestic reservoir host.** For example, one type of human filariasis is caused by a filarial worm, *Brugia malayi,* which is transmitted to humans by a mosquito. Although infections are usually transmitted from one person to another via the mosquito, *B. malayi* can also be transmitted to humans from cats (domestic reservoirs) or monkeys (sylvatic reservoirs). Often, the reservoir host tolerates the parasitic infection better than the human host does. Thus, the reservoir host, by definition, shares the same stage of the parasite with humans.

The term **zoonosis** can be used in various contexts; it is used here to denote a disease of humans that is caused by a pathogenic parasite normally found in wild and domestic vertebrate animals. Person-to-person transmission does not normally occur in zoonosis. An example of a zoonotic disease of significant medical importance is trichinellosis, caused by the nematode *Trichinella spiralis*. The worm is found in a variety of sylvatic and domestic reservoirs, notably pigs, bears, and rodents. Humans become infected by consuming raw or undercooked meat from infected animals.

**Mutualism.**    The fourth category of symbiosis, mutualism, is an association in which the **mutualist** and the host depend on each other physiologically. A classic example of this type of relationship occurs between certain species of flagellated protozoans and the termites in whose gut they live. The flagellate, which depends almost entirely on a carbohydrate diet, acquires nutrients from wood chips ingested by the host termite. In return, the flagellate synthesizes and secretes cellulases, cellulose-digesting enzymes, the endproducts of which the termite utilizes. Incapable of synthesizing its own cellulases, the termite is, thus, dependent on the mutualist and, in turn, provides developmental stimuli to the mutualist and a hospitable environment for reproduction. If the termite is defaunated, it will die; and, conversely, the flagellate cannot survive outside the termite.

**Figure 1–2**
**Schematic drawing illustrating the overlapping between the major categories of symbiosis.**
Note that there is less overlapping between commensalism/phoresis and parasitism and mutualism than between parasitism and mutualism.

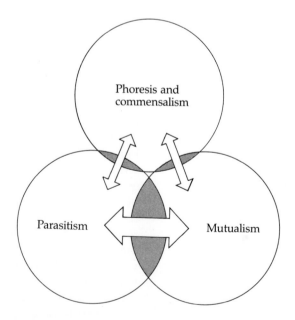

Following definition of symbiosis and the subcategories of heterospecific relationships, it is important to note that definitions are often arbitrary. They are useful in many cases for categorizing natural symbiotic associations; however, in certain instances, there is considerable overlap. Figure 1–2 illustrates, for example, that some associations qualify as both phoretic and commensalistic or as both commensalistic and parasitic. Such overlapping relationships may be regarded as transitional stages that may reflect evolutionary shifts from one category to another. It has been suggested that, theoretically at least, a complete and progressive gradation exists among the various types of symbiosis. This may come about when, for example, in the shift from parasitism to mutualism, the parasite initially gives off some nonessential metabolic by-product that can be utilized by the host; eventually, the host becomes physiologically dependent not only on this by-product of parasite origin but on other factors as well, and the relationship evolves into a mutualistic one.

## ECOLOGY OF PARASITISM

Conceptually, the body of a host constitutes the environment on or in which the parasite spends some or all of its life. Further, the host's environment, whether tropical jungle or freshwater pond, also affects the parasite via the host. In recent years, some parasite ecologists have proposed the use of techniques employed in quantitative life-history studies of free-living populations (i.e., r- and K-selection analysis) for determining certain quantitative aspects of the population biology of parasites. By definition, **r-selection** is the effective process when selective forces upon organisms (r-strategists) are unstable and environmental conditions are variable. **K-selection,** on the other hand, is the process that prevails when forces influencing the organisms (K-strategists) remain relatively stable over a period of time. R-strategists are characterized by high fecundity and, frequently, high, density-independent mortality rates, short life spans, effective dispersal mechanisms, and population sizes that vary over time and are usually below the carrying capacity of the environment. K-strategists are characterized by relatively low rates of fecundity and, generally, low, density-dependent mortality, longer life spans, and relatively stable population sizes. It can be seen, then, that mechanisms that regulate populations of r-strategists are independent of population density, whereas those for populations of K-strategists are density-dependent.

As an example, in the context of parasite ecology, digenetic trematodes are considered r-strategists since both their biotic potential and their mortality rates are high as a result of selective pressures in their unstable environments—unstable in that their habitats differ at practically every phase of their complex life cycles.

It should be emphasized that r- and K-strategy designations are relative. Species B, for example, may be an r-strategist when compared to species C, but a K-strategist when compared to species A.

A number of influences, such as the presence or absence of certain biological, chemical, and physical factors, dictate the geographic distribution of a parasite. For instance, the ability of a particular species of parasite to survive depends upon the availability of all hosts needed to complete its life cycle; therefore, factors governing survival of hosts indirectly govern the presence of parasites. Another feature governing distribution of a parasite is **host specificity,** or the adaptability of a species of parasite to a certain host or group of hosts. The degree of specificity varies from species to species. Host specificity is determined by genetic, immunological, physiological, and/or ecological factors.

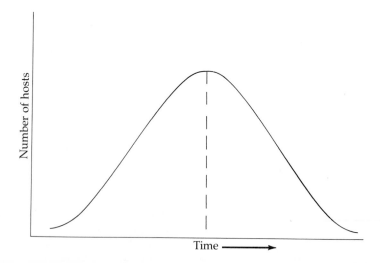

**Figure 1–3**
**Hypothetical scheme showing an increase in the number of obligatory hosts in the evolution of parasites.**
However, as time increases, the number of obligatory hosts decreases.

Many of these ecological aspects play important roles in defining the **epidemiology** of a disease-producing parasite. Epidemiology is the study of factors responsible for the transmission and distribution of disease. The distribution and characteristics of various hosts (including vectors), host specificity, cultural patterns of human hosts (such as diet, often influenced by religion, economic status, etc.), and density of host and parasite populations all influence the epidemiology of pathogenic parasites.

# EVOLUTION OF PARASITISM

When and how did parasites arise? While there is no definitive answer, it is agreed that parasites have evolved among very diverse groups of free-living progenitors. One of these earlier organisms probably formed an initially casual association with another organism, and one member of the pair, perhaps due to **preadaptation,** developed a gradually increasing dependency on the other. The term *preadaptation,* in the context of parasitism, denotes the potential in a free-living organism for adaptation to a parasitic (symbiotic) lifestyle. The predisposition may never become operational as long as the organism remains free-living; however, if for some reason it becomes associated with a potential host, this latent ability becomes critically important for survival should hostile environmental conditions develop. Preadaptations can be structural, developmental, and/or physiological.

Parasites of the alimentary tract probably became such after having been swallowed, either accidentally or intentionally, by the host. If they were preadapted to withstand the environment or were capable of subsequent adaptation to it, they might have become progressively more dependent upon the new environment or might even have migrated to other areas, such as the lungs or the liver. It is evident that parasites requiring two or more hosts developed their multi-host life cycles sequentially. For instance, blood-inhabiting flagellates first parasitized the alimentary tracts of insects and, when introduced into vertebrate blood while the insect was feeding, adapted to that environment secondarily. Thus, present intermediate hosts once may well have been definitive hosts. Recent studies suggest, however, that the advancement to parasitism is best represented by a bell-shaped curve (Fig. 1–3) in which the increasing number of intermediate hosts signifies higher adaptability only up to a point. Thereafter, elimination of certain hosts is considered a more successful state because simplification of the life cycle may enhance the parasite's chance of reaching the definitive host.

## SUGGESTED READINGS

Anderson, R. M., and May, R. M. 1982. Coevolution of hosts and parasites. *Parasitology* 85, 411–426.

Canning, E. U., and Cright, C. A. 1972. Behavioral aspects of parasite transmission. *Linnaean Society of London,* London.

Cheng, T. C. 1986. *General Parasitology,* 2nd ed. Academic Press, Orlando, FL.

Read, C. P. 1970. *Parasitism and Symbiosis.* The Ronald Press, New York.

Force, D. C. 1974. Succession of *r* and *k* strategists in parasitoids. In *Evolutionary Strategies of Parasitic Insects and Mites* (P. W. Price, ed.), pp. 112–129. Plenum Press, New York.

# CHAPTER TWO

## PARASITE–HOST INTERACTIONS

An integral part of modern parasitology is the study of host–parasite relationships. A knowledge of how the parasite survives in its host may serve as the basis for the eventual control of the parasite. For instance, new chemotherapeutic agents may be synthesized if biochemical differences are found to exist between the parasite and its host, or the elaboration of vaccines may be accomplished if the immunological responses of the host to the parasite and the parasite's evasion of these responses are known. Other avenues involving genetic engineering and the like may open as additional knowledge is gathered.

## EFFECTS OF PARASITES ON HOSTS

Parasites trigger varying degrees of change within their hosts. Although not inevitably, disease often results. As previously noted, parasitic diseases, especially when caused by metazoan parasites, are usually functions of parasite density. Two factors commonly influence the onset of recognizable disease symptoms: the number of parasites and the physiological condition of the host. Small numbers of parasites often elicit no clinical symptoms. Several of the conditions that most often develop in parasitic diseases are discussed below.

### Tissue Damage

Beyond the erosion caused by ingestion or by mechanical disruption of cells by the parasite, three major types of histopathological cell damage occur in parasite-injured tissues.

*Parenchymatous or Albuminous Degeneration.*    Swollen cells packed with albuminous or fatty granules, indistinct nuclei, and pale cytoplasm. This type of damage is often seen in infected liver, cardiac muscle, and kidney cells.

*Fatty Degeneration.*    Deposition of abnormal amounts of fat in cells. This type of degeneration imparts a yellowish color to the cells and is common among parasite-laden liver cells.

*Necrosis.*    Death of cells or tissues resulting from persistent cell degeneration of any type. The dead cells give tissues an opaque appearance. Encystment and calcification of *Trichinella spiralis* larvae in mammalian skeletal muscle cells cause necrosis of the surrounding tissue.

## Tissue Changes

Cell and tissue parasites sometimes evoke changes in the growth pattern of the affected tissue. Some of these changes are very deleterious; others are merely structural with no serious systemic consequences to the host organism. Tissue changes of parasitic origin are of four major types.

*Hyperplasia.*    An increase in cell number resulting from accelerated cell division resulting from an elevated cell metabolic rate. This condition, when associated with parasitism, is precipitated by the marked increase in host body repair activity that commonly follows inflammation. For example, inflammation caused by the liver fluke *Fasciola hepatica* stimulates excessive division of epithelial cells lining the bile duct, with a resultant thickening of the duct wall.

*Hypertrophy.*    An increase in cell or organ size usually due, in parasitism, to the presence of intracellular parasites. For example, during the erythrocytic phase in the life cycle of the malaria-producing organism *Plasmodium vivax*, the parasitized red blood cells and the spleen commonly become enlarged.

*Metaplasia.*    Conversion of one type of tissue into another without the intervention of embryonic tissue. This can be seen in patients infected with the lung fluke *Paragonimus westermani*, which is surrounded by a host capsule consisting of cells—for example, fibrocytes—transformed from other types of cells.

*Neoplasia.*    Abnormal cell growth in a tissue, producing an entirely new entity, such as a tumor. The neoplastic tumor is not inflammatory, is not required for the repair of organs, and does not conform to the normal growth pattern. Neoplasms may be **benign,** that is, may remain localized with no invasion of adjacent tissues, or **malignant,** that is, may invade adjacent tissues or spread (metastasize) to other parts of the body through the blood or lymph. Cancers are malignant neoplasms. The human blood fluke *Schistosoma haematobium* is sometimes associated with malignant neoplasia of the urinary bladder.

# BIOLOGICAL ADAPTATIONS OF PARASITISM

The intimacy of parasite–host associations invariably involves physiological, biochemical, morphological, and immunological adaptations. In this section, aspects of physiology, biochemistry, and immunology will be addressed briefly; morphological adaptations will be considered in subsequent chapters.

## Physiology and Biochemistry of Parasitism

The study of parasitism deals with such basic questions as "How are parasites physiologically dependent upon their hosts?" "How do parasites affect their hosts?" and "How do hosts affect the parasites?" Also, since the antigenicity of parasites has somatic as well as physiologic origin, increasing attention is being focused upon the chemical composition of parasite bodies and metabolites. Consequently, it is important for anyone interested in parasitism and parasites to understand the enzymatic activities, pathways associated with energy production, protective mechanisms, secretions and excretions, respiration, and general metabolism of parasites.

From a practical viewpoint, the primary requisite in modern chemotherapeutic research as it relates to parasitic diseases is the identification of some metabolic process vital to a pathogenic parasite that does not occur in the host or that can be chemically impaired or halted in the host with no adverse effect. After such identification, potential therapeutic agents can be developed to inhibit the process, killing the pathogen without harming the host.

The discussion of chemotherapy in subsequent sections includes the information available about targets within the parasite toward which such agents are directed. Chemotherapy must be upgraded continuously as parasites evolve resistance to a particular drug or family of drugs and as research suggests new, more effective targets for drug action.

## Immunology

The guiding principle in immunology is the recognition by animals of *self* and *nonself*. Immunoparasitological implications of this principle are manifested in one of two ways:

either the host recognizes the parasite as foreign (nonself) and reacts against it, or the parasite camouflages itself so that it is accepted by the host as a part of self and, therefore, elicits little or no reaction. In one highly successful type of immunologic camouflage, known as **molecular mimicry,** the parasite produces hostlike molecules on its body surface or its surface becomes covered with host molecules and, as a result, the host is duped into accepting them as its own.

A parasite, whether protozoan or metazoan, is a mosaic of various molecules that when recognized by the host as nonself are known as **antigens.** An antigen is any substance, usually proteinaceous, that is capable, under appropriate conditions, of inducing the host to synthesize **antibodies.** The two substances interact to form an antigen–antibody complex. Antibodies are proteins synthesized in response either to an antigen or, in varying degrees, to molecules of similar structure. A parasite or any portion thereof recognized by the host as antigenic generally elicits one of two responses—either a **cellular** (or **cell-mediated**) **reaction** or a **humoral reaction.** In a cellular reaction, specialized cells are mobilized to arrest and, usually, to eventually destroy the parasite; in a humoral reaction, specialized molecules in the circulatory system interact with the parasite, usually immobilizing or destroying it, or with excretory–secretory products (ESP) of the parasite, forming a precipitate of antigen–antibody complexes.

When a host is immunologically challenged, it signals a functionally specialized type of lymphocyte, a **receptor cell,** to produce a specific antibody (Fig. 2–1). This signal originates from the binding of either the antigen or an antigenically sensitized cell (such as a macrophage) to specific receptors on the receptor cell surface. Each receptor cell carries only one type of specific receptor and will, therefore, respond to only a few closely related antigenic determinants, which may be thought of as chemically distinguishable regions of the surface of the antigen molecule. Once the antigen is bound to the receptor site, the receptor cell is stimulated to proliferate and differentiate into clones. Each cloned cell displays surface receptors of the same configuration (or **idiotype**) as the originally stimulated cell. Receptor cells originate from bone marrow and are of two types: **B cells** (= **B lymphocytes**) and **T cells** (= **T lymphocytes**). B cells are so designated because they were originally recognized by their dependence upon processing through the bursa of Fabricius, an avian lymphoid tissue attached to the intestine

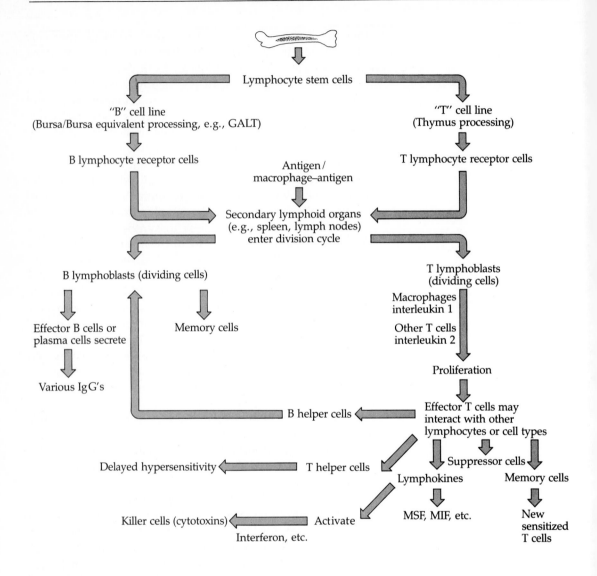

**Figure 2–1**
**Generalized scheme showing the basic patterns of lymphocyte development and differentiation to become immunocompetent.**

near the cloaca. In mammals, processing of B cells is believed to occur in gut-associated lymphoid tissue (GALT) and bone marrow. T cells, on the other hand, are so designated because they must be processed through the thymus. B cells produce humoral, or circulating, antibodies, while T cells elicit cell-mediated reactions usually independent of circulating antibodies. In certain situations, however, humoral antibodies also elicit cell-mediated reactions, as in the case of antibody-dependent, cell-mediated cytotoxicity, described below.

The introduction of parasite antigen into a vertebrate sometimes triggers a series of events involving T cells. After the antigen is phagocytosed by macrophages, the macrophage surface exhibits specific antigenic determinants. T cells, processed through the thymus and equipped with complementary surface receptors, enter lymph tissues, such as spleen and lymph nodes, and come in contact with sensitized macrophages. Or the antigen may bind directly to a complementary receptor site of a T cell. In either case, the sensitized T cells, now known as **T lymphoblasts,** proliferate and differentiate into **effector T cells** that possess antibody on the surface. On entering the general circulation, these specialized T cells function in several ways. For example, one type, called **memory cells,** reverts to a "resting state" and serves as a source of new, sensitized T cells whenever the same antigen enters the body again. Most T cell activity, however, is concentrated in the synthesis and release of various chemical mediators called **lymphokines.** Lymphokines react with other cells essential to the inflammatory process. For instance, lymphokines regulate the activity of macrophages **(macrophage stimulating factor, macrophage inhibitory factor),** attract other types of cells to the inflamed site **(chemotactic factor),** or delay or totally inhibit cell proliferation **(cytostatic factor).**

Two other types of effector T cells are **killer T cells,** which eliminate foreign cells either directly or through lymphokines, and **helper T cells,** which facilitate B cell differentiation and proliferation. It is possible that killer T cells are activated by the lymphokine called **interferon,** which also is known to act directly upon a number of viruses.

An example of T cell action against a specific parasite is seen in the mammalian host reaction in schistosomiasis (see pp. 205–208). Much of the pathology in this disease results from granuloma formation, an immunological response to parasite eggs trapped in host tissues. Antigenic molecules, released through the porous shells of trapped eggs, sensitize T cells, which in turn release lymphokines. The lymphokines attract macrophages to the trapped egg and stimulate phagocytosis. Other cell participants in the inflammatory reaction include eosinophils, neutrophils, and fibroblasts, which accumulate at the site of antigen production. Finally, intercellular collagenous fibers are deposited to form a granuloma, sealing off the egg from surrounding tissue. This reaction to the parasite's antigen also illustrates **delayed hypersensitivity,** an increased reactivity to specific antigens that is mediated by cells rather than antibodies. It is termed *delayed* because of its slow onset; it requires 24 hours to reach maximum intensity.

The B cell follows basically the same pattern of sensitization described for T cells—that is, processing in lymph tissues, transformation to B lymphoblasts, and proliferation as effector B cells or **plasma cells** (Fig. 2–2). The plasma cell, which has a half-life of only a few days, secretes into the circulation large numbers of antibodies of the same idiotype and antigen-recognition specificity as its cell surface receptors. These antibodies, of which there are five classes, are

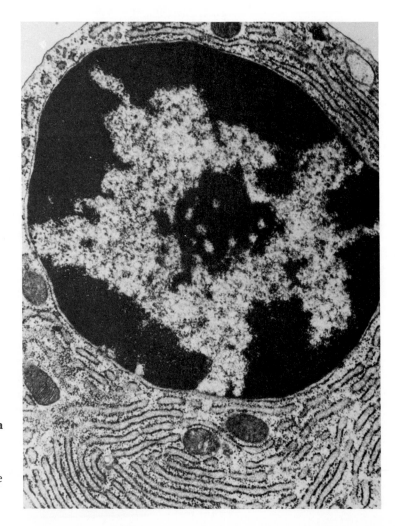

**Figure 2–2**
**Electron micrograph of plasma cell from guinea pig bone marrow.**
Note the extensive rough endoplasmic reticulum and the finely granular contents in the cisternae.

**Table 2–1    Classes of Immunoglobulins**

| Class | Molecular Weight | Biological Function |
|-------|------------------|---------------------|
| IgG | 150,000 | Fix complement<br>Bind to amine-containing cells (e.g., mast cells and basophils)<br>Bind to macrophages and granulocytes<br>Cross placenta |
| IgA | 170,000 | Secreted across mucus surface |
| IgM | 890,000 | Fix complement<br>Secreted across mucus surface |
| IgD | 150,000 | ? |
| IgE | 196,000 | Bind to amine-containing cells (e.g., mast cells and basophils) |

known collectively as **immunoglobulins** (Ig's) (Table 2–1). The first Ig formed is usually IgM (mu), but, with the aid of helper T cells, the B cell can shift to production of any of the other four classes: IgG (gamma), IgE (epsilon), IgA (alpha), or IgD (delta). Except for IgD, the function of which is not totally understood, all classes of Ig's are found in blood and tissue fluids. IgM and IgA are also the primary Ig's in the intestinal lumen. IgE levels are often elevated in helminth infections. In inflammatory reactions they, as well as some subclasses of IgG, can bind via their Fc regions to the surfaces of mast cells and basophils, inducing these cells to release vasoactive substances—such as histamines, which increase capillary permeability.

The currently accepted concept of synthesis and secretion of immunoglobulins by B cells with specific idiotypes is known as the **clonal selection theory.** Briefly, this theory states that B lymphocytes are committed to the production of a particular antibody (immunoglobulin) by genetically determined cell surface receptors. There is a huge population of receptor lymphocytes, each bearing a surface receptor of different antigenic specificity. When an antigen of appropriate idiotype is introduced to the B cell surface and combines with the specific receptor, the combination stimulates the B cell to differentiate and proliferate into a clone of plasma cells, each of which synthesizes Ig's that have the same specificity as the parent cell. The cells of one portion of the clone remain small, serving as memory cells.

**Figure 2–3
IgG molecule.**

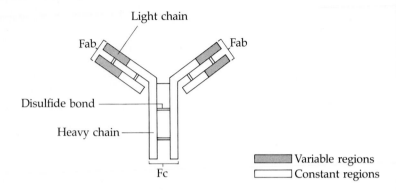

The IgG molecule (Fig. 2–3) illustrates the basic molecular structure of immunoglobulins. The molecule is composed of two identical light chains and two identical heavy chains held together by disulfide bonds. Antigenic specificity lies in regions of the chains susceptible to variation in amino acid sequences (**Fab portions**). Regions where the amino acid sequences remain constant (**Fc portions**) determine the biological properties of the particular class of immunoglobulins.

Reactions of immunoglobulins with antigens vary according to the kind and size of the antigen or the antigen-carrying structure. One such reaction is **antibody-dependent cell-mediated cytotoxicity**, referred to earlier. This interaction usually involves particulate antigens typically associated with parasite surfaces. In the diagram in Fig. 2–4, one class of immunoglobulins, IgE, recognizes and attaches to the parasite surface antigens by means of its Fab ends, exposing Fc portions to the environment. White blood cells—for example, eosinophils with surface IgE–Fc receptor sites—attach to the parasite surface and destroy it by releasing lysosomal hydrolases or other cytotoxic factors onto the parasite.

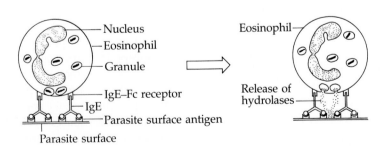

**Figure 2–4
Antibody-dependent cell-mediated cytotoxicity.**

# Resistance

Defined as the ability of a host to withstand infection by a parasite, **resistance** may develop in several ways. (1) It may result from the presence of some physical or chemical barrier that prevents the parasite from penetrating or migrating in the host. Such a barrier is thought to prevent the larval form of avian blood flukes from entering the circulatory system of abnormal hosts, for example, humans. (2) Resistance may also be due to **natural** or **innate immunity.** This type of immunity is conferred when, for example, certain proteins that are naturally present within an organism display structural properties of antibodies to specific antigens even though the organism (i.e., the potential host) has had no previous exposure to those antigens. Natural immunity may also be influenced by such factors as the host's genetic makeup, age, nutritional status, receptor molecules on cells, and gender. (3) **Acquired immunity** is a host's immune response to previous parasitic infection. This type of resistance, like natural immunity, is attracting a great deal of attention in the development of vaccines. **Premunition,** a form of acquired immunity, is resistance to reinfection dependent upon retention of the infectious agent. This type of resistance is seen in regions where malaria is endemic and low parasitemia is maintained in the victim when the disease is left untreated.

## SELECTED READINGS

Bloom, B. R. 1979. Games parasites play: How parasites evade immune surveillance. *Nature* 279, 21–26.

Campbell, W. C. 1986. The chemotherapy of parasitic infections. *Journal of Parasitology* 72, 45–61.

Damian, R. 1964. Molecular mimicry: Antigen sharing by parasite and host and its consequences. *American Naturalist* 98, 129–149.

Leder, P. 1982. The genetics of antibody diversity. *Scientific American* 246, 102–115.

Trager, W. 1986. *Living Together.* Plenum Press, New York.

Wakelin, D. 1984. *Immunity to Parasites: How Animals Control Parasitic Infections.* Edward Arnold Publishers, Baltimore.

# PART ONE
# THE PROTOZOA

# CHAPTER THREE

# GENERAL CHARACTERISTICS OF THE PROTOZOA

Despite immense diversity, organisms of the kingdom Protista share a number of characteristics. Perhaps the most distinctive of these characteristics are that the organisms (1) are all single-celled or colonial and (2) are eukaryotic. Despite these broad criteria, however, sufficient diversity exists, even within the subkingdom Protozoa, to give rise to frequent confusion in taxonomy. The taxonomic scheme adopted for this text is one whereby protozoans parasitic to humans are assigned to three phyla—Sarcomastigophora, Apicomplexa, and Ciliophora—with method of locomotion being one basis for identification. For example, within the phylum Sarcomastigophora, the amoebae (subphylum Sarcodina) move by means of pseudopodia; the flagellates (subphylum Mastigophora) use flagella as their primary locomotor apparatus; and the ciliates (phylum Ciliophora) propel themselves by cilia. Members of the phylum Apicomplexa are primarily intracellular parasites and, except at some stages of their life cycles (flagellated gametes in some species), do not possess locomotor organelles. In some species limited movement is accomplished by contraction of intracellular microfilaments.

A terminology unique in many ways to the protozoans has developed, based on light microscopy studies. Increased use of electron microscopy, however, has shown that many of these structures are ubiquitous to all eukaryotic cells. To preclude confusion resulting from the use of two sets of terms, those used in cell biology are adopted herein with attempts to correlate them to their older counterparts.

## LOCOMOTOR ORGANELLES

### Flagella

The Mastigophora, commonly known as flagellates, include all protozoans usually exhibiting in their **trophozoite** (motile) stage one or more flagella (Fig. 3–1). The ability to swim has facilitated the flagellates' adaptation to a variety of habitats in their hosts. Unlike amoebae, which require a substrate on which to move, flagellates thrive in a liquid medium and thus are well adapted for survival in the blood, lymph, and cerebrospinal fluid of the host. Their elongate, torpedo-shaped form enables them to swim in the host's

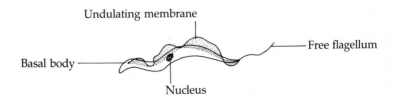

**Figure 3–1**
**A typical flagellate showing**
**relationship among flagella,**
**nucleus, basal bodies, and**
**undulating membrane.**

body fluids with little resistance, a further adaptation for life in a liquid medium.

While flagella are also found in the developmental stages of some amoebae and in the microgametes of some members of the phylum Apicomplexa, they are an invariable characteristic of the trophozoite stage of all flagellates. The number of flagella per organism varies widely according to species.

The single flagellum is a filamentous cytoplasmic projection. When examined with an electron microscope, this projection is seen to be a sheath consisting of a cytoplasmic matrix enclosed by a **plasma membrane** within which is embedded an axial filament or **axoneme** (Fig. 3–2). The axoneme, extending the length of the flagellum, consists of a series of regularly oriented microtubules arranged in a specific pattern of two central microtubules surrounded by an

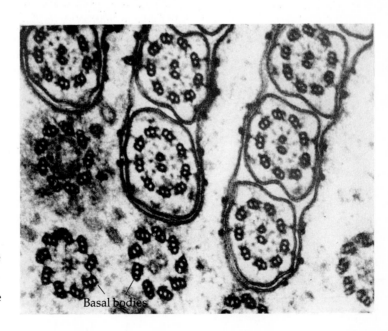

**Figure 3–2**
**Electron micrograph of cross-sections of flagella of**
***Pseudotrichonympha* from the gut of a termite.**
Note that the median fibrils are single and the marginal ones are double. Sections through basal bodies are seen below the flagella.

**Figure 3–3**
Schematic representation of flagellar organization.

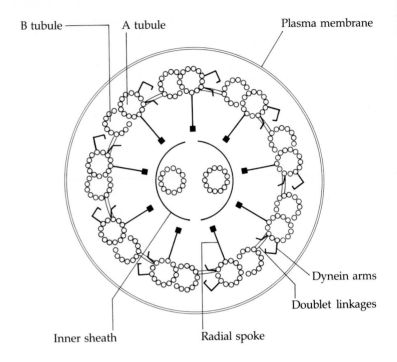

outer circle of nine pairs of microtubules or doublets (Fig. 3–3). Each flagellum is anchored in the cytoplasm by a **basal body** (also called a **blepharoplast** or **kinetosome**) (Fig. 3–4a). Recent ultrastructural studies demonstrate that the basal body is morphologically identical to the centriole of the cell, and it is from this organelle that the flagellum (or cilium) originates. The centriole and basal body consist of microtubules arranged in a circle of nine triplets, with two members of each triplet probably giving rise to and extending distally as one of the peripheral doublets of the flagellum (Fig. 3–4b).

In most flagellated cells, the flagellum extends from the basal body to the exterior; in some, however, one or more flagella may loop back in a complete reversal of their original direction. A flagellum of this type is known as a **recurrent flagellum** (Fig. 3–1). A recurrent flagellum may extend into a cytostome, where it aids in the procurement of food. Or it may be attached to the plasma membrane by a series of desmosomes, in which case, during the beating process, it pulls the plasma membrane and a portion of the cytoplasm away from the body of the cell, producing an **undulating membrane** (Figs. 3–1, 3–5).

**Figure 3–4**
**General cilium structure.**
(a) Longitudinal aspect of
flagellum and basal body.
(b) Cross-section through basal
body.

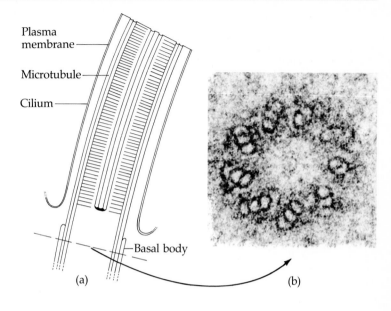

Plasma
membrane

Microtubule

Cilium

Basal body

(a)                    (b)

**Figure 3–5**
**Transmission electron
micrograph of** *Trypanosoma
brucei rhodesiense* **(slender
form) in transverse section.**
The surface coat (small arrows)
is seen as a dense layer
covering the plasma membrane
of both body (below) and
flagellum (above). Large
arrowhead points to
desmosome-like attachment of
flagellar membrane to surface
membrane. On the left, also in
transverse section, is one of the
streamer-like extensions that
may represent a mechanism for
shedding the variable antigen
coat.

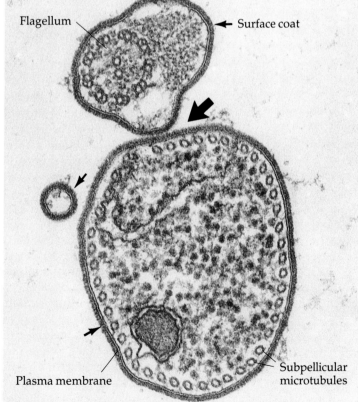

Flagellum                    Surface coat

Plasma membrane

Subpellicular
microtubules

**Figure 3–6**
**Representation of sliding-filament mechanism of ciliary and flagellar bending.**
(a) No resistance to sliding, and doublets slide past one another. (b) Cross-links cause a resistance to sliding at one region. Displacement of doublets in nonlinked regions is accommodated by bending.

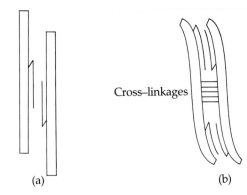

Cross–linkages

(a)                              (b)

It is seen, then, that flagellar movement propels and directs the organism and at times assists in procuring food. The movement may also promote tactility and secretion of mating substances.

The so-called "beat" of a flagellum (or cilium) is actually the propagation of a series of wavelike bends along the length of the organelle that are associated with the connections between outer microtubules and the inner sheath containing the two central microtubules. Energy to fuel this movement comes from the ATPase activity of the **dynein** arms associated with one member of each of the outer doublets (Fig. 3–3). This energy allows the doublet microtubules to slide past each other; however, since this action is restricted by chemical cross-links between the two microtubules, a bending occurs, which becomes a wave as the cross-links are broken and reformed along the axoneme (Fig. 3–6). When this phenomenon occurs sequentially, a regular beat pattern emerges, resulting in directional movement of the cell.

## Cilia

The fine structure of the axoneme of flagella and cilia is identical. Cilia may therefore be considered miniature flagella. In addition to noticeable differences in length, however, there are other fundamental differences between these two types of organelles, the most obvious of which is their number. Flagella usually number no more than ten on a given cell surface, while there may be literally thousands of cilia on a surface. An exception is seen in the flagellate order Hypermastigida, whose members possess greater numbers of flagella. In ciliates the numerous basal bodies are also interconnected by a series of subpellicular **microfilaments** or **neurofibrils,** forming an **infraciliature** believed to be responsible for either coordinating the ciliary beat of the cell or providing support for the ciliary beat. Nevertheless, the exact control mechanism of this coordination is not presently understood.

## Pseudopodia

Amoebae are usually capable of producing **pseudopodia,** which are used as locomotor and food-acquiring organelles. These transitory body extensions depend for their function on the association of actin and myosin. These two molecules function in a manner similar to their roles in the contraction of vertebrate muscle. Activated by ATP-derived energy and certain cations, such as calcium and magnesium, actin and myosin become intimately associated at the tip of the forming pseudopodium. This association produces a localized contractile response in the cytoplasm, whereupon the cytoplasm everts at the plasma membrane and moves posteriad in the cell, forming an outer zone of cytoplasm known as the **ectoplasm.** At the rear of the cell, actin and myosin become dissociated; the ectoplasm reverts to the relaxed state, becoming more fluid, and moves inward to form **endoplasm.** When the endoplasm streams forward under the pressure of the contractile ectoplasm, actin again becomes associated with myosin, producing anew the contractile state. The overall effect, then, is a recurrent outward and posteriad flow of ectoplasm away from the direction of movement and a concomitant movement of the endoplasm from the rear of the cell in the direction of the forming pseudopod (Fig. 3–7).

**Figure 3–7**
**One type of amoeboid motion.** The extension of a pseudopod by an amoeba is accompanied by constant flowing of cytoplasm in the direction of extension and probably by continual transformation from gelated ectoplasm, or *cortex* (outer region of cytoplasm), to fluid endoplasm at the posterior end, with the reverse transformation at the anterior end.

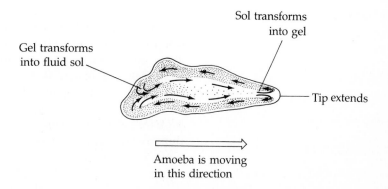

Gel transforms into fluid sol

Sol transforms into gel

Tip extends

Amoeba is moving in this direction

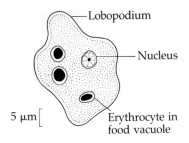

**Figure 3–8**
**Lobopodial type of**
**pseudopodium.**
*Entamoeba histolytica*
trophozoite.

Morphologically, pseudopodia can be assigned to one of four types: **filopodia, lobopodia, rhizopodia,** and **axopodia.** Lobopodia (Fig. 3–8) the most common form among parasitic amoebae, are blunt and may be composed of both ectoplasm and endoplasm or of ectoplasm only. In most species, lobopodia form slowly. Observation of living specimens clearly shows the gradual flow of granular endoplasm, when present, into the broad projection. *Entamoeba histolytica,* an important parasite of the human intestine, is exceptional in that the lobopodia are produced abruptly and withdrawn almost as quickly. Another exception is observed among some amoebae that appear to move on a substratum with no obvious cytoplasmic protrusions. Such amoebae are termed **limax forms** after the slug, *Limax* spp., whose movement they appear to mimic.

Although the formation of pseudopodia by trophozoites usually is considered a distinguishing characteristic of amoebae, some flagellates also are capable of pseudopodial movement at some stage during their life and, conversely, some amoebae possess flagella during their developmental stages (*Naegleria,* for example). As a general rule, however, among flagellates the principal means of locomotion is flagellar, while among amoebae it is pseudopodial.

Most amoebae cannot swim because pseudopodial locomotion requires a substrate on which these organisms can glide. Parasitic species, therefore, are commonly found in the alimentary tracts of their hosts, intimately associated with the epithelial lining.

## OTHER ORGANELLES

### Nucleus

Structurally, protozoa are unicellular organisms with each cell a self-sufficient unit capable of carrying out all the metabolic functions of which multicellular organisms are capable. Each protozoan is surrounded by a unit membrane chemically similar to the plasma membranes common to all eukaryotic cells—a bilipid layer associated with a variety of proteins. Among the sarcodinans, this tends to be a very thin, flexible layer often called the **plasmalemma.** On the other hand, a more rigid body wall, usually supported by microtubules and characteristic of some flagellates and most ciliates, is termed a **pellicle.** It results in a more constant and uniform shape than that of the more amorphic amoebae.

The cytoplasm is usually divided into two areas: the peripheral ectoplasm and the medullary endoplasm. The consistency, extent, and appearance of these two zones differ among species. Typically, the semisolid ectoplasm is a **gel** containing the basal bodies of cilia or flagella, microfilaments, and, in some protozoa, microtubules for rigidity and/ or contractility. The semiliquid endoplasm, or **sol,** is more fluid than ectoplasm and contains such organelles as nuclei, mitochondria, and vacuoles and vesicles of various types.

Well-defined nuclei bounded by nuclear envelopes are a feature of all protozoa. Some protozoa have a single nucleus, others have two or more essentially identical nuclei, and still others, such as the ciliophorans, have two different types of nuclei: a **macronucleus** and one or more **micronuclei.** As the name indicates, the macronucleus of ciliophorans is larger than the micronuclei and is involved with trophic activities of the cell. Micronuclei, whether one or more, are concerned with reproductive activities, both asexual and sexual.

In addition to distinctions as macro- or micronuclei, nuclei may be defined morphologically as either **vesicular** or **compact.** This classification is often used to aid in the identification of species infecting humans, since such species are commonly characterized as having the vesicular type.

**Vesicular Nucleus.**    The nuclear envelope of a vesicular nucleus, although delicate in appearance, is visible by light microscopy. The term *vesicular* denotes numerous clear areas resulting from the irregular distribution of chromatin, creating the impression of many small sacs or vesicles. The chromatin areas may be concentrated peripherally or internally. The nucleoplasm contains one or more **endosomes** or **karyosomes,** which are DNA-negative and are probably analogous to metazoan nucleoli; unlike nucleoli, however, they do not disappear during mitosis.

**Compact Nucleus.**    The compact nucleus appears to contain a larger amount of more densely packed chromatin than does the vesicular nucleus. A nucleus of this type is generally larger than a vesicular nucleus and may vary in shape from round to ovate. Compact nuclei are found in the ciliophorans, where they are involved in the sexual process called **conjugation.** During this process, one micronucleus of each cell undergoes meiosis, and some of the resulting haploid micronuclei are exchanged between the two individuals. Following meiosis and exchange, fusion of the micronuclei occurs, resulting in a genetically new set of micronuclei for each partner cell. During the meiotic division, exchange, and fusion of micronuclei, the macronuclei disappear and subsequently reform. They seem to serve as directors of the phenotypic expressions of the cells. Following conjugation, the two cells separate and then usually divide mitotically.

## Mitochondria

These double-unit membrane-bound organelles serve as the sites of intracellular aerobic metabolism and are similar in ultrastructure to those of most eukaryotes. One feature peculiar to protistan mitochondria is the tubular shape of the cristae (Fig. 3–9). Similar cristae are observed in mitochondria of multicellular eukaryotes but not as consistently as in those of protists. The significance of this structural variation is presently not understood. It should be noted that a number of parasitic protozoans (such as *Entamoeba histolytica*) do not possess mitochondria. Such a deficiency is associated with anaerobic metabolism.

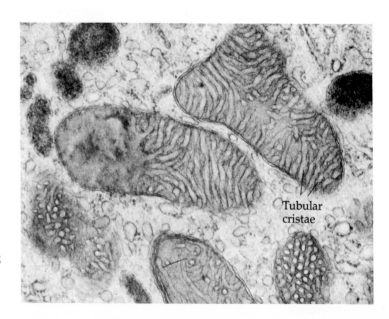

Tubular cristae

**Figure 3–9**
**Several mitochondria showing profiles of tubular cristae, from hamster suprarenal cortex.**

# Golgi Complex

The Golgi complex is another cytoplasmic structure whose specific function in protozoans is essentially identical to that observed in other eukaryotes. The Golgi is the seat of glycosylation of a number of secretory products of the cell. It is in the cisternae of the Golgi complex, for instance, that the final carbohydrate moieties are added to the particular cell coat associated with the plasma membrane. The arrangement and number of Golgi complexes vary during the life cycle of many protozoans. Thus, cyst-forming protozoans may lose their Golgi complexes during encystation, only to resynthesize them when they excyst. The so-called **parabasal body** of protozoans is homologous to the Golgi complex of other eukaryotic cells but with several morphological differences, the most notable of which is the frequent presence of a fibril, the **parabasal filament,** running from the cisternae of the Golgi complex to one or more basal bodies.

# Lysosomes

**Figure 3–10**
**Electron micrographs of lysosomes.**
(a) A cluster of lysosomes.
(b) Two secondary lysosomes enclosing dense inclusion.

The lysosome, an organelle ubiquitous among eukaryotes, is bounded by a single-unit membrane enclosing various hydrolytic enzymes whose optimum activities occur in the acid pH range (Fig. 3–10). Such enzymes, therefore, are designated **acid hydrolases.** Lysosomes, with their battery of acid

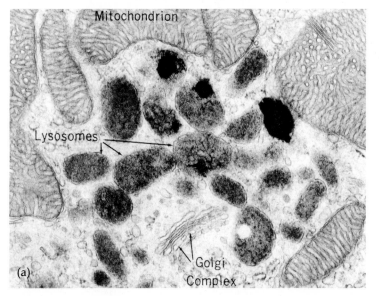

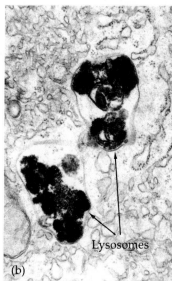

hydrolases, function in autophagy as well as in intracellular digestion of exogenous foodstuffs. In amoebae, for instance, **food vacuoles** are formed by the engulfment of exogenous food—including host cells, in certain parasitic species. Then the food vacuoles fuse with lysosomes, forming a **digestive vacuole,** and the lysosomal enzymes mix with and degrade the ingested material. Among a number of protozoans, ingestion occurs at a specialized site on the plasma membrane called the **cytostome** (Fig. 3–11). After digestion, undigested residues are egested through the plasma membrane. Among amoebae such egestion may occur anywhere on the plasmalemma, while in ciliates a permanent pellicular site, the **cytopyge,** exists through which undigested residues are emitted.

## Cytoplasmic Food Storage

Reserve food inclusions are seen in various species of parasitic protozoa. The nature and amount of stored nutrients vary with the environment and the species involved. For example, glycogen and/or amylopectin are sometimes found in cysts of amoebae that inhabit the human intestine. This stored food, accumulated shortly before encystation and used during the nonfeeding stage, is usually completely exhausted by the time of excystation. In addition to these polysaccharides, lipid droplets and nucleic acid reserves may be observed in both trophozoites and cysts.

## Ribosomes

These organelles, the sites of cellular protein synthesis, are part of the organelle population of all eukaryotes and occur abundantly in those cells that actively synthesize protein for either secretion or internal use. They may be seen in association with the endoplasmic reticulum or free, either singly or in clusters (**polyribosomes**), in the cytoplasm. During encystation, much of the ribosomal constituency of the cell is exhausted.

## Costa, Axostyle, and Vacuoles

Associated with the basal bodies of many flagellates is a prominent, striated rod, the **costa.** This structure usually courses from one of the basal bodies along the base of the

**Figure 3–11**
**A uninucleate trophozoite of**
*Plasmodium cathemerium*
**ingesting host cell cytoplasm**
**through a cytostome**
**(micropore) (arrow).**

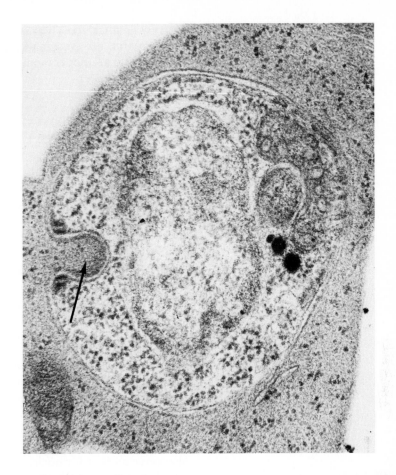

undulating membrane. It can best be described as a modi-fied, striated **rootlet.** Rootlets are found at the bases of many cilia and flagella in other eukaryotes, penetrating deep into the cytoplasm where they are believed to serve as anchors. In addition to the costa, a sheath of microtubules in the shape of a tube, the **axostyle,** is observed in many flagel-lates. This structure extends posteriorly from the basal body and may actually appear to protrude through the plasma membrane. The function of this organelle is unknown, and it has no counterpart in other eukaryotic cells.

Some parasitic protozoans, such as the ciliate *Balantid-ium coli*, possess fluid-filled vesicles sometimes called **con-tractile vacuoles.** In protozoans in general, these are consid-ered osmoregulatory organelles, ridding the cell of excess water; some dissolved metabolic wastes are also eliminated.

However, since most parasitic protozoa, like their marine counterparts, are isoosmotic to their environment, contractile vacuoles are not common in parasitic protozoa.

## ENCYSTATION

Many parasitic protozoa are capable of encystation, during which the rounded cytoplasmic mass is surrounded by a rigid or semirigid cyst wall secreted by the organism. The cyst wall may be single- or multilayered. Cysts of parasitic protozoa serve three primary functions: (1) as protection against unfavorable external environmental conditions, (2) as the site of morphogenesis and nuclear division, and (3) as means of transmission from one host to another.

Examples of the first function are seen in the human pathogens *Entamoeba histolytica,* an amoeba, and *Giardia lamblia,* a flagellate, which form cysts in the intestinal tract and pass out in fecal material. Such cysts may remain viable for many weeks under normal conditions and for days at higher and lower temperatures and during periods of dessication. Further, the cyst wall protects the ingested organism as it passes through the host's hostile gastric fluids.

As previously stated, cysts of many parasitic protozoa also serve as sites for nuclear and cytoplasmic reorganization and division. Shortly after the trophozoite encysts, cytoplasmic reorganization occurs, sometimes followed by nuclear divisions—after which the mature cyst may enclose from one (in the absence of nuclear division) to eight vesicular nuclei. In *E. histolytica,* for instance, two consecutive mitotic divisions result in four vesicular nuclei (see Fig. 4–2, page 53). If mature cysts are reintroduced into a suitable host, excystation occurs, and the escaping motile trophozoite usually divides once more, resulting in eight small trophozoites produced from the single, tetranucleated mass of cytoplasm encased within the cyst wall. Following excystation, the newly excysted trophozoites begin a period of active feeding, followed by rapid growth and binary fission.

Finally, intestinal protozoa are transmitted to a new host (or become reestablished in the same host) when that host swallows the cysts. Thus, the cysts serve as a means of transmission.

The precise environmental conditions that cause encystation are not totally defined. In many species, the process often occurs in response to a deficiency in the host of nutrients useful to the parasite. In addition, increased osmotic pressure, temperature changes, low pH's, accumulation of waste products in the medium, and crowding all appear to stimulate encystment.

# REPRODUCTION

Parasitic protozoa most commonly reproduce by means of an asexual process called **fission,** a form of mitosis whereby each parent forms two progeny. The plane of division is random among amoebae, usually longitudinal in flagellates, and transverse in ciliates. The sequence of division in a typical protozoan is as follows: organelles, nucleus, and, finally, cytoplasm.

In apicomplexans, **multiple fission** or **schizogony** occurs. This type of asexual reproduction is characterized by rapid organelle and nuclear divisions, followed by multiple cytokinesis. The multinucleated cell is called the **schizont** or **segmenter.** After cytoplasmic division, each nucleus, with its attendant cytoplasm, forms a separate organism, a **merozoite,** which usually breaks away from the aggregate to infect a new host cell. Once a merozoite enters a new host cell, it may either enter another schizogonic cycle or become a macro- or microgametocyte. **Syngamy,** the union of gametes derived from the gametocytes, initiates the sexual cycle. The resulting zygote undergoes **sporogony,** which results in the production of **sporozoites.** The organisms that produce malaria are apicomplexans capable of both schizogonic (asexual) and sporogonic (sexual) reproduction. In fact, the apicomplexans are considered unique among protists in displaying alternation of generations, a characteristic more commonly encountered in plants and some invertebrate animals, for example, cnidarians.

Conjugation, the specialized sexual mechanism in the ciliates, has already been discussed; it is distinguishable from syngamy in that conjugation involves nuclear exchange and union, whereas syngamy involves the union of entire cells (e.g., gametes).

◇
## SELECTED READINGS

Allen, R. D. 1961. A new theory of ameboid movement and protoplasmic streaming. *Experimental Cell Research* 8, 17–31.

Jahn, T. L., Bovee, E. C., and Jahn, F. F. 1979. *How to Know the Protozoa*, 2nd ed. William C. Brown, Dubuque, IA.

Pitelka, D. R. 1963. *Electron-microscopic Structure of Protozoa*. Pergamon Press, Elmsford, NY.

Satir, P. 1974. How cilia move. *Scientific American* 231, 45–52.

# CLASSIFICATION OF THE PROTOZOA*

## PHYLUM SARCOMASTIGOPHORA

Single type of nucleus; sexuality, when present, essentially syngamy; with flagella, pseudopodia, or both types of locomotor organelles.

### Subphylum Mastigophora

One or more flagella typically present in trophozoites; asexual reproduction basically by intrakinetal (symmetrogenic) binary fission; sexual reproduction known in some groups.

#### CLASS PHYTOMASTIGOPHOREA

Typically with chloroplasts; if chloroplasts lacking, relationship to pigmented forms clearly evident; mostly free living.

ORDER CRYPTOMONADIDA

ORDER DINOFLAGELLIDA

ORDER EUGLENIDA

ORDER CHRYSOMONADIDA

ORDER HETEROCHLORIDA

ORDER CHLOROMONADIDA

ORDER PRYMNESIDA

ORDER VOLVOCIDA

ORDER PRASINOMONADIDA

ORDER SILICOFLAGELLIDA

#### CLASS ZOOMASTIGOPHOREA

Chloroplasts absent; one to many flagella; amoeboid forms, with or without flagella, in some groups; sexuality known in few groups; a polyphylectic group.

ORDER CHOANOFLAGELLIDA

ORDER KINETOPLASTIDA

One of two flagella arising from depression; flagella typically with paraxial rod in addition to axoneme; single mitochondrion (nonfunctional in some forms) extending length of body as a single tube, hoop, or network of branching tubes, usually containing conspicuous Feulgen-positive (DNA-containing) kinetoplast located near flagellar kinetosomes; Golgi apparatus typically in region of flagellar depression, not connected to kinetosomes and flagella; parasitic (majority of species) and free living.

---

*Only those taxa that include parasitic species are defined.

*Suborder Bondonina*

*Suborder Trypanosomatina*
Single flagellum either free or attached to body by undulating membrane; kinetoplast relatively small and compact; parasitic. (Genera mentioned in text: *Leishmania, Trypanosoma.*)

## ORDER PROTERMONADIDA

## ORDER RETORTAMONADIDA
Two to four flagella, one turned posteriorly and associated with ventrally located cytostomal area bordered by fibril; mitochondria and Golgi apparatus absent; intranuclear division spindle; cysts present; parasitic. (Genera mentioned in text; *Chilomastix, Retortamonas.*)

## ORDER DIPLOMONADIDA
One or two karyomastigonts; genera with two karyomastigonts with twofold rotational symmetry or, in one genus, primarily mirror symmetry; individual mastigonts with one to four flagella, typically one of them recurrent and associated with cytostome, or, in more advanced genera, with organelles forming cell axis; mitochondria and Golgi apparatus absent; intranuclear division spindle; cysts present; free living or parasitic.

*Suborder Enteromonadina*

*Suborder Diplomonadina*
Two karyomastigonts; body with twofold rotational symmetry, or bilateral symmetry in one genus; each mastigont with four flagella, one of them recurrent; with variety of microtubular bands; cysts present; free living or parasitic. (Genus mentioned in text: *Giardia.*)

## ORDER OXYMONADIDA

## ORDER TRICHOMONADIDA
Typically karyomastigonts with four to six flagella, but with only one flagellum in one genus and no flagella in another; karyomastigonts and akaryomastigonts in one family with permanent polymonad-organization; in mastigont(s) of typical genera, one flagellum recurrent, free or with proximal or entire length adherent to body surface; undulating membrane, if present, associated with adherent segment of recurrent flagellum; pelta and noncontractile axostyle in each mastigont, except for one genus; hydrogenosomes present; true cysts infrequent, known in very few species; all or nearly all parasitic. (Genera mentioned in text: *Dientamoeba, Trichomonas, Pentatrichomonas.*)

## ORDER HYPERMASTIGIDA

### Subphylum Sarcodina
Pseudopodia, or locomotive protoplasmic flow without discrete pseudopodia; flagella, when present, usually restricted to developmental or other temporary stages; body naked or with external or internal test or skeleton; asexual reproduction by fission; sexual-

ity, if present, associated with flagellate or, more rarely, amoeboid gametes; most species free living.

### SUPERCLASS RHIZOPODA
Locomotion by lobopodia, filopodia, or reticulopodia, or by protoplasmic flow without production of discrete pseudopodia.

### CLASS LOBOSEA
Pseudopodia lobose or more or less filiform but produced from broader hyaline lobe; usually uninucleate; multinucleate forms not flattened or much-branched plasmodia.

#### Subclass Gymnamoebia
Without test.

##### ORDER AMOEBIDA
Typically uninucleated; mitochondria typically present; no flagellate stage.

*Suborder Tubulina*
Body a branched or unbranched cylinder; no bidirectional flow of cytoplasm; nuclear division mesomitotic. (Genera mentioned in text: *Hartmannella, Entamoeba, Endolimax, Iodamoeba.*)

*Suborder Thecina*

*Suborder Flabellina*

*Suborder Conopodina*

*Suborder Acanthopodina*
More or less finely tipped, sometimes filiform, often furcate hyaline pseudopodia produced from a broad hyaline lobe; not regularly discoid; cysts usually formed; nuclear division mesomitotic or metamitotic. (Genus mentioned in text: *Acanthamoeba.*)

##### ORDER SCHIZOPYRENIDA
Body with shape of monopodial cylinder, usually moving with more or less eruptive, hyaline, hemispheric bulges; typically uninucleate, nuclear division promitotic; temporary flagellate stages in most species. (Genus mentioned in text: *Naegleria.*)

#### Subclass Testacealobosia
##### ORDER ARCELLINIDA
##### ORDER TRICHOSIDA

### CLASS ACARPOMYXEA
##### ORDER LEPTOMYXIDA
##### ORDER STEREOMYXIDA

### CLASS ACRASEA
##### ORDER ACRASIDA

### CLASS EUMYCETOZOEA
#### Subclass Protosteliia

ORDER  PROTOSTELIIDA

**Subclass Dictyosteliia**

ORDER  DICTYOSTELIIDA

**Subclass Myxogastria**

ORDER  ECHINOSTELIIDA

ORDER  LICEIDA

ORDER  TRICHIIDA

ORDER  STEMONITIDA

ORDER  PHYSARIDA

**CLASS PLASMODIOPHOREA**

ORDER  PLASMODIOPHORIDA

**CLASS FILOSEA**

ORDER  ACONCHULINIDA

ORDER  GROMIIDA

**CLASS GRANULORETICULOSEA**

ORDER  ATHALAMIDA

ORDER  MONOTHALAMIDA

ORDER  FORAMINIFERIDA

Suborder Allogromiina

Suborder Textulariina

Suborder Fusulinina

Suborder Miliolina

Suborder Rotaliina

**CLASS XENOPHYOPHOREA**

ORDER  PSAMMINIDA

ORDER  STANNOMIDA

**SUPERCLASS ACTINOPODA**

**CLASS ACANTHAREA**

ORDER  HOLACANTHIDA

ORDER  SYMPHYACANTHIDA

ORDER  CHAUNACANTHIDA

ORDER  ARTHRACANTHIDA

Suborder Sphaenacanthina

Suborder Phyllacanthina

ORDER  ACTINELIIDA

*CLASS POLYCYSTINEA*

*ORDER SPUMELLARIDA*

Suborder Sphaerocollina

Suborder Sphaerellarina

*ORDER NASSELLARIDA*

**CLASS PHAEODAREA**

*ORDER PHAEOCYSTIDA*

*ORDER PHAEOSPHAERIDA*

*ORDER PHAEOCALPIDA*

*ORDER PHAEOGROMIDA*

*ORDER PHAEOCONCHIDA*

*ORDER PHAEODENDRIDA*

**CLASS HELIOZOEA**

*ORDER DESMOTHORACIDA*

*ORDER ACTINOPHYRIDA*

*ORDER TAXOPODIDA*

*ORDER CENTROHELIDA*

**Subphylum Opalinata**
Numerous cilia in oblique rows over entire body surface; cytostome absent; nuclear division accentric; binary fission generally interkinetal; known life cycles involve syngamy with anisogamous flagellated gametes; all parasitic.

*CLASS OPALINATEA*
With characters of the subphylum.

*ORDER OPALINIDA*

**PHYLUM APICOMPLEXA**
Apical complex (visible with electron microscope), generally consisting of polar ring(s), rhoptries, micronemes, conoid, and subpellicular microtubules present at some stage; micropore(s) generally present at some stage; cilia absent; sexuality by syngamy; all species parasitic.

*CLASS PERKINSEA*
Conoid forming incomplete cone; zoospores (sporozoites?) flagellated, with anterior vacuole; no sexual reproduction; homoxenous.

*ORDER PERKINSIDA*

*CLASS SPOROZOEA*
Conoid, if present, forming complete cone; reproduction generally both sexual and asexual; oocysts generally containing infective sporozoites with result from sporogony; locomotion of mature organisms by body flexion, gliding, or undulation of

longitudinal ridges; flagella present only in microgametes of some groups; pseudopods ordinarily absent, but if present, used for feeding, not locomotion; homoxenous or heteroxenous.

### Subclass *Gregarinia*

ORDER *ARCHIGREGARINIDA*

ORDER *EUGREGARINIDA*

ORDER *NEOGREGARINIDA*

### Subclass *Coccidia*
Gamonts ordinarily present; mature gamonts small, typically intracellular, without mucron or epimerite; syzygy generally absent, but if present, involves markedly anisogamous gametes; life cycle characteristically consists of merogony, gametogony, and sporogony; most species in vertebrates.

ORDER *AGAMOCOCCIDIIDA*
Merogony and gametogony absent.

ORDER *PROTOCOCCIDIIDA*
Merogony absent; in invertebrates.

ORDER *EUCOCCIDIIDA*
Merogony present; in vertebrates and/or invertebrates.

Suborder *Adeleina*

Suborder *Eimeriina*
Macrogamete and microgamont developing independently; no syzygy; microgamont typically producing many microgametes; zygote nonmotile; sporozoites typically enclosed in sporocyst within oocyst; homoxenous or heteroxenous. (Genus mentioned in text: *Toxoplasma*.)

Suborder *Haemosporina*
Macrogamete and microgamont developing independently; no syzygy; conoid usually absent; microgamont producing eight flagellated microgametes; zygote motile (ookinete); sporozoites naked, with three-membraned wall; heteroxenous, with merogony in vertebrates and sporogony in invertebrates; transmitted by blood-sucking insects. (Genus mentioned in text: *Plasmodium*.)

### Subclass *Piroplasmia*
Piriform, round, rod-shaped, or amoeboid; conoid absent; no oocysts, spores, and pseudocysts; flagella absent; usually without subpellicular microtubules, with polar ring and rhoptries; locomotion by body flexion, gliding or, in sexual stages (in Babesiidae and Theileriidae, at least), by large axopodium-like organelle; asexual and probably sexual reproduction; parasitic in erythrocytes and sometimes also in other circulating and fixed cells; heteroxenous, with merogony in vertebrates and sporogony in invertebrates; sporozoites with single-membraned wall; vectors are ticks, but vectors of dactylosomatids unknown.

*ORDER PIROPLASMIDA*
With characters of the subclass. (Genus mentioned in text: *Babesia*.)

## PHYLUM MICROSPORA

Unicellular spores, each with impertorate wall, containing one uninucleate or dinucleate sporoplasm and simple or complex extrusion apparatus always with polar tube and polar cap; without mitochondria; often, if not usually, dimorphic in sporulation sequence; obligatory intracellular parasites in nearly all major animal groups.

## PHYLUM ASCETOSPORA

Spore multicellular (or unicellular?); with one or more sporoplasms; without polar capsules or polar filaments; all parasitic.

## PHYLUM MYXOZOA

Spores of multicellular origin, with one or more polar capsules and sporoplasms; with one, two, or three (rarely more) valves; all species parasitic.

## PHYLUM CILIOPHORA

Simple cilia or compound ciliary organelles typical in at least one stage of life cycle; with subpellicular infraciliature present even when cilia absent; two types of nuclei, with rare exception; binary fission transverse, but budding and multiple fission also occur; sexuality involving conjugation, autogamy, and cytogamy; nutrition heterotrophic; contractile vacuole typically present; most species free living, but many commensal, some parasitic, and a large number found as phoronts on a variety of hosts.

### CLASS KINETOFRAGMINOPHOREA

Oral infraciliature only slightly distinct from somatic infraciliature and differentiated from anterior parts, or other segments, of all or some of somatic kineties; cytostome often apical (or subapical) or midventral, on surface of body or at bottom of atrium or vestibulum; cytopharyngeal apparatus commonly prominent; compound ciliature, oral or somatic, typically absent.

#### Subclass Gymnostomatia

Cytostomal area superficial, apical or subapical; circumoral infraciliature without kinetosomal differentiation other than closer packing of kinetosomes; cytopharyngeal apparatus of rhabdos type; toxicysts common; somatic ciliation usually uniform.

*ORDER PROSTOMATIDA*

*ORDER PLEUROSTOMATIDA*

*ORDER PRIMOCILIATIDA*

*ORDER KARYORELICTIDA*

#### Subclass Vestibuliferia

Apical or near-apical (occasionally at posterior pole) vestibulum commonly present, equipped with cilia derived from anterior parts of somatic kineties and leading to cytostome; cytopharyngeal apparatus resembling rhabdos; free living or parasitic, especially in digestive tract of vertebrates and invertebrates.

## ORDER TRICHOSTOMATIDA

No reorganization of somatic kineties at level of vestibulum other than more packed alignment of kinetosomes or addition of supernumerary segments of kineties; many species endosymbiotic in vertebrate hosts.

### Suborder Trichostomatina

Somatic ciliature not reduced. (Genus mentioned in text: *Balantidium*.)

## ORDER ENTODINIOMORPHIDA

## ORDER COLPODIDA

## CLASS OLIGOHYMENOPHOREA

Oral apparatus, at least partially in buccal cavity, generally well defined, although absent in one group; oral ciliature, clearly distinct from somatic ciliature, consisting of paroral membrane on right side and small number of compound organelles (membranelles, etc.) on left side; cytostome usually ventral and/or near anterior end, situated at bottom of buccal cavity; cysts common; various species loricate; colony formation common in some groups.

## CLASS POLYMENOPHOREA

Dominated by well-developed, conspicuous adoral zone of numerous buccal or peristomial organelles, often extending out onto body surface; on right side, one or seven lines of paroral ciliature; somatic ciliature complete or reduced, or as cirri; cytostome at bottom of buccal cavity; somatic infraciliature rarely including kinetodesmata; cytoproct often absent; cysts, and especially loricae, very common in some groups; often large and commonly free-living, free-swimming forms in great variety of habitats.

# CHAPTER FOUR

# VISCERAL PROTOZOA I: AMOEBAE AND CILIATES

## AMOEBAE

This category of parasites consists of members of the sub-phylum Sarcodina. All species in this subphylum that are parasitic in humans belong to the order Amoebida and, with few exceptions, are nonpathogenic or produce only mild disease; however, they require special emphasis in order to distinguish them from the potentially highly pathogenic *Entamoeba histolytica* (Table 4–1). Such attention is amply justified since *E. histolytica* can produce extreme illness and even death. Furthermore, since side effects from chemotherapy may be pronounced, it is of great importance that diagnosis of the condition be precise and accurate in order to assure treatment only when absolutely necessary, not merely to eliminate a protozoan that resembles *E. histolytica*.

At least seven species of amoebae belonging to three genera are known to parasitize humans. These are *Entamoeba histolytica, E. hartmanni, E. coli, E. polecki, E. gingivalis, Endolimax nana,* and *Iodamoeba butschlii.* All inhabit the large intestine except *E. gingivalis,* which is found in the mouth. In addition, amoebae belonging to at least three genera—*Naegleria, Acanthamoeba,* and *Hartmannella*—normally free-living, have been shown on occasion to parasitize humans by accident.

### Entamoeba histolytica

Undoubtedly, the best known species of amoebae parasitizing humans is *E. histolytica* (Fig. 4–1), the causative agent of amoebic dysentery or amoebiasis. First discovered in Russia by Lösch in 1875, it is global in distribution, although its prevalence varies markedly from one area to another. For

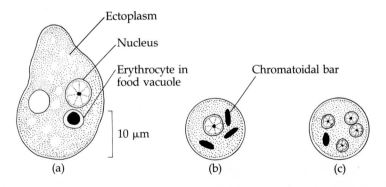

**Figure 4–1**
*Entamoeba histolytica.*
(a) Trophozoite. (b) Early cyst with chromatoidal bars.
(c) Later cyst.

Ectoplasm

Nucleus

Erythrocyte in food vacuole

Chromatoidal bar

10 μm

(a)    (b)    (c)

**Table 4-1    Some Important Enteric Amoebae of Humans**

| | *Entamoeba histolytica* | *Entamoeba coli* | *Endolimax nana* | *Iodamoeba butschlii* | *Entamoeba gingivalis* | *Dientamoeba fragilis*\* |
|---|---|---|---|---|---|---|
| **Trophozoite** | | | | | | |
| Size (range) | 25 μm (15–60) | 25 μm (15–40) | 9 μm (5–14) | 10 μm (6–25) | 15 μm (5–35) | 10 μm (6–25) |
| Motility | active, directional, progressive | sluggish, nondirectional, nonprogressive | similar to E. coli | similar to E. coli | moderately active, progressive | active, progressive |
| Pseudopodia | fingerlike, explosive | short, blunt, broad, slow | similar to E. coli | similar to E. coli | blunt, rapidly formed | thin, leaflike, multiple, rapidly formed |
| Nucleus (stained) | delicate envelope & chromatin; central endosome | coarse envelope & chromatin, eccentric endosome | large endosome; no peripheral chromatin | large endosome surrounded by granules | similar to E. hystolytica | similar to E. hystolytica; endosome divided into 4–6 granules |
| **Cyst** | | | | | | |
| Size (range) | 12 μm (10–20) | 17 μm (10–33) | 9 μm (5–14) | 10 μm (5–18) | none | none |
| Inclusions | | | | | | |
| Glycogen | diffuse in young cysts; | ill defined in young cysts; | absent | large mass | | |
| Chromatoidal bars | rounded ends | splintered ends | occasionally as granules | usually absent | | |
| Number of nuclei | 1–4 | 1–8 | 1–4 | 1 | | |

\*Mastigophora

example, it has been reported to infect 85% of the population of Mérida, Yucatán, Mexico, but no more than 13.6% (range, 0.8–38%) of several populations surveyed in the United States. It is, nevertheless, important to remember that amoebiasis is not restricted to the tropics and subtropics; it is found also in temperate and even in arctic and antarctic zones. The usual mode of infection—ingestion of cysts from contaminated hands, food, or water—causes the incidence to increase considerably in densely populated areas where contact with infected individuals is more likely. Children's homes and mental health institutions often produce conditions favorable to transmission of these organisms.

**Life Cycle** (Fig. 4–2).   The uninucleate trophozoite of *E. histolytica* inhabits the colon and rectum and, at times, the lower end of the small intestine of humans and other primates. The motile trophozoite measures 25 μm in diameter (range, 15–60 μm) and is typically monopodial, producing one large, fingerlike pseudopodium at a time (Fig. 4–1a). The single pseudopodium erupts and is withdrawn so rapidly that, in prepared slides, trophozoites with pseudopodia extended are rarely seen. The cytoplasm is differentiated into two zones: a clear, refractile ectoplasm and a finely granular endoplasm in which food vacuoles are situated. Such vacuoles may contain host erythrocytes, leukocytes, and epithelial cells, as well as bacteria and other intestinal material. Trophozoites proliferate mitotically (binary fission) within the host's gut.

The nucleus is of special importance in differentiating *E. histolytica* from other intestinal amoebae. In saline preparations, the nucleus has a barely discernible nuclear envelope. However, in stained preparations, the vesicular nucleus is clearly visible. Ideally, it has a well-defined envelope lined on the inner surface with fine, peripheral, chromatin granules and a minute, centrally located endosome. Unfortunately, this "ideal" morphology is not confined to *E. histolytica*. Oftentimes, other species of *Entamoeba* may show similar nuclear morphologies.

Under certain adverse environmental and/or physiological circumstances, trophozoites assume precystic characteristics by becoming more spherical and, as food vacuoles are extruded, shrinking in size. Pseudopodia, if formed, are sluggishly extended, and there appears to be no progressive movement. Encystation begins with the secretion by the precyst trophozoite of a thin, surrounding hyaline membrane to

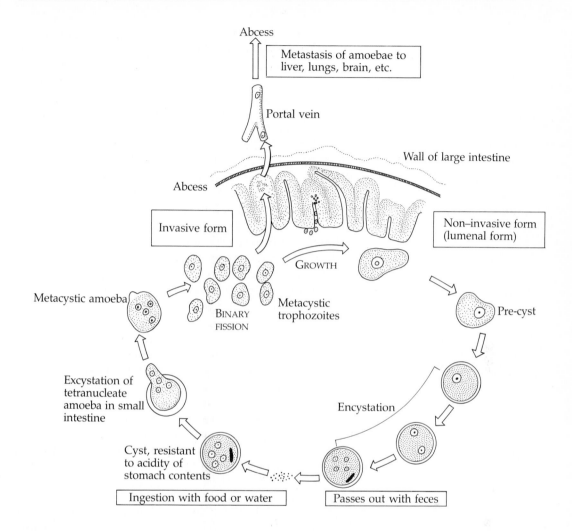

**Figure 4–2**
**Life cycle of *Entamoeba histolytica*.**

form a cyst. At this stage the cyst is usually spherical, 12 μm in diameter (range, 10–20 μm), with a single nucleus. At times, glycogen masses and **chromatoidal bars** may be observed (Fig. 4–1b). The latter structures are considered to be deposits of nucleic acids that may vary in shape but always have smoothly rounded ends in *E. histolytica*. This characteristic distinguishes *E. histolytica* cysts from those of *E. coli*, in which the chromatoidal bars have jagged or splintered ends. The nucleus undergoes two mitotic divisions to produce four vesicular nuclei in the mature cyst of *E. histolytica* (Fig. 4–1c). Such cysts represent the infective form and pass out of the host in feces, after which the glycogen and chromatoidal substance are slowly metabolized and disappear.

Cysts of *E. histolytica* are highly resistant to dessication and even to certain chemicals. Cysts in water can survive for a month, while those in feces on dry land can survive for more than 12 days; they tolerate temperatures up to a thermal death point of 50°C.

When food or water contaminated with *E. histolytica* cysts is ingested by a host, the cysts pass through the stomach (protected by the cyst wall) to the ileum, where excystation occurs. The neutral or slightly alkaline environment afforded by the small intestine is apparently requisite for this phenomenon. However, *in vitro* studies suggest that excystation does not occur immediately; cysts placed in fresh culture medium at body temperature require 5 or 6 hours for excystation. Upon excystation, a single tetranucleate organism immediately undergoes mitosis, giving rise to eight small, uninucleate **metacystic trophozoites,** which pass downward to the large intestine where they feed, grow, and reproduce. Reduction in intestinal peristalsis often allows the trophozoites to become established in the caecal area of the colon. The greater the number of organisms, the greater the likelihood that they will attain a foothold in the intestinal epithelium. Conversely, greater intestinal motility and/or large volumes of ingested food reduce the potential for establishment of the amoebae.

Multiplication of this species is thus seen to occur at two stages during the life cycle: by binary fission in the intestine-dwelling mature trophozoite stage and by nuclear division followed by binary fission in the metacystic stage.

**Epidemiology.**   *Entamoeba histolytica* is cosmopolitan, with an estimated incidence of human infection exceeding 400 million cases. Although the prevalence of infection varies widely, certain groups appear more susceptible than others, for example, patients in mental institutions. Transmission depends upon ingestion of contaminated food and drinking water. Areas with low standards of sanitation and those in which night soil is used as fertilizer display the highest prevalence of human infections. The main source of infection is the cyst-passing, asymptomatic carrier or chronic patient. The infection in these individuals is called **luminal amoebiasis.** Acutely ill patients, those with **invasive amoebiasis,** are not significant transmitters since they pass the noninfective trophozoite (noninfective because, unlike the cyst, it is unable to survive outside the intestinal environment) in their diarrheic feces. In addition, flies and cockroaches have been implicated as mechanical vectors in the spread of this and other amoebae since cysts can survive for lengthy periods in their digestive tracts, later to be regurgitated or passed out in feces upon human food.

The explanation for the apparent nonpathogenicity in certain human hosts remains elusive. In humans living in temperate zones, the organism often produces the nonpathogenic, luminal form of the disease, while in the tropics and subtropics the invasive form of the disease is more common.

Under pathogenic conditions, the food vacuoles of *E. histolytica* trophozoites characteristically contain host erythrocytes along with leukocytes and epithelial cells. At the height of its pathogenicity, the trophozoite secretes proteolytic enzymes that enable the organism to invade submucosal tissue. In the infected individual who develops dysentery, the mucosal ulceration may penetrate deeper into the intestinal tissue, causing vast areas of tissue to be destroyed. The overlying mucosal epithelium then may be sloughed off, exposing these necrotic areas (Fig. 4–3). This destructive process is usually followed by a regenerative period, resulting in a thickening of the intestinal wall as a result of the

**Figure 4–3**
**Section of human colon showing chronic amoebic ulcer.**

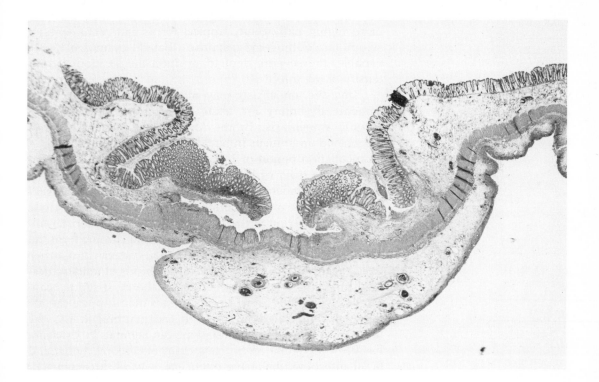

deposition of fibrous connective tissue. Trophozoites also may be carried to the liver, chiefly by the hepatic portal system, causing **hepatic amoebiasis** and even amoebic hepatitis. The first sign of hepatic involvement is the formation of an early hepatic abcess containing a matrix of necrosed hepatic cells, which eventually become liquified. Hepatic abcesses may be single or multiple (Fig. 4–4). While the liver appears to be the visceral organ most often affected (about 5% of all cases), other organs such as the lungs, heart, brain, spleen, gonads, and skin may also be invaded, resulting in **secondary amoebiasis.** The reaction in the liver is believed to be due not only to the trophozoite and its secretions but also to emanation of toxic material due to the ulcerative changes in the intestine.

Next to the liver in frequency as an extraintestinal site are the lungs. Pulmonary amoebiasis is relatively rare, however, and is probably a direct result of hepatic infection. Unlike most amoebic abcesses, which are commonly bacteriologically sterile, the pulmonary abcess is often vulnerable to secondary bacterial infections.

**Symptomatology and Diagnosis.**    Among victims of amoebiasis, symptoms vary widely; in some individuals even the more highly pathogenic, tropical forms can occur without symptoms. Pathogenic responses that do occur are highly variable, the severity depending upon the location and intensity of the infection.

Invasive amoebiasis may manifest itself in two ways: **amoebic dysentery** (= **acute intestinal amoebiasis**) and **chronic amoebiasis.** In the former type, severe diarrhea (i.e., blood and mucus in liquid feces) usually develops after an incubation period of 1 to 4 weeks and is usually accompanied by a fever of 100 to 102°F. Diagnosis requires differentiation of amoebic dysentery from other types of dysentery and, ultimately, identification of the parasite; one diagnostic criterion is the presence of the characteristic trophozoites and/or cysts in the stools. In the chronic form, on the other hand, there may be continuous attacks of diarrhea or recurrent attacks with intervening periods of milder intestinal problems. Hepatic amoebiasis is the most serious consequence of either form, since abcesses may rupture the abdominal wall or extend through the diaphragm into the lungs. Any of these manifestations can be fatal. *E. histolytica* has been incriminated in a few cases of cerebral, optic, and facial infections that have often had severely damaging or

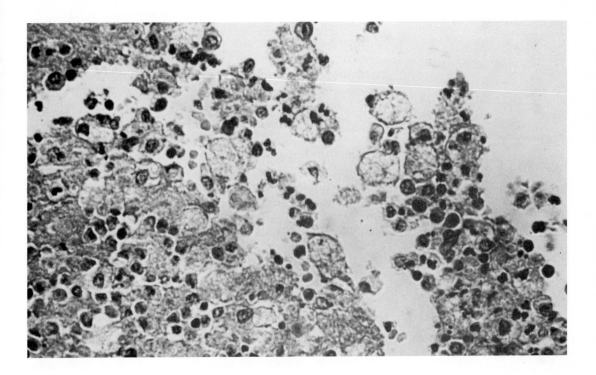

**Figure 4–4**
**Abcess in human liver due to**
*Entamoeba histolytica.*

even fatal consequences. In such cases, transmission of the organism is through direct, fecal contamination of the skin, eye socket, etc., rather than metastasis from the intestine or liver.

Laboratory diagnosis of amoebiasis depends upon identification of trophozoites or cysts of *E. histolytica.* Examination of stools for intestinal forms requires both direct smears and concentration procedures such as zinc sulfate flotation or formalin–ether. Such examinations should be performed for three consecutive days unless positive results are obtained in a shorter period. The chance of finding cysts in infected persons almost triples after three days. Combining direct smears with concentration methods of detection doubles the diagnostic effectiveness of a single examination. Different diagnostic procedures are required for patients with extraintestinal amoebiasis since stool specimens may not disclose the presence of the parasite. Trophozoites may be detected in sputum samples and tissue biopsies. Serological tests and X-ray scans may prove useful in revealing abcesses of the liver. It should be reemphasized at this point that direct demonstration of the parasite is requisite for a positive diagnosis before chemotherapy is undertaken.

**Treatment.** Appropriate chemotherapy should be used to destroy trophozoites, relieve symptoms, and control secondary bacterial infections. The drug of choice for the entire spectrum of symptoms is metronidazole or diiodohydroxyquin. Common sense dictates complete bed rest in cases of severe diarrhea accompanied by fever, regardless of the cause. In addition, a bland diet, low in carbohydrates such as sugar and high in liquids and proteins, is recommended. In symptomless carriers, it is essential that the trophozoites be destroyed since they are the precursors of cysts that pass out of the host. Metronidazole is contraindicated for pregnant women, especially those in their first trimester, since it is a known carcinogen and mutagen in rodents and bacteria.

To combat secondary bacterial infections, antibiotics such as tetracycline are used in combination with either metronidazole or, more recently, diiodohydroxyquin. The latter combination produces a high rate of cure for intestinal amoebiasis and may supplant the use of metronidazole. However, in cases of iodine sensitivity, diiodohydroxyquin is contraindicated.

Hepatic amoebiasis also responds well to metronidazole, although the treatment is not totally effective. Emetine or dehydroemetine is used in instances when metronidazole treatment has been unsuccessful. Chloroquine can be used where there are contraindications for either of these two drugs, if it is kept in mind that chloroquine has no effect upon trophozoites in the intestine. Two drugs closely akin to metronidazole—ornidazole and tinidazole—are reported to have cured hepatic amoebiasis with a single dose.

**Physiology.** Knowledge of the physiology of *E. histolytica* is fragmentary and incomplete. When the metabolism of the organism is better understood, perhaps more effective chemotherapeutic methods will be developed. Since it grows best in an oxygen-free atmosphere, *E. histolytica* was once considered an obligate anaerobe. However, it has recently been shown that the organism can use oxygen in low concentrations even though it does not possess the usual organelles (i.e., mitochondria) or metabolic pathways, such as the cytochrome system or a functional Krebs cycle, normally associated with oxygen utilization. *In vitro*, an oxygen concentration of 10% or higher is lethal to the organism, while carbon dioxide is required for growth, a characteristic *E. histolytica* shares with most intestine-dwelling organisms.

Glucose and galactose are the major carbohydrates used by the organisms, from which they produce ethanol, acetate, and carbon dioxide. In the presence of oxygen, the same end-products are produced but in different proportions.

**Prevention.** Food and water contaminated with feces containing the cysts of *E. histolytica* are the most common vehicles for transmission. Prevention, therefore, depends upon interruption of the contamination–ingestion cycle. One such measure is the boiling or iodination (1.25 grams iodine/liter drinking water, allow to stand 2–3 hours) of drinking water in endemic areas. In many areas, fruits and vegetables become contaminated when human excrement (night soil) is used as fertilizer. The rule of thumb for Westerners travelling in Third World countries is to drink bottled water and avoid ice cubes, salads, and those fruits not peeled by the person consuming them. Broad education to improve sanitation coupled with a ban on the use of untreated human excrement as fertilizer are perhaps the most efficient means for curbing transmission of pathogenic protozoa such as *E. histolytica*.

The role of infected food handlers in the transmission of *E. histolytica* can be controlled by local ordinances requiring periodic physical examinations, including stool examinations, for all food handlers.

## Entamoeba hartmanni

Following verification of the fact that of the species of intestinal amoebae in humans only one, *E. histolytica*, can cause disease, it was reported that this amoeba occurred in two sizes—one ("small race") with trophozoites measuring 12–15 $\mu$m in diameter and cysts 5–9 $\mu$m in diameter, the other ("large race") with trophozoites measuring 20–30 $\mu$m in diameter and cysts 10–20 $\mu$m in diameter. About one-third of the patients infected with intestinal amoebae harbor the small race, and these individuals display no disease. Current thinking is that the small race of *E. histolytica* is a separate species, *E. hartmanni*, whose life cycle and overall morphology are very similar to those of *E. histolytica*. However, *E. hartmanni* is considerably smaller and nonpathogenic, so no erythrocytes, etc., are to be found in vacuoles. It is important, therefore, that diagnosticians differentiate between the two organisms to preclude unnecessary chemotherapy.

## *Entamoeba coli*

This widely distributed intestinal amoeba (Fig. 4–5) is generally considered nonpathogenic in humans. The trophozoite measures 25 μm in diameter (range, 15–40 μm), and it forms a cyst 17 μm in diameter (range, 10–33 μm). The prevalence of infection, like that for all parasites, varies in different localities, seasons, etc. For example, one report shows 31.7% of a sampling of Tennesseans harboring *E. coli;* one survey has revealed that 26.1% of the inhabitants of Wise County, Virginia, harbor this amoeba, while another, involving an extensive study of all sections of the United States, found infection rates exceeding 19%, making *E. coli* possibly the most common intestinal amoeba in the United States.

The *Entamoeba coli* trophozoite does not ingest or invade host tissues. The food vacuoles observed in its heavily granulated cytoplasm usually contain bacteria, yeast, and fragments of intestinal debris. The nucleus may be visible in saline preparations. When stained, the nuclear envelope appears coarse with irregularly dispersed, peripheral chromatin on its inner surface, and there is a large, eccentric endosome. However, there is a wide variation in this morphology. As in *E. histolytica*, cysts are the usual means of identification. The mature cyst characteristically contains eight vesicular nuclei with eccentrically situated endosomes. Younger cysts may contain one, two, or four nuclei. Chromatoidal bodies, when present in cysts, may be needlelike or irregular with distinctly splintered terminals. Cysts are found frequently in diarrheic stools, but there is no evidence that this amoeba is the cause of the diarrhea.

The life cycle of *E. coli* parallels that of *E. histolytica* (Fig. 4–2), including the precystic, metacystic, and trophozoite stages, with infection of the host initiated by ingestion of cysts.

**Figure 4–5**
*Entamoeba coli.*
(a) Trophozoite. (b) Mature cyst with eight nuclei and splintered chromatoidal bars.

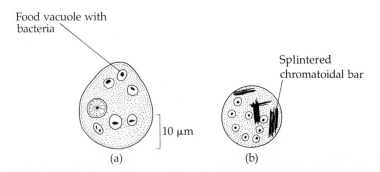

Food vacuole with bacteria

Splintered chromatoidal bar

10 μm

(a)                    (b)

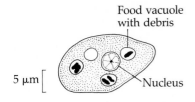

Food vacuole
with debris

5 μm

Nucleus

**Figure 4–6**
*Entamoeba gingivalis*
**trophozoite.**

## Entamoeba polecki

An intestinal amoeba rarely found in humans but usually reported in pigs, goats, monkeys, and dogs, this parasite can be confused with *E. histolytica*. In size, its trophozoite and cyst are intermediate between *E. histolytica* and *E. coli*, with the cyst stage being almost always uninucleate. Some investigators consider the parasite identical to *E. coli*, while others place it in a separate species; hence its inclusion here. It is generally believed to be nonpathogenic.

## Entamoeba gingivalis

*Entamoeba gingivalis* (Fig. 4–6) is cosmopolitan in distribution, commonly found in the tartar and debris associated with the gingival tissues in the mouth. It was the first parasitic amoeba reported in humans (Gros, 1849). There is little indication that it is pathogenic, and, while it abounds in people with unhealthy oral conditions (i.e., gingivitis or peridontitis), a cause and effect relationship has not been established. Food vacuoles may contain oral epithelial cells, leukocytes, occasionally erythrocytes, and various microbial organisms. No cyst is formed by *E. gingivalis*, and it is transmitted either directly (kissing) or indirectly via trophozoite-contaminated food, chewing gum, toothpicks, etc.

## Iodamoeba butschlii

*Iodamoeba butschlii* (Fig. 4–7) also is transmitted by a cyst that is very distinctive, facilitating identification. It varies from a rounded to a somewhat angular shape, usually 10 μm in greatest diameter (range, 5–18 μm). The nucleus is large with a large, ovoid, usually eccentric endosome. Within the cyst is a large glycogen body, which stains deeply with iodine. The cyst and the emerged trophozoite are uninucleate. The amoeba escapes through a pore in the cyst wall and

**Figure 4–7**
*Iodamoeba butschlii.*
(a) Trophozoite. (b) Cyst.

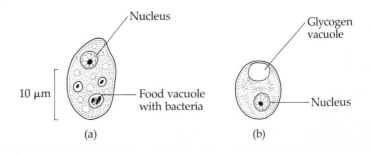

Nucleus

10 μm

Food vacuole
with bacteria

Glycogen
vacuole

Nucleus

(a)

(b)

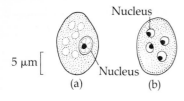

**Figure 4–8**
*Endolimax nana.*
(a) Trophozoite. (b) Cyst.

moves rapidly. Moisture and warmth are the only known requirements for excystation. Mature trophozoites measure 10 μm in diameter (range, 6–25 μm) and reside in the large intestine, feeding on bacteria and yeast, as is evident from the contents of their food vacuoles. This species is not considered a pathogen. In the trophozoite, as in the cyst, the large, vesicular nucleus is a prominent feature.

## Endolimax nana

*Endolimax nana* (Fig. 4–8) is the smallest of the intestine-dwelling amoeba infecting humans, and its trophozoite measures only 8 μm in diameter (range, 6–15 μm). The trophozoite lives in the host's colon and is generally considered to be nonpathogenic. According to some surveys, prevalence may be as high as 30% in some populations. The life cycle is identical to that of other cyst-forming amoebae, with the cyst being the infective stage. *E. nana* cysts can be identified and differentiated from other cysts by their smaller size (9 μm in greatest diameter; range, 5–14 μm), ovoid shape, and one to four vesicular nuclei, each usually with a large, eccentric endosome. The nuclear envelope is very thin and is difficult to see even in stained preparations. A tetranucleate metacystic amoeba escapes through a pore in the cyst wall and undergoes a series of cytoplasmic divisions in which a portion of cytoplasm is passed on to each uninucleate product. Trophozoites actively feed upon bacteria and multiply rapidly by binary fission.

## PATHOGENIC FREE-LIVING AMOEBAE

In recent years, there has been a great deal of interest in a group of small, free-living amoebae belonging to the genera *Naegleria*, *Acanthamoeba*, and *Hartmannella*. These amoebae, normally free-living in fresh water and soil, are capable of facultative parasitism in humans. Those belonging to the genus *Hartmannella* are typically nonpathogenic to humans, but certain strains of *Naegleria* and *Acanthamoeba* are highly pathogenic. Their pathogenicity to humans was first noted in 1965 when fatal cases of primary amoebic meningoencephalitis (PAM) were diagnosed simultaneously in Australia and Florida. Since then, 150 cases have been reported worldwide, including cases from many of the United States.

Most victims have a history of recent exposure to warm, fresh or brackish water, such as in swimming pools, ponds, lakes, and streams.

## *Naegleria fowleri*

*Naegleria fowleri* (Fig. 4–9) appears to be the principal causative agent for PAM. Its life cycle includes flagellated and amoebic trophozoites and cysts, with rapid transformation from one form to the other. The flagellated trophozoites are capable of rapid movement through the water, and transmission to humans most likely occurs when the nasopharyngeal mucosa is invaded by these forms. The amoebic trophozoite migrates through the nervous system to the brain, where inflammation occurs and death usually ensues. No cyst stage occurs in the human host, and flagellated trophozoites are observed only during the invasive stage. The disease progresses rapidly to an acute stage. Diagnostic confirmation requires identification of the motile amoebic trophozoite in cerebrospinal fluid, but since death may occur in 5 to 7 days, most cases are diagnosed at autopsy.

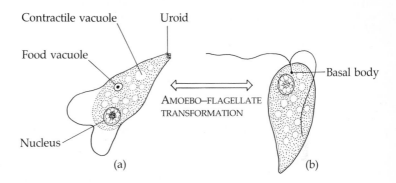

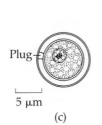

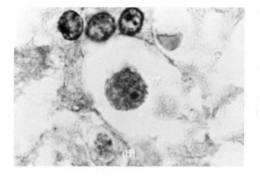

**Figure 4–9**
*Naegleria gruberi,* **a soil amoeba sometimes pathogenic in humans.**
Under certain physiological conditions, the amoeboid form undergoes transformation into a flagellated form.
(a) Amoeboid phase.
(b) Flagellated form. (c) Cyst. Scale only approximate.
(d) Amoeboid form from cerebrospinal fluid (phase contrast).

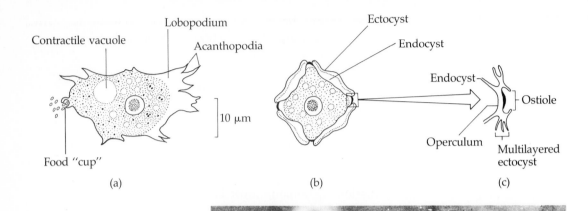

Contractile vacuole

Lobopodium

Acanthopodia

Food "cup"

10 μm

(a)

Ectocyst

Endocyst

Endocyst

Ostiole

Operculum

Multilayered ectocyst

(b)

(c)

**Figure 4–10**
*Acanthamoeba castellanii,* **a potentially pathogenic soil amoeba.**
(a) Trophozoite. (b) Cyst.
(c) Ostiole enlarged.
(d) Trophozoite from eye
(phase contrast).

## *Acanthamoeba* spp.

Four species of *Acanthamoeba* (Fig. 4–10) (*A. culbertsoni, A. polyphaga, A. castellanii,* and *A. rhysodes*) cause chronic PAM and have been positively implicated in human cases. It is possible that some of these may represent strains of a single species rather than separate species. Except for the absence of a flagellated trophozoite stage, the life cycle of *Acanthamoeba* is very similar to that of *Naegleria.* The amoeboid trophozoites of the two genera can be identified by their distinctive pseudopodia. Those of *Naegleria* form a single, lobose pseudopodium and move rapidly; *Acanthamoeba* amoebic trophozoites, on the other hand, form pointed pseudopodia and move sluggishly. *Acanthamoeba* infections can be distinguished from those of *Naegleria* by the characteristic cysts of *Acanthamoeba* found in affected tissues. Less common than *Naegleria, Acanthamoeba* is a facultative parasite of humans responsible for symptoms similar to but less severe than those of *Naegleria* infections. Central nervous system involvement is relatively rare, but usually fatal.

While there is no effective treatment for *Naegleria* infections, in a few cases there has been favorable response to intravenous administration of amphotericin B. New infections of *Acanthamoeba* respond favorably to sulfonamides, and established infections appear to respond to amphotericin B. Corneal ulcers attributed to *Acanthamoeba* infecting contact lens wearers are refractory to these drugs.

# CILIATES

Members of the phylum Ciliophora are protozoans possessing cilia in at least one stage of their life cycle and having two different types of nuclei: one macronucleus and one or more micronuclei. Only one ciliate, *Balantidium coli*, infects humans.

## *Balantidium coli*

A distinctive feature of *Balantidium coli* (Fig. 4–11) is the presence of a depression, or **peristome,** leading into the cytostome. *B. coli* is commonly considered a pathogen of humans that also parasitizes pigs and monkeys. Some investigators, however, classify the organism parasitic to pigs as a distinct species, *B. suis.*

**Life Cycle.**    Both a motile trophozoite stage and a cyst stage occur in the life cycle of *B. coli.* The trophozoite inhabits the caecum and colon of humans and is the largest

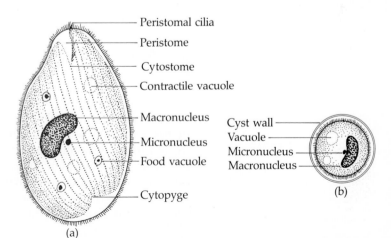

Peristomal cilia
Peristome
Cytostome
Contractile vacuole
Macronucleus
Micronucleus
Food vacuole
Cytopyge

Cyst wall
Vacuole
Micronucleus
Macronucleus

(a)
(b)

**Figure 4–11**
*Balantidium coli,* **an intestinal parasite of pigs, monkeys, and humans.**
(a) Trophozoite. (b) Cyst.

known protozoan parasite of humans, measuring 50–130 μm by 20–70 μm. The conspicuous vestibulum leads into a large cytostome at the anterior end of the cell, opposite to which lies a cytopyge. Coarse cilia line the peristomal area. The macronucleus is typically elongate and kidney-shaped, while the vesicular micronucleus is spherical. There are two prominent contractile vacuoles: one in the middle of the cell and the other near the posterior end. The presence of contractile vacuoles, unique among parasitic protozoa, indicates a degree of osmoregulatory capability. Food vacuoles in the cytoplasm contain debris, bacteria, starch granules, erythrocytes, and fragments of host epithelium. While the organism typically reproduces asexually by transverse fission, with the posterior daughter cell forming a new cytostome after division, conjugation also occurs in this species.

Transmission of *B. coli* from one host to another is accomplished via the cyst. The cysts are round, measuring 40–60 μm in diameter, with a heavy cyst wall consisting possibly of two membranes. Cilia, the large macronucleus, and contractile vacuoles are readily visible within the cyst wall. Encystation usually occurs in the large intestine but may also occur outside the body of the host. Cysts are common in the feces of infected hosts and are generally not considered sites of reproduction, although cysts containing two individuals sometimes occur. Infection occurs when cysts are ingested by the host. Excystation occurs in the small intestine.

**Epidemiology.**    Balantidiosis is most often found in tropical regions throughout the world; however, with an infection rate of less than 1%, it is not a common human disease. The parasite, while nonpathogenic in pigs, is far more common among these animals than among humans in these regions, with a prevalence among pigs ranging from 20 to 100%. Human infection is most common where malnutrition is widespread, where pigs share habitation with human families, and where fecal contamination of food and water occurs.

**Symptomatology and Diagnosis.**    The trophozoite resides in the caecal area and throughout the large intestine. It thrives in an environment rich in starch, such as the small intestine; however, in such an environment, the trophozoite does not invade the intestinal mucosa. This proclivity for starch may be the reason for the trophozoite's invasive character once it becomes established in the human caecal region, a region of low starch content; in the pig's intestine, where starch is more abundant, the organism remains in the lumen. It is believed that the trophozoite secretes proteolytic enzymes that act upon the mucosal epithelium, facilitating tissue invasion.

Results of infection range from asymptomatic to severe. Parasitic invasion of the mucosal lining is followed by hemorrhage and ulceration; hence the name **balantidine dysentery** often given to this condition. While symptoms such as colitis and diarrhea may resemble amoebiasis in many respects, extraintestinal disease is rare. Occasionally, *B. coli* is transported by the blood into the spinal fluid. Fatalities are rare, although one case of fatal myocarditis in the USSR has been attributed to *B. coli*. A few deaths have been reported from Mexico and Central America.

The usual diagnostic procedure consists of stool examination for the presence of trophozoites and cysts. The trophozoites are readily identified by their large size and the fact that *B. coli* is the only ciliate parasitic in humans. Cysts can be identified by their large size, heavy cyst wall, large macronucleus, and the presence of cilia within the cyst.

**Treatment.**    The infection may disappear spontaneously, or the host may become asymptomatic, remaining as a carrier. Drug treatment usually consists of oral administration of oxytetracycline or, in some cases, diiodohydroxyquin. The usual course of treatment lasts about 10 days.

# SELECTED READINGS

Elsdon-Dew, R. 1968. The epidemiology of amoebiasis. *Advances in Parasitology* 6, 1–62.

Martinez-Palomo, A. 1987. The pathogenesis of amoebiasis. *Parasitology Today* 3, 111–118.

Warhurst, D. C. 1985. Pathogenic free-living amoebae. *Parasitology Today* 1, 24–28.

Reeves, R. E. 1984. Metabolism of *Entamoeba histolytica* Schaudinn, 1903. *Advances in Parasitology* 23, 106–142.

# CHAPTER FIVE

# VISCERAL PROTOZOA II: FLAGELLATES

Members of the subphylum Mastigophora, the flagellates, infecting the digestive and reproductive systems of humans, belong to seven species of the orders Retortamonadida, Diplomonadida, and Trichomonadida. As in the case of amoebae, only a few are pathogenic, but it is important to distinguish the nonpathogenic from the pathogenic forms. The nonpathogenic species are *Chilomastix mesnili, Retortamonas intestinalis, Enteromonas hominis, Trichomonas tenax, Pentatrichomonas hominis,* and *Dientamoeba fragilis;* forms pathogenic in humans are *Giardia lamblia* and *Trichomonas vaginalis.* Of the eight species listed above, all but two—*T. tenax* and *T. vaginalis*—are intestinal parasites.

## NONTRICHOMONAD FLAGELLATES

### *Giardia lamblia*

The bilateral symmetry of members of this genus (Figs. 5–1, 5–2) is distinctive among the protozoa. The trophozoite is rounded at the anterior end, tapered posteriorly, and flattened dorso-ventrally. It is 14 μm long (range, 8–16 μm) by 10 μm wide (range, 5–12 μm) (Fig. 5–1). The dorsal surface is convex; the ventral surface is usually concave but occasionally flat and is dominated by a large adhesive disc with a nucleus in the center of each half (Fig. 5–2a). The rim of the adhesive disc is supported by microtubules and fascicles of microfilaments (Fig. 5–2b), and four pairs of flagella arise from basal bodies clustered between the two nuclei. One

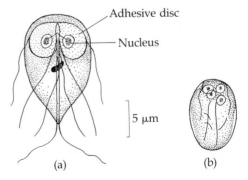

**Figure 5–1**
*Giardia lamblia.*
(a) Trophozoite. (b) Cyst.

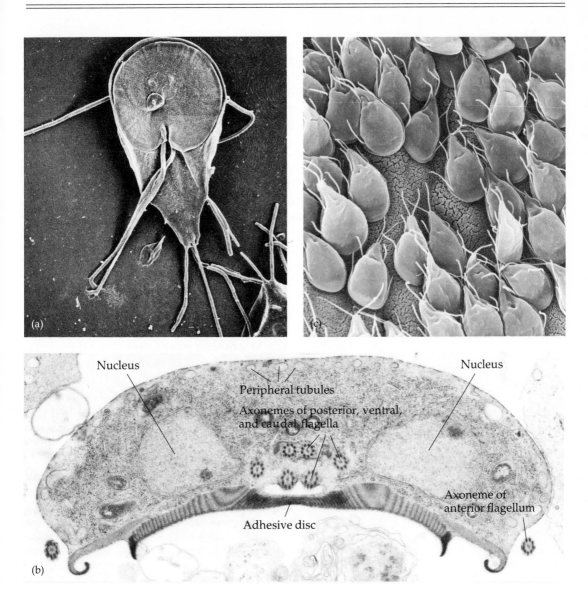

**Figure 5–2**
*Giardia.*
(a) Trophozoite of the *Giardia duodenalis* type. Scanning electron micrograph of the ventral surface showing the attachment organelle. Bar: 1 μm. (b) Transmission electron micrograph of a cross-section of a *Giardia muris* trophozoite in the small intestine of an infected mouse. The marginal groove is the space between the striated rim of cytoplasm and the lateral ridge of the adhesive disc. The beginning of the ventral groove can be seen dorsal to the central area of the adhesive disc. This specimen bears endosymbionts, which are apparently bacteria. (× 15,350) (c) Scanning electron micrograph of an intestinal villus. The microvillus border of the epithelial cells is almost obscured by attached trophozoites. Bar: 5 μm.

pair extends down the midline of the cell, emerging posteriorly as trailing flagella; the ventral pair emerges at the posterior edge of the adhesive disc. Of the remaining two pairs, one emerges anteriolaterally and one laterally. Trophozoites are approximately 15 μm long. Two prominent, slightly curved transverse bodies, the function of which is unknown, are another distinctive morphological feature for identification of *Giardia*.

**Life Cycle.**    The trophozoite of *G. lamblia* reproduces by longitudinal fission. Its organelles undergo division in the following order: nuclei, adhesive disc, and cytoplasm. In the duodenum and bile duct of its host, the trophozoite can either maintain position by attaching its large adhesive disc to the epithelial cells (Figure 5–2c) or use its flagella to swim rapidly in the lumen. Attachment is facilitated by the two ventral flagella working with the flexible rim of the disc. As trophozoites pass through the digestive tract, they usually encyst in the colon. The cystic transmission stage is typically ovoid and averages 11 μm long (range, 9–12 μm) (Fig. 5–1). In saline smears, refractile granules can be seen in the cysts and, at times, the cytoplasm appears to be detached from the cyst wall in several places. In cysts stained with iodine or hematoxylin, two to four nuclei are visible in addition to numerous fibrils (probably flagellar remnants) and transverse bodies.

In victims of giardiasis, massive infection is common. The presence of up to several billion trophozoites in a single diarrheic stool sample is not unusual. Cysts are rarely encountered in such stools, being found instead in either formed or partially formed stools. Infection results from ingestion of cyst-contaminated food or water or from direct hand-to-mouth contact. Ingestion of 100 or more cysts is considered infective. Following ingestion, cysts pass through the stomach to the small intestine where they excyst and begin the cycle anew.

**Epidemiology.**    *Giardia* is the most prevalent intestinal parasite in humans. It is cosmopolitan and is common in children 6–10 years of age but is also seen often in older children and adults, with a high incidence in homosexual males. Outbreaks are frequent in day-care nurseries and other institutions where sanitation may be inadequate. An outbreak of giardiasis occurred in the ski resort town of Aspen, Colorado, when a water supply line was inadvertently crossed with a sewage line, and 11% of the skiers present that season became infected. Among 59 persons whose stools were positive, 56 experienced clinical symptoms of the disease. Giardiasis is common among tourists (an infection rate of approximately 23%) returning from the USSR. Recently, an increase in *Giardia* infection has been noted among wilderness campers in the United States, probably due to the drinking of water polluted beyond the line above which human contamination is unlikely. Such outbreaks have led epidemiologists to suspect that wild animals may harbor species of *Giardia* capable of infecting humans. Surveys have implicated beavers, dogs, and sheep as potential reservoirs for human infections. Significant differences in size and structure among species of the genus *Giardia* have led to the assumption that each different host species has a different parasite species. It now appears more likely that the variable morphology of *Giardia* is due to host diet rather than genetic variation, so that many of the described "species" are invalid distinctions.

**Symptomatology and Diagnosis.**    *Giardia lamblia* infection causes severe intestinal disorders, most commonly diarrhea and others due to malabsorption. Attachment of the trophozoite to the mucosal surface by means of its adhesive disc (Figure 5–2c) causes shortening of the villi of the small intestine, inflammation of the crypts and lamina propria, and lesions on mucosal cells. Occasionally, trophozoites penetrate the mucosa, but this is rare. Since *Giardia* is known to produce no toxins, it appears that symptoms result from combined mechanical and chemical factors. Severe *Giardia* infections produce a malabsorption syndrome characterized by the inability of the small intestine to absorb such essential, fat-soluble substances as carotene, vitamin $B_{12}$, and folate. These absorptive abnormalities may be accompanied by reduced secretion of a number of small-intestinal digestive enzymes, such as disaccharidase. Additional symptoms of infection are diarrheic stools, steatorhea, abdominal distension, nausea, flatulence, and eventual weight loss. Occasionally, bile duct and gall bladder involvement may produce jaundice and colic.

Identification of characteristic cysts in the stool is used in diagnosis of this parasite. Either saline or iodine smears can be employed for initial diagnosis, but a concentration method is commonly used to enhance detection. Examination for trophozoites is rare since their detection depends upon almost immediate inspection or fixation of diarrheic stool samples. Duodenal aspiration, either by intubation or by the enteric capsule method, is another satisfactory technique for trophozoite detection, especially in early stages of infection.

**Treatment.**    Treatment with either quinacrine hydrochloride or metronidazole is recommended. Complete cure usually results within a week after treatment begins. However, if the bile duct or gall bladder is infected, "relapses" may occur for years. Tinidazole is a one-dose treatment that is highly effective but is not approved for use in the United States at this time. Because of the ease with which the cyst is transmitted, all members of a household should be treated simultaneously.

**Physiology.**    Little is known of the physiology of *Giardia*, due in large measure to the inadequancy of *in vitro* culture methods. An *in vivo* study to determine the method of uptake of macromolecular markers such as ferritin by *Giardia* indicates rapid transfer of the marker from the host's intestinal lumen into vacuoles close to the surface of the protozoan, suggesting a means by which *Giardia* obtains nutrients. Other studies using radiolabeled sugars show *Giardia* capable of incorporating certain monosaccharides into glycogen. There is little conclusive evidence pertaining to biochemical pathways, but the organisms are probably anaerobic, relying on glycolysis as their major means of obtaining ATP.

**Prevention.**    Generally, preventive measures recommended for *E. histolytica* are applicable to *G. lamblia* as well. The prescribed amount of iodine added to drinking water should be doubled to insure killing of *G. lamblia* cysts.

## *Chilomastix mesnili*

Cosmopolitan in distribution, this organism (Fig. 5–3) infects about 6% of the world's human population. Usually considered nonpathogenic, *C. mesnili*, like most protozoan parasites, when present in sufficient numbers may cause intestinal disorders, most commonly diarrhea. The stage found in the human colon—the motile, pyriform trophozoite, 12 μm long (range, 5–20 μm)—has a blunt anterior end from which extend three free flagella. A spiral groove extends the length of the cell, terminating at the pointed posterior end. A prominent cytostome enclosing a fourth,

**Figure 5–3**
*Chilomastix mesnili.*
(a) Trophozoite. (b) Cyst.

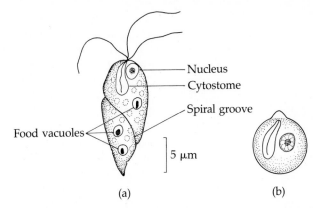

Nucleus

Cytostome

Spiral groove

Food vacuoles

5 μm

(a)                    (b)

recurrent flagellum is located in the anterior portion of the cell, as is the large nucleus. A prominent, curved, supporting fibrillar structure, the so-called Shepherd's Crook, lies just under the cytostome wall.

Since the trophozoite is unable to withstand the gastric juices of the host, the parasite utilizes a resistant cyst stage for transmission. The lemon-shaped, relatively thick-walled cyst, approximately 8 μm in diameter, is identifiable by its single nucleus and the cytostome containing the remnant of the recurrent flagellum and Shepherd's Crook. When the cyst is stained, basal bodies, one for each of the four flagella, may be seen.

## Retortamonas intestinalis

Although only about one-third its size, this nonpathogen (Fig. 5–4) closely resembles *Chilomastix mesnili*. The trophozoite has one free, anterior flagellum and a recurrent, cytostomal flagellum that emerges as a free, posteriorly trailing flagellum. As in *C. mesnili*, the trophozoite resides in the colon, and a cyst, approximately 6 μm long by 3 μm wide, serves as the transmission stage.

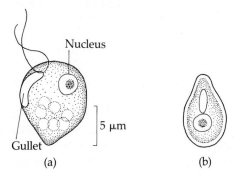

Nucleus

5 μm

Gullet

(a)                    (b)

**Figure 5–4**
*Retortamonas intestinalis.*
(a) Trophozoite. (b) Cyst.

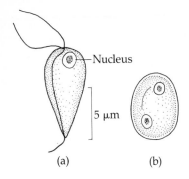

Figure 5–5
*Enteromonas hominis.*
(a) Trophozoite. (b) Cyst.

## Enteromonas hominis

This rare human intestinal parasite (Fig. 5–5) also has trophozoite and cyst stages, but human hosts experience no clinical symptoms with the infection. The pyriform trophozoite, 4–10 μm long by 3–6 μm wide, has three anterior flagella and one recurrent flagellum, the latter extending posteriorly along one side and trailing free. The mature cyst, approximately 7 μm by 4 μm, is ovoid with two to four nuclei, which are usually situated at the ends of the cyst. Most cysts are binucleate.

## Dientamoeba fragilis

The current system of classification of the Protozoa places *Dientamoeba fragilis* (Fig. 5–6) in the class Zoomastigophorea, which includes certain amoeboid forms that may or may not possess flagella. Although *D. fragilis* exists only in the amoeboid form, it is assigned to this class on the basis of ultrastructural and immunological affinities.

*D. fragilis* occurs worldwide. While this organism is often considered nonpathogenic and intestinal lesions attributable to the organism have never been demonstrated, patients with gastrointestinal disturbances experience relief from discomfort when the organism is destroyed by chemotherapy. Fibrosis of the appendiceal wall in all *Dientamoeba fragilis* infections of the appendix constitutes further strong evidence of the pathogenic potential of *D. fragilis*. Also, *D. fragilis* shows a decided preference for erythrocytes when they are available.

The trophozoite moves sluggishly by means of thin, leaf-like pseudopodia. It is frequently binucleate, with a thin nuclear envelope visible only after staining. The prominent endosome is surrounded by minute clumps of chromatin, giving it a beaded appearance. Since no cyst form has been reported, the mechanism of transmission is unknown, although the eggs of the intestinal nematode *Trichuris* have been suggested as possible carriers. While the trophozoite is highly viable and is capable of motility up to 48 hours after leaving the host in feces, it cannot survive the digestive juices in the upper regions of the digestive tract.

From 20 to 80% of the trophozoites recovered from human feces are binucleate, a condition that may represent merely an arrested telophase stage of mitosis. Identification of the trophozoite in feces serves as diagnosis of infection.

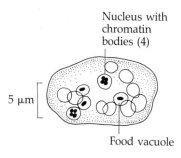

Figure 5–6
**Binucleate form of**
***Dientamoeba fragilis.***

When placed in water, the trophozoite swells and then return to normal size. In the swollen state, numerous cytoplasmic granules exhibit Brownian movement. This feature, called the "Hakansson Phenomenon," is peculiar to *D. fragilis* and occasionally is used in its identification.

## THE GENUS *Trichomonas* AND RELATED FORMS

Of the trichomonads that infect humans, two species, *Trichomonas tenax* and *T. vaginalis*, possess four free, anterior flagella. A third species, formerly called *T. hominis*, has five free, anterior flagella and is accordingly placed in the genus *Pentatrichomonas* as *P. hominis*. All trichomonads possess certain common features (Fig. 5–7), among which are three to five anterior flagella, an undulating membrane of varying length, and a recurrent flagellum fused to the edge of the undulating membrane. All flagella in these forms originate from anteriorly situated basal bodies. The costa also originates from the region of the basal bodies and extends along

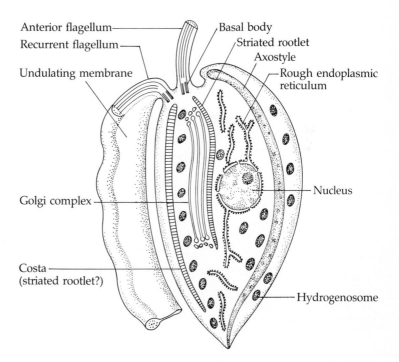

**Figure 5–7**
**Ultrastructural morphology of a generalized trichomonad.**

the base of the undulating membrane. In all three species, associated with the costa and/or the axostyle is a row of granules, the **hydrogenosomes** (paracostal or paraxostylar granules). An axostyle extending the length of the trichomonad appears to protrude from its posterior end, although it is covered by the plasma membrane. A prominent Golgi complex (parabasal body) lies anteriorly near the single nucleus. There are no known cyst stages in the life cycles of these organisms; while venereal or oral contact are obvious methods of transmission for *T. vaginalis* and *T. tenax*, that of *P. hominis* remains obscure.

## Trichomonas tenax

This flagellate (Fig. 5–8a) is commonly found in the tartar and gums of the mouth, as well as in the nasopharyngeal region. Trophozoites are very small (5–16 μm by 2–15 μm), with four free flagella and a fifth fused to the undulating membrane that extends about two-thirds of the length of the cell. Transmission is necessarily by direct contact, usually kissing or using contaminated eating utensils. Drinking contaminated water from a community source may be another means of transmission since some investigators have shown

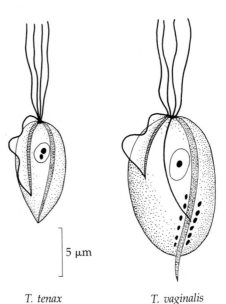
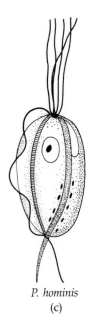

**Figure 5–8**
**(a) *Trichomonas tenax*.**
**(b) *Trichomonas vaginalis*.**
**(c) *Pentatrichomonas hominis*.**

5 μm

*T. tenax*
(a)

*T. vaginalis*
(b)

*P. hominis*
(c)

that this flagellate can live in drinking water for several hours. The organism is not considered pathogenic and can be avoided through proper oral hygiene. Like *Entamoeba gingivalis*, it tends to flourish in unhealthy environments fostered by poor oral hygiene and is most easily found in patients who practice such poor hygiene.

## *Trichomonas vaginalis*

Of the three human-infecting trichomonads, *T. vaginalis* (Fig. 5–8b) is the only pathogen, although a heavy infection of *Pentatrichomonas hominis* may cause diarrhea. *T. vaginalis* inhabits the vagina in the female and the urethra, epididymis, and prostate gland in the male. Morphologically, it is distinguishable from the other two trichomonads by its larger size (7–32 μm by 5–12 μm) and its shorter undulating membrane, which extends only one-third the length of the cell. The trophozoite occasionally produces pseudopodia. Clusters of hydrogenosomes extend along both the costa and the axostyle.

**Life Cycle.**    Typical of flagellates, *T. vaginalis* reproduces by longitudinal binary fission. The optimum pH range for the organism to reproduce is approximately 5 or 6. While the normal pH of the vagina is 4 to 4.5, when the level of acidity is disturbed, an environment is created in which *T. vaginalis* thrives. Normally, the pH of the vagina is maintained by the activity of a group of lactic acid-producing bacteria, but *T. vaginalis* can disrupt such bacteria, causing the pH to rise above 4.9.

**Epidemiology.**    The prevalence among women is approximately 10 to 25%, varying inversely with the level of hygiene practiced. While about 15% of women with trichomoniasis complain of symptoms, altered vaginal secretions are evident in many more. In infected households, the recorded incidence of infection among men is much lower than among women from the same household. This statistic is misleading, however, since the flagellate is much more difficult to detect in men; in fact, positive identification sometimes requires the examination of prostate exudate. Transmission is by direct contact, usually through sexual intercourse. Damp wash cloths and similar items also are sources of infection among children and adults, viable trophozoites having been recovered from wet wash cloths 24 hours after contamination. Trichomoniasis among newborns indicates that the fetus can acquire the organism while passing through the birth canal.

**Symptomatology and Diagnosis.**    *Trichomonas vaginalis* produces deterioration of the cells of the vaginal mucosa, resulting in low-grade inflammation and persistent vaginitis. The condition is characterized by a yellowish discharge accompanied by persistent itching and burning. In males, symptoms are much less noticeable, although there may be urethritis and swelling of the prostate gland. These symptoms are sometimes confused with gonorrhea.

Diagnosis in females is confirmed by microscopic identification of motile trophozoites in vaginal discharge smears. Examination of the urine of both sexes and examination of prostate secretions of the male following prostate massage are also useful diagnostic procedures.

**Treatment.**    Metronidazole is the most effective drug, although it is contraindicated in pregnant patients. Restoration of the normal pH of the vagina by periodic vinegar douches is an effective preventive method and can control mild infections. It is recommended that sexual partners be treated simultaneously.

**Physiology.**    While trichomonads are anaerobic organisms, deriving much of their energy from the metabolism of simple sugars accompanied by the production of organic acids such as acetic acid, the presence of oxygen has little effect on this process. Glucose and maltose are the most effective growth stimuli *in vitro*. One of the products of carbohydrate metabolism is acetic acid, which is anaerobically produced from pyruvic acid via acetyl coenzyme A. This conversion occurs in the hydrogenosome and is accompanied by the formation of molecular hydrogen and ATP by substrate phosphorylation. While trichomonads lack mitochondria, it has been suggested that the hydrogenosome may be a modified mitochondrion since it shows morphological and functional similarities to such organelles, such as a double membrane and regulation of cell calcium. However, this organelle is also considered by some to be a specialized microbody.

In culture, *T. vaginalis* feeds on bacteria and, occasionally, erythrocytes. The predilection for bacteria suggests a mechanism for the breakdown of the normal pH of the infected vagina, since the lactic acid bacilli act to maintain normal pH levels.

## *Pentatrichomonas (= Trichomonas) hominis*

This trichomonad (Fig. 5–8c) is a smaller, highly motile organism (5–14 μm by 7–10 μm) with an anterior cytostome and three to five free flagella. Typically, four flagella beat synchronously, while the fifth beats independently. The sixth, a recurrent flagellum fused to the undulating membrane, extends the length of the cell, protruding beyond the posterior end as a trailing flagellum. *P. hominis* is generally considered a nonpathogen of the human colon, and while it is often associated with diarrhea, there is no definite evidence that it causes the condition. *P. hominis* has no cyst stage, so transmission must occur via trophozoites, and flies may be implicated as mechanical vectors. The ability of trophozoites to survive for at least 24 hours in feces-contaminated milk suggests that transmission may occur through contaminated food and drink and that trophozoites are able to withstand the acidic environment of the stomach en route to the intestine. Reproduction is by longitudinal fission. *P. hominis* infects dogs, cats, and mice and other rodents, with such hosts serving as reservoirs in nature.

Identification of trophozoites in fresh fecal preparations provides the most accurate means of diagnosis. It is important that only fresh samples be used since old stools may contain atypical or degenerating trophozoites resembling amoebae, which could result in their misidentification.

## SELECTED READINGS

Camp, R. R., Mattern, C. F. T., and Honigberg, B. M. 1974. Study of *Dientamoeba fragilis* Jepps and Dobell. I. Electron-microscopic observations of the binucleate stages. II. Taxonomic position and revision of the genus. *Journal of Protozoolgy* 21, 69–82.

Honigberg, B. M. 1978. Trichomonads of importance in human medicine. In *Parasitic Protozoa* (Kreier, J. P., ed.), vol. 3. Academic Press, New York.

Kavousi, S. 1979. Giardiasis in infancy and childhood: A prospective study of 160 cases with comparison of quinacrine (Atabrine) and metranidazole (Flagyl). *American Journal of Tropical Medicine and Hygiene* 28, 19–23.

Meyer, E. A., and Radulescu, Z. 1979. Giardia and giardiasis. *Advances in Parasitology* 17, 1–47.

# CHAPTER SIX

# BLOOD AND TISSUE PROTOZOA I: HEMOFLAGELLATES

Hemoflagellates belonging to two genera—*Leishmania* and *Trypanosoma*, of the family Trypanosomatidae—infect humans. Both require blood-feeding insect vectors as transmitters for completion of their life cycles. The term **hemoflagellate** denotes the protozoan's site of residence in the human host: the blood and/or closely related tissues such as spleen and liver. During their life cycle, hemoflagellates may assume as many as four distinct morphologic forms. While these forms appear to be successive stages, there is no specific sequential pattern of progression from one form to the next. Indeed, it appears that any of the forms is capable of developing into any other. Each of the forms is discussed in detail below.

## MORPHOLOGIC FORMS

### Amastigote

The amastigote (Fig. 6–1) is ovoid in form and usually develops in vertebrate host cells. It is characterized by a single prominent nucleus and a very short flagellum projecting barely (if at all) beyond the cell surface. The flagellum arises from a basal body next to a prominent **kinetoplast,** a structural characteristic of members of the order Kinetoplastida. This organelle is rich in DNA that resembles mitochondrial DNA of other organisms, being composed of a limited num-

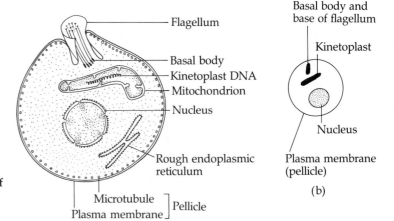

**Figure 6–1**
**(a) Diagram of ultrastructure of a hemoflagellate amastigote. (b) Amastigote as it would appear under a light microscope.**

ber of nucleotides arranged in linked circlets. Kinetoplast DNA appears to be responsible for the elaboration of the mitochondrion in succeeding forms as well as for the metamorphosis of one stage to another. Underlying the plasma membrane of the amastigote is a system of microtubules, the **pellicular microtubular network,** which forms a spiral framework just beneath the surface of the pellicle and provides limited structural support.

## Promastigote

The promastigote (Fig. 6–2), which occurs only in the insect vector, differs morphologically from the amastigote in two significant aspects: (1) it is more elongated and (2) its long flagellum is free anteriorly and serves the functions of both locomotion through the medium and attachment to the insect gut wall. In addition, protruding from the kinetoplast of promastigotes are two mitochondrial branches: a prominent posterior one, often extending the length of the cell, and a shorter, anterior one.

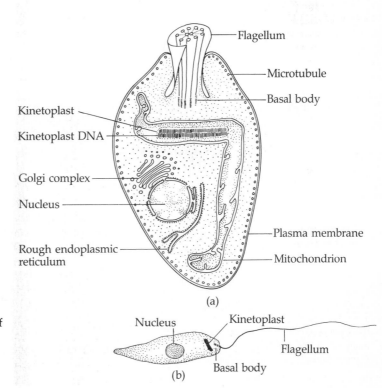

Figure 6–2
(a) Diagram of ultrastructure of hemoflagellate promastigote. (b) Promastigote as it would appear under a light microscope.

## Epimastigote

In this form (Fig. 6–3), the kinetoplast–basal body complex is situated more posteriorly but remains anterior to the nucleus. From its point of origin near the kinetoplast–basal body complex to its emergence at the anterior tip of the cell, the flagellum is enclosed by and attached to the pellicle, producing an undulating membrane. The distal, free portion of the flagellum projects anteriorly, and anterior and posterior mitochondrial branches remain well developed.

## Trypomastigote

The fourth morphological form (Fig. 6–4) discernible among hemoflagellates, the trypomastigote, exhibits varying degrees of polymorphism. One type, the **long, slender trypomastigote** (Fig. 6–5), is characterized by (1) lengthening of the body, (2) elongation of the undulating membrane and flagellum, and (3) migration of the kinetoplast–basal body complex to a site posterior to the nucleus. In this form, mitochondria are greatly diminished in function, and **glycosomes**—membrane-bound, microbody-like organelles con-

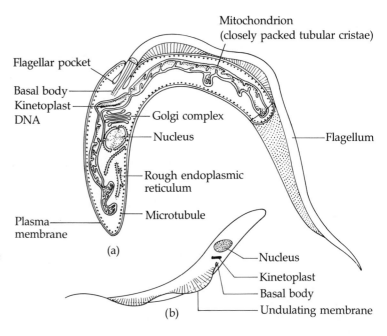

Figure 6–3
(a) Diagram of ultrastructure of a hemoflagellate epimastigote.
(b) Epimastigote as it would appear under a light microscope.

**Figure 6–4**
**(a) Diagram of ultrastructure of a hemoflagellate trypomastigote of *Trypanosoma congolense*.**
The flagellate is seen cut in sagittal section except for most of the shaft of the flagellum and the anterior extremity of the body. **(b) Trypomastigote as it would appear under a normal laboratory light microscope.**

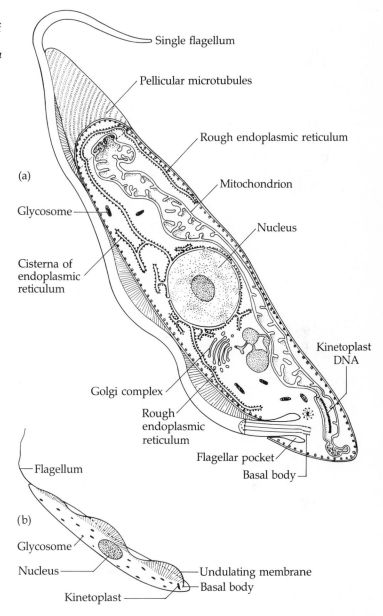

(a)

Single flagellum

Pellicular microtubules

Rough endoplasmic reticulum

Mitochondrion

Nucleus

Kinetoplast DNA

Glycosome

Cisterna of endoplasmic reticulum

Golgi complex

Rough endoplasmic reticulum

Flagellar pocket

Basal body

Flagellum

(b)

Glycosome

Nucleus

Kinetoplast

Undulating membrane

Basal body

taining at times crystalline cores—occur in the cytoplasm. Another type, the **stumpy trypomastigote** (Fig. 6–5), is relatively shorter and thicker in form and has either a shorter or no free flagellum. The significance of polymorphism in the trypomastigote will be treated later.

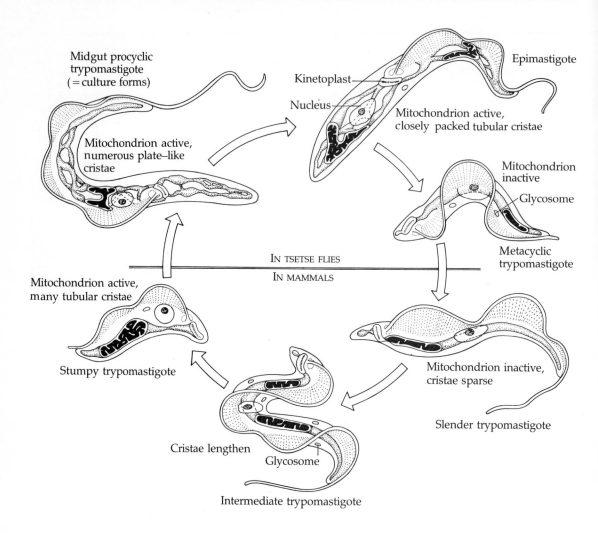

**Figure 6–5**
**Form and metabolic activity of the mitochondrion in *Trypanosoma brucei* at various stages of the life cycle.**

## GENUS *Leishmania*

A number of species of this genus infect humans and are responsible for a condition known as leishmaniasis (Table 6–1). While their life cycles are identical and they are morphologically indistinguishable, they differ in the type and location of primary lesions they produce in the human host.

**Table 6–1**     *Leishmania* **Species and Forms of Human Leishmaniasis**

**Old World forms**
   *L. major* "wet" cutaneous: widespread in rural areas of Asia and Africa
   *L. tropica* "dry" cutaneous: uncommon; urban areas of Europe, Asia, and North Africa
   *L. aethiopica* "diffuse" cutaneous: Ethiopia and Kenya, associated with rock rabbits
   *L. donovani donovani* visceral (kala-azar): Africa and Asia
   *L. donovani infantum* infantile visceral: Mediterranean region

**New World forms**
   *L. donovani chagasi* cutaneous: South America
   *L. braziliensis braziliensis* mucocutaneous: South America, especially Brazil
   *L. braziliensis guyanensis* cutaneous: South America
   *L. braziliensis panamensis* cutaneous: South and Central America
   *L. mexicana mexicana*
   *L. mexicana amazonensis* } cutaneous: South and Central America
   *L. mexicana pifanoi*
   *L. peruviana* cutaneous: South America, mainly Andean region

# Life Cycle

For all species of *Leishmania* (Fig. 6–6), the portion of the life cycle spent in mammalian hosts is paradoxical in that the amastigote infects macrophages, the very cells of the mammalian host that constitute its primary defense against invasion by foreign organisms. The parasite, upon entering the macrophage, establishes itself in an endocytotic vacuole called a **parasitophorous vacuole.** Lysosomes fuse with this vacuole, producing a variation of a secondary lysosome (= digestive vacuole). The amastigote, impervious to the lytic action of the lysosomal enzymes, lives and reproduces within the parasitophorous vacuole. A number of mammals act as natural reservoir hosts for the parasite, the most common being canines, both wild and domestic, and rodents. Leishmaniasis in humans is then a **zoonosis.**

In the course of obtaining a blood meal from a mammalian host, any of a wide variety of species of sandflies belonging to the genera *Phlebotomus* and *Lutzomyia* ingests infected cells containing the amastigotes. Following ingestion by the vector, the amastigote transforms into the promastigote stage in the gut of the insect; the promastigote

**Figure 6–6**
**Life cycle of *Leishmania donovani* and *L. tropica*.**

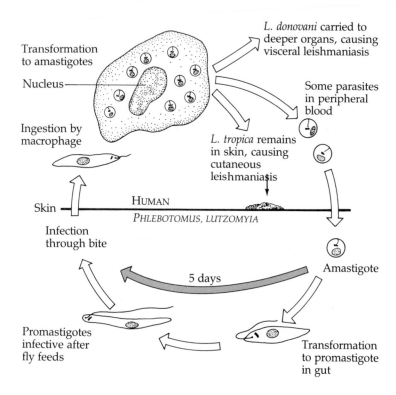

then reproduces by longitudinal binary fission. The reproductive rate is so rapid that after 1 to 3 weeks the anterior gut and the pharynx of the insect become clogged with promastigotes, some of which attach to the walls of the gut by their flagella. When the sandfly feeds again, some promastigotes are dislodged and deposited in the skin of the mammal. Macrophages of the mammalian host quickly engulf the promastigotes, which then transform back into the intracellular amastigote form. Reproduction of the amastigotes by longitudinal binary fission, followed by rupture of the infected host cells, produces large numbers of amastigotes, which are engulfed by other phagocytic cells, thus spreading the infection. Factors such as the species of *Leishmania* involved, temperature, immune status of the host, and even behavioral characteristics of the insect vector may determine the extent and site of infection in the mammalian host.

Reservoir hosts play an important role in the prevalence of leishmaniasis. In many regions of the world, domestic reservoir hosts such as dogs serve as a link between the sylvatic, or wild, reservoir hosts and the human population, via the sandfly vector. The reservoir hosts are usually unaffected by the parasites, and thus they serve as a constant source of infection for the human population. Where reservoir hosts occur, human infection usually results from infected reservoir hosts via the bite of the sandfly vector rather than human-to-human transmission.

## Physiology

Carbohydrate metabolism among members of the genus *Leishmania* is inextricably linked to the kinetoplast, the mitochondrion, and glycosomes of the amastigote and promastigote forms. For example, since the poorly developed mitochondrion of the amastigote includes neither a cytochrome system nor a functional Krebs cycle, the amastigote metabolizes carbohydrates incompletely by anaerobic metabolism in glycosomes and cytosol, producing organic acids as endproducts. When the amastigote is ingested by the sandfly or subjected to *in vitro* culture conditions simulating conditions within the vector, the mitochondrion grows, the number of cristae increases, and the amastigote becomes functionally and morphologically well developed with an active cytochrome system and functional Krebs cycle. Under such conditions, the cell undergoes aerobic metabolism, producing ATP by oxidative phosphorylation. Such mitochondrial proliferation is controlled by kinetoplastic DNA.

The chemical structure of the amastigote pellicle apparently protects the cell from the hydrolytic action of the macrophage lysosomal enzymes. Knowledge of the physiology of these organisms has not, to date, led to the development of effective chemotherapeutic agents or vaccines. An agent currently in use is the pentavalent antimony compound antimony sodium gluconate (Pentostam). It is most effective against most forms of cutaneous leishmaniasis. Its mode of action is not understood at this time.

## *Leishmania donovani*

*Leishmania donovani* is the causative agent for **visceral leishmaniasis,** also known as **dumdum fever** or **kala-azar,** an often fatal disease of humans. In the mammalian host, amastigote-infected cells can be found in many sites: for example, spleen, liver, bone marrow, lymph glands, and intestinal mucosa.

**Epidemiology.**    Recent epidemiologic and clinical studies reveal the existence of at least three varieties or strains of *L. donovani*. The Mediterranean–Middle Asian variety occurs throughout the Mediterranean Basin and extends through the southern USSR to China. The common sandfly vectors are *Phlebotomus major*, *P. chinensis*, *P. perniciosus*, and *P. longicuspis*. A number of canines serve as both sylvatic and domestic reservoir hosts, and, since young children are the most frequent human victims, the disease is known as **infantile kala-azar.**

A second variety, classic kala-azar, occurs in northeast India and Bangladesh. The usual vector for this strain is *Phlebotomus argentipes*. The amastigote mainly infects adult and adolescent humans and involves no reservoir hosts. A more virulent, but clinically similar, variety is transmitted by different *Phlebotomus* species in east Africa and employs wild rodents as reservoirs.

A third variety is widespread in Central and South America, using *Phlebotomus longipalpis* as the vector and both sylvatic and domestic canines as reservoir hosts.

**Symptomatology and Diagnosis.**    Since leishmaniasis is primarily a disease of the reticulo–endothelial system (macrophage system), replacement of infected cells produces hyperplasia and consequent enlargement of visceral organs associated with the system, such as the spleen and liver (splenomegaly and hepatomegaly). A concomitant decrease in red and white blood cell production results in anemia and leukopenia, facilitating secondary bacterial infection. Without medical treatment, the condition is usually fatal. Surviving individuals, however, will commonly demonstrate long-lasting immunity.

In India, a **post–kala-azar dermal leishmanoid** may develop in which numerous parasite-laden nodules appear in the skin. Such nodules are found in no more than 10% of fully recovered kala-azar patients.

In endemic areas, classic initial symptoms of kala-azar are fever and chills, which may persist for several weeks. The fever chart typically shows two fever spikes per day (a "dromedary" curve), a pattern that is valuable in the diagnosis of kala-azar. In more advanced cases, enlargement of the liver and spleen causes abdominal distention. Ultimate diagnosis is made by positive identification of intracellular amastigotes from blood or tissue smears. When such smears are inconclusive, other diagnostic techniques must be employed. One technique is **xenodiagnosis,** that is, the direct inoculation of laboratory animals, such as hamsters, with tissue homogenates from the patient. Signs of infection in the animal within one month constitute positive diagnosis. Biopsy and punctures of such organs as the spleen, liver, or sternum to reveal parasites are also employed for diagnosis. Immunological tests are used, but these are difficult to evaluate since post-recovery cases are indistinguishable from active cases. Further, such tests cannot differentiate among the various species of *Leishmania* and *Trypanosoma cruzi.*

**Treatment.**    Proper nursing care and complete bed rest are essential, especially in more acute cases; blood transfusions are frequently required. Chemotherapy consists of closely monitored intramuscular or intravenous injection of pentavalent antimony compounds such as antimony sodium gluconate. Extreme caution is essential in the administration of such treatment since not only can antimony produce serious side effects, but insufficient treatment may result in relapses or post–kala-azar dermal leishmanoid.

## *Leishmania tropica*

**Cutaneous leishmaniasis,** a relatively mild skin disease commonly known as **oriental sore,** is caused by *Leishmania tropica.* Unlike the amastigote of *L. donovani,* that of *L. tropica* is found primarily in macrophages around cutaneous sores. Sandflies must feed at these sites in order to acquire the infective amastigotes.

**Epidemiology.**    Endemic to those countries of Europe and north Africa bordering the Mediterranean Sea and to the Asian countries of Syria, Israel, the southern USSR, China, Vietnam, and India, *L. tropica* has also been reported from Peru, Bolivia, Brazil, the Guianas, and Mexico. A variant, clinical form of cutaneous leishmaniasis occurring in South and Central America and Ethiopia is referred to as **diffuse cutaneous leishmaniasis.**

The vectors for *L. tropica* are *Phlebotomus sergenti, P. major, P. papatasii, P. caucasicus,* and a few lesser known species of sandflies. The life cycle of *L. tropica* parallels that of *L. donovani.* In addition to humans, this species infects dogs and cats in China and in a few Mediterranean countries. Natural infections are known to occur in monkeys, bullocks, and brown bears in the mideast, as well as horses and gerbils. In some areas of the Middle East, the infection is endemic among rodents in whose burrows the sandflies live and breed. Humans, intruding in these areas, are readily infected. In the Western Hemisphere, dogs serve as the primary domestic reservoir.

**Symptomatology and Diagnosis.**    In humans, the initial sign of the infection is the appearance of a vascularized papule or nodule on the skin at the feeding site of the insect. The papule becomes ulcerated after a few weeks, erupts, and spreads, forming cutaneous lesions most commonly on the hands, feet, legs, and face (Fig. 6–7). The usual incubation period varies from 1 to 2 weeks up to several months or even, in rare instances, several years. Two types of oriental sores are produced by different strains of the protozoan: (1) the chronic, dry (or urban) type (*L. minor*, which is often considered a different species), producing delayed ulceration with numerous amastigotes; and (2) the acute, moist (or rural) type (*L. major*), characterized by early ulceration with few amastigotes.

In the absence of secondary bacterial contamination, sores tend to heal within a year, but disfiguring scars often remain. The lesions in diffuse cutaneous leishmaniasis, however, differ from those accompanying the usual infection in that they are disseminated as multiple nodules under the skin and contain numerous parasites in the associated macrophages, in this manner resembling lepromatous lep-

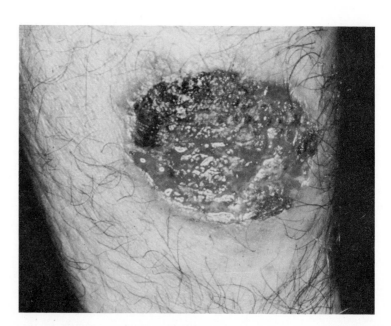

**Figure 6–7**
**Oriental sore, or cutaneous leishmaniasis.**

rosy. This form of cutaneous leishmaniasis is found in patients with specific deficiency in their cell-mediated immune processes.

Characteristic features of the lesions of cutaneous leishmaniasis, such as elevated and hardened rim of the ulcer, are useful in diagnosis. Positive diagnosis requires identification of amastigotes in infected cells. The most reliable diagnosis is achieved by *in vitro* culturing of lesion scrapings or aspirates and subsequent identification of promastigotes in the medium. An immunological test is available, but, as in *L. donovani*, its diagnostic value is limited.

**Treatment.** Healing may eventually occur without chemotherapy, but the process is long and can produce disfiguring scars, especially if proper hygienic practices are not strictly observed. Secondary microbial infections are a constant danger as long as the ulcer is open. Treatment of choice is a daily intramuscular injection of pentavalent antimony compounds for approximately one week. A second or third course of treatment may be required. Concomitant topical antibiotic treatment is employed in cases of microbial contamination of skin lesions.

## *Leishmania braziliensis*

*Leishmania braziliensis* causes **mucocutaneous leishmaniasis.** Amastigotes are found in macrophages in ulcerations at mucocutaneous junctures of the skin. This disease is also known by various other names, including **American leishmaniasis, espundia, uta, pian bois,** and **chiclero ulcer.**

**Epidemiology.** The disease is common in humans in an area extending from the Yucatán peninsula in Mexico south to Argentina. While human infections have occurred in the Sudan, Kenya, Italy, China, and India, the disease is far more common in the Western Hemisphere; hence the name **American leishmaniasis.** Interestingly, its vector is not found in the high Andes mountains, so the disease is not present in this region.

A primary skin lesion appears following the bite of an infected sandfly of the genus *Lutzomyia*. Geographic location determines the site of secondary lesions. For instance, in Mexico and Central America the secondary lesion usually appears on the ear, causing chiclero ulcer, a condition common among the chicleros, forest-dwelling natives who harvest the gum of chicle trees. Recent investigations suggest that the variety of the parasite that causes chiclero ulcer may be a separate species, *L. mexicana*. This variation of the disease, like many forms of leishmaniasis, is zoonotic, and various forest rodents, dogs, cats, and kinkajous serve as reservoirs. Mucocutaneous involvement is seldom seen in the geographic region where *L. mexicana* is acknowledged as the causative agent.

In its southern range, the disease caused by *L. braziliensis* follows a different course. The secondary lesions erupt at the mucocutaneous junctures of the skin, with nasal and buccal tissues most often affected. In these geographic areas the disease is commonly called espundia or uta.

**Symptomatology and Diagnosis.**    As indicated earlier, clinical manifestations in the Western Hemisphere vary so widely that considerable confusion exists concerning the identity of the parasite responsible (Table 6–1). Some investigators attribute the entire battery of symptoms occurring at multiple loci to a single species, *L. tropica;* others list four or more species. Regardless, introduction of promastigotes into humans by the sandfly typically results in a small red papule on the skin, the **primary lesion** (Fig. 6–8), which ulcerates in 1 to 4 weeks and heals within 6 to 15 months. In Venezuela and Paraguay, primary lesions often appear as flat, ulcerated plaques that remain open and ooze. The disease is termed **pian bois** in these areas. A **secondary lesion** invariably appears elsewhere on the body. The sites of secondary lesions are usually distinctive. For instance, chiclero ulcer is associated with degeneration of the pinna of the ear, while degeneration of the cartilaginous and soft tissues of the nasal and buccal areas is characteristic of espundia and uta. Occasionally, infections metastasize to adjacent tissues, forming satellite lesions. Secondary bacterial and fungal infections are common.

Distinguishing the lesions of leishmaniasis from those of other skin diseases, such as yaws, syphilis, and chronic skin diseases, is essential for accurate diagnosis. The surest diagnosis is identification of the protozoan in infected cells and in cultures. Material collected by either aspiration or scrapings from edges of the lesions is suitable for such diagnostic studies. The most efficient method providing the most accurate results is histological examination of biopsy material. When possible, it is preferable to examine early lesions since they yield more parasites than older lesions. The

**Figure 6–8**
**Mucocutaneous leishmaniasis.**
Lesions caused by *Leishmania tropica.*

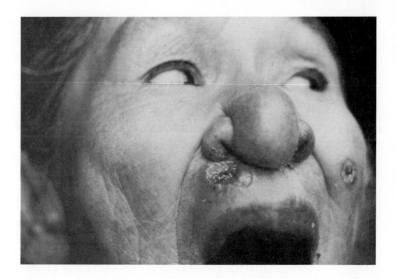

same problems exist with immunological diagnostic procedures for this form of leishmaniasis as are encountered in *L. donovani* and *L. tropica* infections.

**Treatment.**   Generally, the treatment with pentavalent antimony compounds used for the other forms of leishmaniasis is also used for this form. When there is mucocutaneous involvement, more extensive chemotherapy is indicated, since these lesions are most resistant to the usual regimen. For the most intractible cases, daily intravenous injections of amphotericin B for up to 10 days is recommended. Amphotericin B is toxic to some patients, and its administration should be closely monitored. If treatment is insufficient or is discontinued too soon, the parasite may remain dormant for many years and then cause relapse. Once complete cure is effected, however, lifetime immunity is conferred.

# GENUS *Trypanosoma*

Members of the genus *Trypanosoma* infecting humans can be divided into two major groups according to geographic distribution and characteristic pathogenicity. The African varieties, indigenous to that continent, cause a disease commonly known as **African sleeping sickness.** The other species, confined to the Western Hemisphere, causes **American trypanosomiasis,** or **Chagas' disease.** The New World disease involves intracellular parasitism; however, the parasite also affects blood and tissue fluids.

## AFRICAN TRYPANOSOMIASIS

### *Trypanosoma brucei rhodesiense* and *T. b. gambiense*

The two organisms responsible for African sleeping sickness are subspecies of *Trypanosoma brucei,* namely *Trypanosoma brucei rhodesiense* and *T. b. gambiense.* The life cycles of the organisms are essentially identical, the major differences being (1) which of the 21 species of the insect genus *Glossina* serve as vectors, (2) what animal serves as vertebrate host, (3) what time intervals are required for development within host and vector, and (4) what length of time is required for evolution of the disease in the vertebrate host. The following generalized life cycle therefore can be used for both organisms (Fig. 6–9).

**Life Cycle.**   Introduction of the infective stage of the protozoan into the human host occurs with the bite of an infected tsetse fly vector belonging to the genus *Glossina.* In preparation for its blood meal, the insect secretes parasite-laden saliva into the dermis of its victim to dilate the blood vessels and prevent coagulation of the blood, simultaneously introducing the **metacyclic trypomastigote,** the infective form of the protozoan. Morphology and physiology of the mitochondrion distinguish the metacyclic trypomastigote from the long, slender trypomastigote that occurs in other stages of the life cycle. The mitochondrion of the metacyclic trypomastigote has few cristae and contains no intermediates for electron transport. Also, the metacyclic trypomastigote is blunter, with a short, free flagellum. Once introduced into the mammalian circulatory system, metacyclic trypomastigotes spread rapidly within the host, migrating eventually to the cerebrospinal fluid. In the mammalian bloodstream, trypomastigotes exhibit three forms: (1) a long, slender form with a free flagellum extending from the undulating membrane; (2) a short, stumpy form lacking a free flagellum; and (3) a form intermediate between the two.

**Figure 6–9**
**Life cycle of *Trypanosoma brucei gambiense* and *T. b. rhodesiense*.**
(a) Development of trypanosomes in the peripheral blood of humans: infection of the central nervous system.
(b) Development in tsetse flies (species of *Glossina*).
(c) Development similar to (a) in the peripheral blood of the reservoir host (for example, an antelope).

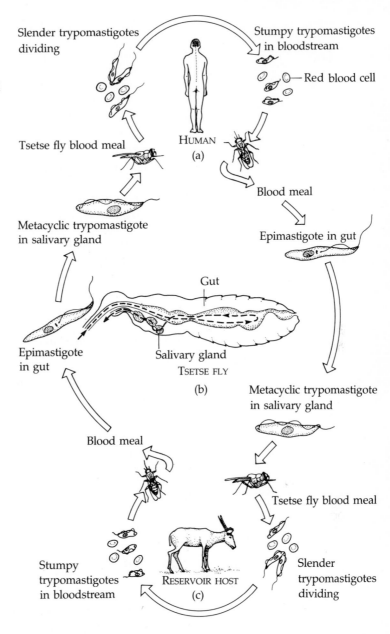

Slender trypomastigotes dividing

Stumpy trypomastigotes in bloodstream

Red blood cell

Tsetse fly blood meal

HUMAN
(a)

Blood meal

Metacyclic trypomastigote in salivary gland

Epimastigote in gut

Gut

Epimastigote in gut

Salivary gland
TSETSE FLY
(b)

Metacyclic trypomastigote in salivary gland

Blood meal

Tsetse fly blood meal

Stumpy trypomastigotes in bloodstream

RESERVOIR HOST
(c)

Slender trypomastigotes dividing

In order for the parasite's life cycle to be completed and for the tsetse fly to transmit sleeping sickness, the insect must ingest in its blood meal the short, stumpy trypomastigote, which is physiologically adapted for existence within the insect vector. The presence of a mitochondrion with prominent cristae and a functional electron transport system enables this form to live in the aerobic environment of the insect midgut. Once ingested by the insect, the stumpy trypomastigotes elongate, lose their surface coat and antigenic identity, and become **procyclic trypomastigotes.** These multiply by longitudinal binary fission and invade the extra-peritrophic spaces. As their numbers increase, they migrate anteriorly, and by the tenth day after ingestion they enter the proventriculus.

Metamorphosis during this migration to the insect's foregut produces the epimastigote, the dominant form in the esophagus and buccal cavity of the fly. By the twentieth day, the epimastigotes move into the salivary gland ducts, attach to the epithelium, multiply, and, by the end of the third week, transform into metacyclic trypomastigotes. Thus, in trypanosomes that produce African sleeping sickness, two distinct forms—the trypomastigote, with its morphological and physiological variations, and the epimastigote—are essential for completion of the life cycle.

**Epidemiology.** African sleeping sickness has probably plagued human inhabitants of Africa since humans first encroached upon the domain of the tsetse fly. Its pathological effects on humans and domestic animals (primarily cattle) have sometimes brought productive activity in certain areas to a virtual standstill. So devastating is the disease that the area of Africa between the fifteenth northern parallel and the fifteenth southern parallel (an area approximately the size of the continental United States), with the potential for supporting 125 million head of livestock, still lies essentially useless (Fig. 6–10). The toll in human victims is staggering: 10,000 new cases diagnosed annually, about 50% fatal and the remaining 50% often resulting in permanent brain damage. Since the disease also affects cattle, sheep, and goats in a region where human diet has historically been acutely deficient in protein, its effects are compounded. A related disease in domestic animals, called **nagana,** is caused by similar organisms—*Trypanosoma brucei brucei, T. vivax,* and *T. congolense.* Authorities disagree as to whether humans are susceptible to *T. b. brucei.* Fortunately for the rest of the world, the tsetse fly appears to be the only insect capable of transmitting African trypanosomes that cause human sleeping sickness, and Africa appears to provide its only habitat.

*Trypanosoma brucei rhodesiense* causes the more virulent, East African or Rhodesian, form of African sleeping sickness

**Figure 6–10**
**Africa's cattle-raising country and tsetse-infested areas show virtually no overlap.**
Tsetse-caused disease has kept 4 million square miles of grazing land out of production.

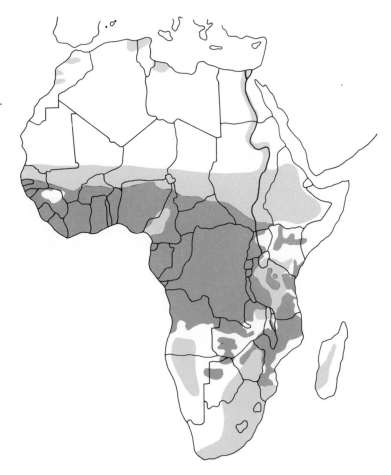

and is usually transmitted by *Glossina morsitans.* In addition to human hosts, wild game and domestic animals in which this parasite is endemic may serve as reservoir hosts and sources of human infection. The disease runs its course so rapidly (2 to 6 months) in humans that person-to-person transmission via the tsetse fly is uncommon.

*Trypanosoma brucei gambiense* causes West African, Equatorial African, or Gambian sleeping sickness, a more chronic form of the disease. Domestic and wild animals, such as pigs, antelopes, buffaloes, and reed bucks, may serve as reservoir hosts. The insect vectors are *Glossina palpalis* and *G. tachinoides.* Human-to-human transmission via the bite of the tsetse fly is common since the trypomastigotes can remain in circulating blood for 2 to 4 years, providing ample opportunity for vectors to transmit them.

In Gambian sleeping sickness, fluctuation in the number of parasites in the blood is common, producing periods of remission alternating with periods when the parasite census is high. These fluctuations are attributed to the ability of the organism to change the chemical composition of its surface coat (glycocalyx), producing a veritable parade of successive **variant antigenic types** (VAT's) in the vertebrate host (Fig. 6–11). It is estimated that more than 1,000 variants are theoretically possible for *T. b. gambiense*. With each alteration of the coat, the immunological mechanism of the vertebrate host is activated, gradually depleting the ability of the host immune system to respond. The antigenic variability of these parasites makes the search for an effective vaccine conferring lasting protection an unpromising avenue for the control of this disease.

**Symptomatology and Diagnosis.**   The diseases caused by the two organisms are very similar except for the interval required for their development in humans. In general, shortly after the introduction of metacyclic trypomastigotes through the bite of the tsetse fly, an inflammatory reaction of 1 to 2 days' duration occurs at the site of the bite. The characteristic reaction, a **trypanosomal chancre,** includes reddening of the skin, a swelling of 2 to 5 cm diameter, and enlargement of adjacent lymph nodes. When the blood and lymph are invaded, headache and irregular fever develop. These symptoms are accompanied by further enlargement of lymph glands, especially in the neck and supraclavicular areas. During this period, the patient may show a number of neurological symptoms, such as tremors of the tongue and eyelids, and some mental dullness manifested as progressive apathy. From this point, neurological symptoms dominate the clinical picture along with increased apathy, loss of appetite, extended daytime sleeping, and concurrent involvement of the muscular system, progressing to paralysis. Classic symptoms are rapid weight loss due to anorexia, anemia induced by malnutrition, drowsiness, and, finally, irreversible coma.

Typically, diagnosis of the disease is a multistep procedure. Step 1 is clinical assessment, especially when there are telltale neurological signs and/or mental dullness accompanied by enlarged and sensitive cervical lymph nodes (known as **Winterbottom's sign**). Step 2 is examination of blood smears, marrow, or cerebrospinal fluid for trypomastigotes.

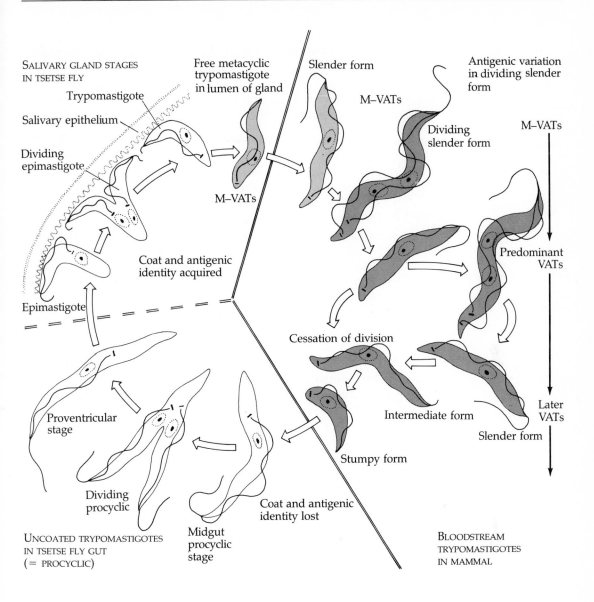

SALIVARY GLAND STAGES
IN TSETSE FLY

Trypomastigote

Salivary epithelium

Dividing
epimastigote

Free metacyclic
trypomastigote
in lumen of gland

M–VATs

Coat and antigenic
identity acquired

Epimastigote

Slender form

M–VATs

Antigenic variation
in dividing slender
form

M–VATs

Dividing
slender form

Predominant
VATs

Cessation of division

Intermediate form

Later
VATs

Slender form

Stumpy form

Proventricular
stage

Dividing
procyclic

Coat and antigenic
identity lost

Midgut
procyclic
stage

UNCOATED TRYPOMASTIGOTES
IN TSETSE FLY GUT
( = PROCYCLIC)

BLOODSTREAM
TRYPOMASTIGOTES
IN MAMMAL

**Figure 6–11**
**Diagram of life cycle of *Trypanosoma brucei* showing phases of multiplication and stages
possessing the variable antigen-containing surface coat (VAT) (shaded).**
The coat is acquired in the salivary glands of the tsetse vector, when free-swimming metacyclic
trypomastigotes arise from vector-attached trypomastigote stages. Only the coated metacyclic stage
can infect the mammal. The coated stumpy and intermediate bloodstream trypomastigotes transform
into uncoated procyclic trypomastigotes after ingestion by the vector, simultaneously losing the
variable antigen coat.

Finally, step 3, if results from the previous two steps are inconclusive, is testing for specific antibodies in the blood. A complete history of the patient is also required for verification of contact with known tsetse fly habitats. It is estimated that this diagnostic regimen produces accurate results in more than 80% of cases.

**Treatment.**   In his search for a successful trypanocidal agent, Paul Ehrlich, a pioneer in therapeutic research and immunology in the early twentieth century, developed a series of compounds such as trypan blue and trypan red. These compounds were used as chemotherapeutic agents for some time until it was discovered that their level of toxicity in humans was too great to justify their continued use. Suramin sodium, one of the current drugs of choice (see below), evolved from these earlier agents. The research by Ehrlich, in spite of its failure at the time to produce a satisfactory drug for curing African sleeping sickness, proved that chemotherapeutic agents could be effective against disease-producing organisms; Ehrlich eventually succeeded in developing salvarsan, one of the first drugs to treat syphilis.

At the present time, therapeutic drugs are most effective against African sleeping sickness when treatment is initiated early in the course of the disease, prior to central nervous system involvement. Chemotherapy begun later becomes increasingly complex with diminished effects. During the hemolymphatic stage, it is recommended that six intravenous injections of suramin sodium be administered over a 3-week interval. For the late, central nervous system stage, melarsoprol is administered intravenously for several weeks. These two drugs, as well as a number of alternatives, can cause various toxic side effects. Severe reactions are rare, however, and the usually mild adverse effects are not sufficient to contraindicate treatment when weighed against the virulence of a disease that is almost invariably fatal when left untreated.

**Physiology.**   The physiology of the long, slender form found in the circulatory system of the vertebrate host differs from the epimastigote observed in the insect vector. Morphological changes related to metabolic characteristics occur in the mitochondrion of each form. For example, the epimastigote, with its well-developed mitochondrion, depends on oxidative phosphorylation for synthesis of ATP. A dearth of metabolizable substrate in the lumen of the insect gut dictates that the epimastigote evolve an efficient system for synthesis of energy-rich compounds. On the other hand, the long, slender form, living in the organic cornucopia of the mammalian blood plasma, derives no selective advantage from substrate conservation; so it can obtain energy-rich compounds by the far less efficient system of substrate phosphorylation via glycolysis. This process occurs in specialized organelles called **glycosomes.** Reduced nicotinamide adenosine dinucleotide (NAD) is oxidized by an α-glycerophosphate oxidase system part of which is localized in the mitochondrion.

# AMERICAN TRYPANOSOMIASIS

## *Trypanosoma cruzi*

In 1909, the Brazilian physician and scientist Carlos Chagas found that thatched-roof huts in a small village in Brazil were infested with large, blood-sucking insects whose digestive tracts were laden with flagellates able to infect laboratory animals. Diseased children inhabiting these infested huts were found later to harbor the same flagellates. Today, this disease is recognized as an American form of trypanosomiasis caused by *Trypanosoma cruzi.* The disease is named Chagas' disease in recognition of its discoverer.

**Life Cycle** (Fig. 6–12).   The stage of *T. cruzi* infective to humans, the metacyclic trypomastigote, develops in the hindgut of the cone-nosed insect, or "kissing bug," *Panstrongylus megistus* and many related hemipteran insects. Since development to infectivity occurs in the hindgut rather than the salivary glands, *T. cruzi* is placed in the section Stercoraria. Metacyclic forms are passed with the feces of the bug, usually as it is taking a blood meal from a vertebrate host, and infection occurs when infected fecal material is rubbed into the bite wound, eyes, or mucous membranes. Mammalian reservoir hosts may become infected by ingestion of infected insects or small mammals.

Upon entering the blood stream of the vertebrate host, trypomastigotes invade a variety of cells, including macrophages, and rapidly transform into the amastigote form. The amastigote evades the lysosome system by escaping into the cytosol of the infected macrophage. The organs most vulnerable to infection are the spleen, liver, lymph glands, and all types of muscle cells. Other areas, such as the nervous and

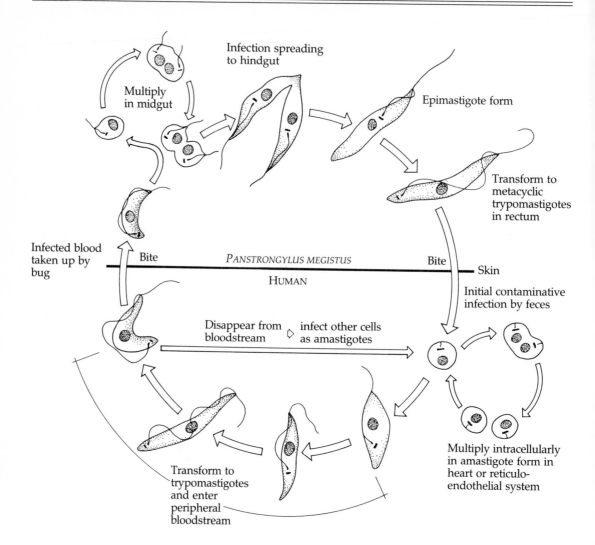

**Figure 6–12**
**Life cycle of *Trypanosoma cruzi* in humans and in the insect *Panstrongylus* ( = *Triatoma) megistus.***

reproductive systems, intestine, and bone marrow, are occasionally invaded. The trypomastigotes actively penetrate the macrophages or are phagocytosed by them. Following the form's repeated longitudinal binary fission, the infected cell ruptures, and the released amastigotes enter other cells. When a cluster of amastigotes occurs in a cardiac muscle fiber, the aggregate is termed a **pseudocyst.** Some of the released amastigotes revert to the trypomastigote form and enter the circulatory system, but, unlike other trypanosomes, the trypomastigote form of *T. cruzi* never reproduces in mammalian blood plasma. In chronic cases, trypomastigotes are rarely observed in the blood since they can be effectively destroyed by circulating antibodies. Unlike salivarian try-panosomes, *T. cruzi* appears unable to produce variable sur-face antigens. Amastigotes in various host cells, on the other hand, are apparently protected thereby from antibody reac-tions. Trypomastigotes of *T. cruzi* differ morphologically from those of African trypanosomes, being shorter (about 20 μm long) and showing a characteristic "U" or "C" shape in stained blood preparations.

Insects become infected by ingesting blood containing trypomastigotes, which then undergo repeated longitudinal fission during passage through the digestive tract of the in-sect. By the time they reach the midgut, they have meta-morphosed to the epimastigote stage. Still replicating, the epimastigotes pass into the insect hindgut. By the tenth day after ingestion, infective, metacyclic trypomastigotes appear in the rectum.

**Epidemiology.** *Trypanosoma cruzi* infection is prevalent throughout Latin America, affecting an estimated 10 million people. Incidence is greatest in rural areas, especially among the poor, whose primitive living conditions facilitate being bitten by the insect vectors. American trypanosomiasis is a typical zoonotic disease that affects cats, dogs, bats, arma-dillos, rodents, and other mammalian reservoir hosts. Ro-dent infections also occur in the southwestern United States and in raccoons as far north as Maryland and Illinois. How-ever, only a few cases of naturally acquired human infec-tions have been reported in the United States and only in Texas and California. Several explanations have been ad-vanced to account for the dearth of human infection in the United States. One maintains that the insect vectors are **zoo-philic;** that is, they prefer animal hosts to human hosts (con-verse = **anthropophilic**). Another suggestion is that per-haps defecation by northern insect vectors occurs not during a blood meal but well afterward, thereby reducing the prob-ability of infection.

**Symptomatology and Diagnosis.**   Upon introduction into the human, the parasites invade macrophages of the subcu-taneous tissue at the site of infection, causing a local, edem-atous swelling called a **chagoma.** In endemic areas, as the disease progresses, human patients often exhibit edematous patches over the body, which occur most frequently on one side of the face. This unilateral edema is oftentimes perior-bital and associated with conjunctivitis, a syndrome known

**Figure 6–13**
**Romaña's sign.**

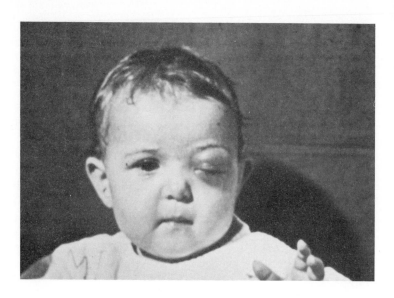

as **Romaña's sign** (Fig. 6–13). In early stages of the disease, parasites abound in infected tissues as well as in the circulating blood. As the infection becomes more chronic, the number of parasites in the circulation diminishes greatly, to the extent that they are almost impossible to find. In acute cases, approximately 1 to 3 weeks after infection, fever, headache, malaise, and prostration may develop. Enlargement of the liver and spleen as well as myocardial damage may follow, but cardiac involvement and gastrointestinal symptoms may not become apparent until many years after the primary infection.

Examination of fresh blood within the first month or two following infection may reveal *T. cruzi* trypomastigotes, particularly if blood is drawn during a fever episode. Blood cultures may also yield incriminating organisms, and serological tests and clinical examinations sometimes provide accurate diagnosis. Direct agglutination tests with the IgM serum fraction are sensitive even in acute cases when infectious organisms are scarce. Normally, however, antibodies do not develop until several months following initial infection, rendering other serological tests, such as complement fixation and immunofluorescence, impractical. Another simple, but practical, method employed in public health surveys is called **xenodiagnosis.** This procedure involves allowing a laboratory-raised vector to feed on a suspected patient, dissecting the insect after 2 to 3 weeks, and examining it for intestinal flagellates.

**Treatment.** Current lack of an effective chemotherapeutic agent makes treatment of Chagas' disease extremely difficult. A Bayer product, Nifurtimox, has shown promise in treating early chronic and acute cases. Once the protozoan invades the host cell, it apparently is shielded from the action of any drug. Limited success against the bloodstream forms has been achieved by treatment with the antimalarial drug primaquine phosphate. It is felt that, even though the intracellular amastigotes are shielded from drug activity, any reduction in the number of circulating infective trypomastigotes is beneficial in that it reduces the number of potential cell invaders.

**Physiology.** *Trypanosoma cruzi* differs physiologically from the African trypanosomes. For instance, the occurrence of well-developed mitochondrial cristae in all stages of the life cycle of *T. cruzi* suggests that there is little difference in oxygen metabolism in the various stages. Indeed, recent data indicate that oxygen consumption is the same in the intracellular amastigote, the bloodstream trypomastigote, and the insect stages. A complete glycolytic pathway has been reported in all stages, with glucose the major carbohydrate. Also, at least some intermediates of a functional Krebs cycle have been reported in all stages. Of the glucose consumed by the organisms, some is degraded entirely to carbon dioxide while some is incompletely degraded to organic acids such as succinic and acetic.

## SELECTED READINGS

Barry, J. D. 1986. Surface antigens of African trypanosomes in the tsetse fly. *Parasitology Today* 2, 143–145.

Bloom, B. R. 1979. Games parasites play: How parasites evade immune surveillance. *Nature* 279, 21–26.

Nantulya, V. M. 1986. Immunological approaches to the control of animal trypanosomiasis. *Parasitology Today* 2, 168–173.

Turner, M. J. 1982. Biochemistry of the variant surface glycoproteins of salivarian trypanosomes. *Advances in Parasitology* 21, 70–153.

Williams, P., and Coelho, M. DeV. 1978. Taxonomy and transmission of *Leishmania*. *Advances in Parasitology* 16, 1–42.

# CHAPTER SEVEN

# BLOOD AND TISSUE PROTOZOA II: APICOMPLEXANS

The organisms that cause human malaria, babesiosis, toxoplasmosis, and *Pneumocystis carinii* pneumonia belong to the phylum Apicomplexa. This taxonomic group was established to accommodate protozoans possessing structures known collectively as the **apical complex** (Fig. 7–1), found in the sporozoite and merozoite stages of the life cycles of these organisms. At the anterior end, immediately beneath the cell membrane, are one or two electron-dense structures called **polar rings** (Fig. 7–1). In certain members of the suborder Eimeriina (including *Toxoplasma gondii*, the causative agent of human toxoplasmosis), a truncated cone of spirally arranged fibrillar structures (the **conoid**) lies within the polar rings. The **rhoptries** (singular, **rhoptry**) are two or more electron-dense bodies located within the polar rings (and the conoid, when present) and extending posteriorly from the plasma membrane.

Except in members of the genus *Babesia*, **subpellicular microtubules** radiate from the polar rings parallel to the long axis of the cell. These organelles probably serve as support elements and possibly facilitate the limited motility of these parasitic cells. A group of smaller, more convoluted structures, called **micronemes,** lies parallel to the rhoptries and

**Figure 7–1**
**(a) Apicomplexan sporozoite showing constituents of apical complex. (b) Cross-section through anterior polar ring.**

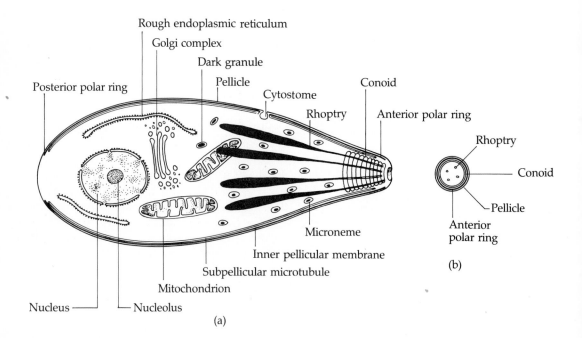

Rough endoplasmic reticulum
Golgi complex
Dark granule
Pellicle
Cytostome
Conoid
Posterior polar ring
Rhoptry
Anterior polar ring
Rhoptry
Conoid
Pellicle
Anterior polar ring
Microneme
Inner pellicular membrane
(b)
Subpellicular microtubule
Mitochondrion
Nucleus
Nucleolus
(a)

appears to merge with them at the apex of the cell. The function of the rhoptries and micronemes has not been elucidated, but they appear to be secretory organelles that may facilitate the parasite's penetration into the host cell.

Located at the lateral edges of the parasite are one or more **micropores.** These organelles are analogous to cytostomes, since they seem to be the sites for endocytosis of nutrients during the intracellular life of the organism. At the edges of the micropore are two concentric, electron-dense rings, situated directly beneath the plasma membrane. Host cytoplasm is drawn through the microporal rings into the parasite, where a food vacuole forms and is pinched off from the plasma membrane—whereupon the process of intracellular digestion begins. Once transformation from the sporozoite or merozoite to the trophozoite stage has occurred following incorporation into a host cell, all the aforementioned organelles lose their physical integrity and disappear—except the micropores, which persist through all succeeding stages.

## *Plasmodium* species AND HUMAN MALARIA

Malaria, one of the most prevalent and debilitating diseases afflicting humans, has played a major role in shaping history and civilizations. Its ravages probably contributed to the fall of the ancient Greek and Roman empires. In medieval times, crusaders often fell victim to malaria during their expeditions, and probably more of their casualties can be attributed to the disease than to the infidels they fought. The manner in which malaria was introduced into the Western Hemisphere is uncertain. Writings from ancient civilizations, such as the Mayan, make no reference to any malaria-like diseases. It appears most likely that the Spanish conquistadors and their African slaves first brought the parasite to the New World. United States troops in both the American Civil War and the Spanish–American War were severely incapacitated by this disease; more than one-quarter of all persons admitted to hospitals during those conflicts were malaria patients. During World War II, malaria epidemics critically affected both the Japanese and the Allied forces in the Pacific Islands and in southeast Asia. It has been claimed that, during the Vietnam conflict, casualties from malaria were the second most important cause for hospitalization among American forces after battle wounds.

While malaria is often regarded as a tropical disease, it is by no means confined to the tropics. As recently as 1937, there were at least 1 million cases of malaria annually in the United States. Elsewhere, the disease has been reported from 52 of 58 countries in Africa, 11 of 18 countries in southwest Asia, all of the 23 political states in the Pacific Basin (Oceania), and 9 of 24 countries in southcentral and southeast Asia. It has been estimated that worldwide incidence in 1982 was 800 million cases, making malaria the most prevalent human parasitic disease, with an annual death toll of about 2 million. Although control programs sponsored by several cooperating nations and the World Health Organization of the United Nations have made great inroads in the fight against this disease, it remains a major health problem in many parts of the world.

The more than fifty species of *Plasmodium* included in the suborder Haemosporina infect a wide variety of animals, but only four—*P. vivax, P. falciparum, P. malariae,* and *P. ovale*—commonly cause malaria in humans. Regardless of the species responsible, certain facets of the disease, such as life cycle of the infective organism, chemotherapy, and epidemiology, are similar enough that the following discussion will make no distinction among the four species except where dissimilarities are medically significant.

## Life Cycle

The entire life span of the four species of *Plasmodium* that infect humans is spent in two hosts: the insect vector, a female mosquito belonging to the genus *Anopheles,* and a human host (Fig. 7–2). Only female mosquitoes serve as vectors: the mouthparts of males cannot penetrate human skin; hence they feed solely on plant juices, while females also feed on blood, which is usually required for oviposition. A significant feature of the life cycle is the alternation of sexual and asexual phases in the two hosts. The asexual cycles, termed **schizogony,** occur in the human, whereas the sexual cycle, **gamogony,** occurs mainly in the mosquito; subsequent to the sexual stage, another asexual phase of reproduction occurs in the mosquito, termed **sporogony.** The infective form in humans is the slender, elongated **sporozoite,** about 10–55 μm in length and about 1 μm in diameter. Its surface, as described earlier, is reinforced by subpellicular microtubules; a single mitochondrion lies posteriorly and a nonfunctional micropore is also present.

During feeding, the mosquito secretes sporozoite-bearing saliva beneath the epidermis of the human victim, thus inoculating the sporozoites into the bloodstream. After approximately 1 hour, the sporozoite disappears from the circulation, reappearing 24–48 hours later in the parenchymal cells of the liver where the **exoerythrocytic schizogonic cycle** begins. Inside the liver cell, the sporozoite develops into a trophozoite, feeding on host cytoplasm with its now functional micropore. There is evidence that additional nutrients enter the trophozoite by pinocytosis. After 1 to 2 weeks (depending upon the species), the nucleus of the trophozoite divides a number of times, followed by division of the cytoplasm. This multiple fission process produces thousands of **merozoites,** each approximately 2.5 μm in length and 1.5 μm in diameter, which rupture from the host cell, enter the blood circulation, and invade red blood cells, initiating the **erythrocytic schizogonic cycle.** Studies of *P. vivax* show that the membrane receptor site for the engulfment phenomenon is determined by the type of antigen present on the surface of the red blood cell. For instance, merozoite penetration requires the presence of at least one of two Duffy antigens ($Fy^{a+}$ or $Fy^{b+}$). Humans lacking the Duffy antigens, practically all West Africans and approximately 70% of American blacks, are resistant to vivax malaria. *P. falciparum* and *P. ovale* malarias, on the other hand, are not influenced by Duffy antigens, thus accounting for their prevalence in West Africa.

Electron microscopy has confirmed that merozoites interact with the erythrocyte plasma membrane and actively invade the cell (Fig. 7–3). During this process, rhoptries and micronemes are believed to secrete surface-active molecules that cause the host erythrocytic plasma membrane to expand and then invaginate to form a **parasitophorous vacuole** which envelops the parasite.

Once in the erythrocyte, the merozoite assumes an early trophozoite shape consisting of a ring of cytoplasm and a dotlike nucleus. Due to its resemblance to a finger ring, this stage is called the **signet ring stage.** These early trophozoites

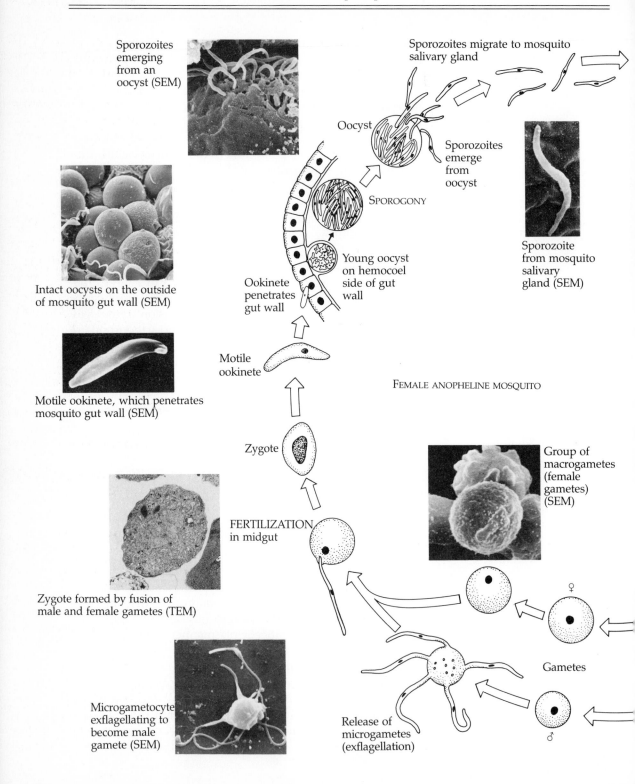

Sporozoites emerging from an oocyst (SEM)

Sporozoites migrate to mosquito salivary gland

Oocyst

Sporozoites emerge from oocyst

Sporogony

Young oocyst on hemocoel side of gut wall

Ookinete penetrates gut wall

Sporozoite from mosquito salivary gland (SEM)

Intact oocysts on the outside of mosquito gut wall (SEM)

Motile ookinete

Female anopheline mosquito

Motile ookinete, which penetrates mosquito gut wall (SEM)

Zygote

Group of macrogametes (female gametes) (SEM)

FERTILIZATION in midgut

Zygote formed by fusion of male and female gametes (TEM)

Gametes

♀

Microgametocyte exflagellating to become male gamete (SEM)

Release of microgametes (exflagellation)

♂

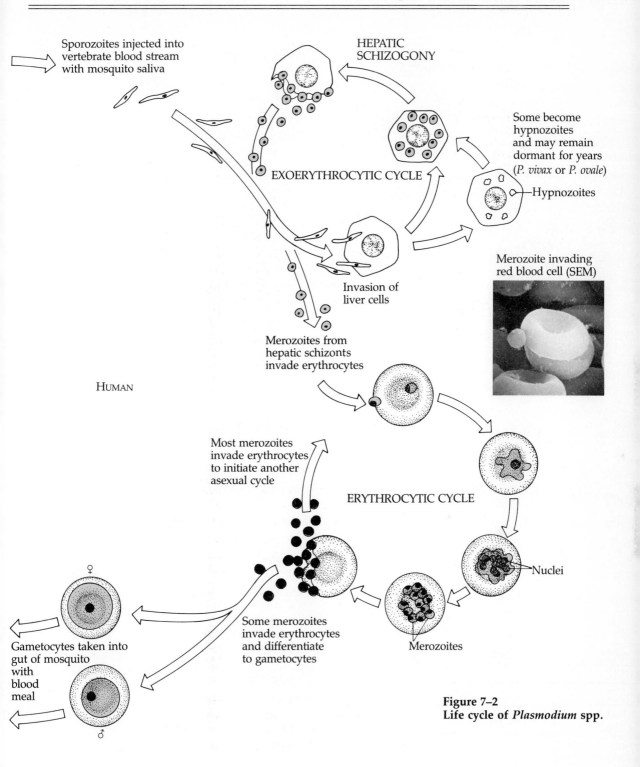

Sporozoites injected into vertebrate blood stream with mosquito saliva

HEPATIC SCHIZOGONY

EXOERYTHROCYTIC CYCLE

Some become hypnozoites and may remain dormant for years (*P. vivax* or *P. ovale*)

Hypnozoites

Invasion of liver cells

Merozoite invading red blood cell (SEM)

Merozoites from hepatic schizonts invade erythrocytes

HUMAN

Most merozoites invade erythrocytes to initiate another asexual cycle

ERYTHROCYTIC CYCLE

Nuclei

Merozoites

Some merozoites invade erythrocytes and differentiate to gametocytes

Gametocytes taken into gut of mosquito with blood meal

♀

♂

**Figure 7–2**
**Life cycle of *Plasmodium* spp.**

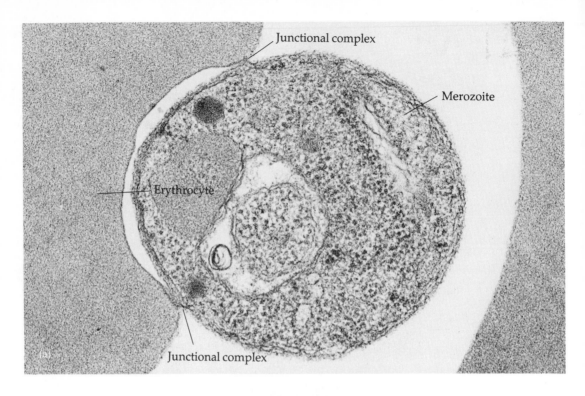

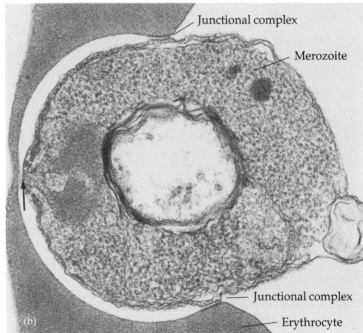

**Figure 7–3**
**(a) Merozoite entering erythrocyte.**
Note junctional complexes at each side of entry. (b) Merozoite further along in penetrating erythrocyte. Arrow points to projection connecting apical end and erythrocyte membrane. Again, note junctional complexes.

feed on host hemoglobin (Fig. 7–4), grow to the **mature trophozoite stage,** and then undergo multiple fission as schizonts, producing a characteristic number of merozoites in each infected erythrocyte. As in the liver, each merozoite is capable of infecting a new erythrocyte. One of two fates await this new penetrant. It can become another signet ring trophozoite and begin schizogony anew, or, later in the cycle, it can become a male **microgametocyte** or a female **macrogametocyte.** The determinants influencing the courses these parasites take have not yet been identified.

The sexual phase occurs in the female *Anopheles* and begins when the mosquito takes a blood meal that contains macrogametocytes and microgametocytes. These stages are

**Figure 7–4**
**An erythrocytic trophozoite of** *Plasmodium gallinaceum* **showing a cytostome that is ingesting host cell hemoglobin.**
The bulge is prominently limited by a double membrane, whereas the food vacuole near the cytostome is limited by a single membrane. The content of the food vacuoles is darker when compared with the host cell contents, indicating that digestion is taking place. A large nucleus with a nucleolus, a mitochondrion, endoplasmic reticulum, and ribosomes are also present on the parasite. ($\times$ 22,500)

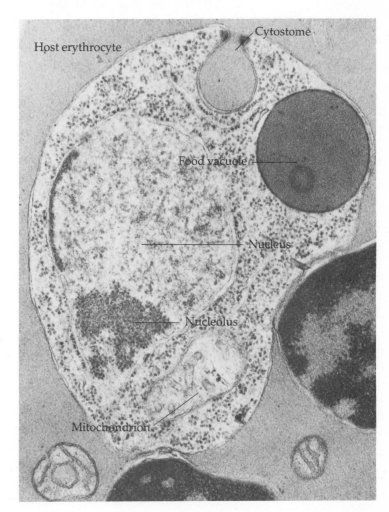

unaffected by the digestive juices of the insect. Once the surrounding erythrocytic material is lysed, gametocytes are released into the lumen of the stomach. There, microgametocytes undergo a maturation process known as **exflagellation**. The nucleus undergoes three mitotic divisions, producing 6 to 8 nuclei that migrate to the periphery of the gametocyte. Accompanying the nuclear divisions are centriolar divisions, following which one portion joins each nuclear segment to become a basal body, providing the center from which the axoneme subsequently arises. Almost simultaneously, the nucleus with the axoneme and a small amount of adhering cytoplasm form a microgamete, which detaches from the mass and swims to the macrogametocyte. During this period the macrogametocytes have developed into female macrogametes, each of which forms a membrane-derived fertilization cone to be penetrated by the microgamete.

The fusion of male and female pronuclei (syngamy) produces a diploid **zygote** that, after 12 to 24 hours, elongates into a motile, wormlike **ookinete.** This ookinete penetrates the gut wall of the mosquito to the area between the epithelium and the basal lamina, where it develops into a rounded **oocyst.** Formation of the oocyst occurs approximately 40 hours after the mosquito has taken its blood meal. Following a period of growth during which its diameter increases 4 to 5 times, the oocyst is seen as a bulge on the hemocoel side of the gut. Growth of the oocyst is due, in part, to the proliferation of haploid cells, called **sporoblasts,** within the oocyst. Sporoblast nuclei undergo numerous divisions, producing thousands of sporozoites enclosed within the sporoblast membranes. As the membranes rupture, sporozoites enter the cavity of the oocyst.

Within 10 to 24 days after the mosquito ingests the gametocytes, the sporozoite-filled oocysts themselves rupture, releasing the sporozoites into the hemocoel. The sporozoites are carried to the salivary gland ducts of the insect and are then ready to be injected into the next person from whom the mosquito draws a blood meal.

## Life Cycle Variations

While the life cycles of the various species of *Plasmodium* that infect humans are basically similar, a number of differences do exist, some of which are important in clinical diagnosis. These differences are summarized in Table 7–1.

**Table 7–1    Diagnostic Differences Among the Four Species of Human-Infecting *Plasmodium***

|  | *Plasmodium vivax* | *Plasmodium malariae* | *Plasmodium ovale* | *Plasmodium falciparum* |
|---|---|---|---|---|
| Duration of schizogony | 48 hours | 72 hours | 49–50 hours | 36–48 hours |
| Motility | Active amoeboid until about half grown | Trophozoite slightly amoeboid | Trophozoite slightly amoeboid | Trophozoite active amoeboid |
| Pigment (hematin) | Yellowish-brown; fine granules and minute rods | Dark brown to black; coarse granules | Dark brown; coarse granules | Dark brown; coarse granules |
| Stages found in peripheral blood | Trophozoites, schizonts, gametocytes | Trophozoites, schizonts, gametocytes | Trophozoites, schizonts, gametocytes | Trophozoites, gametocytes |
| Multiple infection in erythrocyte | Common | Very rare | Rare | Very common |
| Appearance of infected erythrocyte | Greatly enlarged; pale with red Schüffner's dots | Not enlarged; normal appearance with Ziemann's dots | Slightly enlarged; outline oval to irregular, with Schüffner's dots | Normal size; greenish; basophilic Maurer's clefts and dots |
| Trophozoites (ring forms) | Amoeboid; small and large rings with vacuole and usually one chromatin dot | Small and large rings with vacuole and usually one chromatin dot; also young band forms | Amoeboid; small and large rings with vacuole | Very small and large rings with vacuole, commonly with two chromatin dots; amoeboid |
| Segmented schizonts | Fills enlarged RBC; 12–24 merozoites irregularly arranged around mass of pigment | Almost fills normal-sized RBC; 6–12 merozoites regularly arranged around central pigment mass | Fills approx. ¾ of RBC; 6–12 merozoites around centric or eccentric pigment mass | Not usually seen in peripheral blood |
| Gametocytes | Round; fills RBC; chromatin undistributed in cytoplasm | Round; fills RBC; chromatin undistributed in cytoplasm | Round; fills ¾ of RBC; chromatin undistributed in cytoplasm | Crescentic- or kidney-shaped; chromatin undistributed in cytoplasm |

***Plasmodium vivax* and *P. ovale* (benign tertian malaria).**
*Plasmodium vivax* was first described by Grassi and Feletti in 1890 and is the most common species in the Americas. *Plasmodium ovale* was first described by Stephens in 1922. Both

species have a predilection for immature erythrocytes (reticulocytes). A diagnostically significant characteristic is the larger size of these infected erythrocytes, probably due to the fact that the parasites prefer to invade relatively larger reticulocytes. This enlargement of infected cells is less pronounced in ovale malaria than in vivax infections. Cells infected with *P. ovale* also tend to be somewhat ellipsoid in shape. In all *Plasmodium*-infected erythrocytes, two types of granules are found. One type (**Schüffner's dots** in *P. vivax* and *P. ovale*) is distributed throughout the cytoplasm of the erythrocyte and usually stains pink to red when subjected to traditional hematological stains, such as Giemsa, Wright's, or Romanovsky's. Knowledge of the source of these granules in infected cells is speculative; they may be products of degenerative changes in the cytoplasm of the infected erythrocyte. The second type is the coarser, dark **hemozoin** granules, the by-products of hemoglobin degradation by the parasite. Hemozoin is usually found more closely associated with the parasite. Less than 1% of the total erythrocyte population in each victim is parasitized by *P. vivax* or *P. ovale*.

The cytoplasm of the trophozoite stages is very irregular and displays an active amoeboid movement; hence the species name (*P. vivax*, from Latin meaning "vigorous"). During schizogony, 12 to 24 (average, 16) merozoites are produced, each measuring about 1.5 μm in diameter. These rupture from the infected erythrocyte synchronously at 48-hour intervals, with accompanying fever.

Gametocytes begin to appear in approximately 4 days. Macrogametocytes, which outnumber their somewhat smaller male counterparts about 2 to 1, measure about 10 μm in diameter, each almost completely filling the infected erythrocyte.

***Plasmodium malariae* (quartan malaria).** *Plasmodium malariae*, the first parasite to be recognized as a cause of malaria, was described in 1880 by a French army physician, Charles Louis Alphonse Laveran. While *P. vivax* and *P. ovale* selectively parasitize young cells, *P. malariae* shows an affinity for older cells, parasitizing about 0.2% of the victim's total erythrocyte population.

Following incorporation into erythrocytes, early trophozoites begin to accumulate hemozoin and the pink-staining **Ziemann's dots.** The cytoplasm of the trophozoite is compact, often appearing as a band across the infected cell. Morphologically, mature trophozoites resemble macrogametocytes and are, therefore, difficult to distinguish. No change in diameter is evident in the infected erythrocyte, probably due to the parasite's affinity for older erythrocytes.

The number of merozoites, following schizogony, varies from 6 to 12 (average, 8). Hemozoin usually accumulates as a dense mass in the center of the schizont. Merozoites rupture from the infected cell synchronously every 72 hours with an accompanying fever paroxysm. Recrudescences (see pp. 126–127) have been reported as long as 53 years after initial infections.

***Plasmodium falciparum* (malignant tertian malaria).**    *Plasmodium falciparum* is responsible for most cases of human malaria worldwide (80%) and is deeply entrenched in tropical Africa. Examination of blood smears of infected patients, originally described by William Welch in 1897, shows that *P. falciparum* differs significantly from the preceding three species. Only ring trophozoites and gametocytes are usually seen in the peripheral circulation, the later stages of schizogony being trapped in capillaries of muscle and visceral organs. Plasma membranes of infected erythrocytes undergo alteration that causes them to adhere to the walls of capillaries. Infected erythrocytes are not enlarged and represent about 10% of the total erythrocyte population. *P. falciparum* infects erythrocytes of any age indiscriminately. Multiple infections of single erythrocytes are common, and the presence of more than one ring trophozoite in a cell is not unusual. Double nuclei also occur frequently in the ring stage. The schizonts, rarely seen in peripheral blood, produce 8 to 32 (average, 20) merozoites. Rupture of merozoites from infected erythrocytes is erratic, with accompanying fever paroxysms occurring at 48- to 72-hour intervals. Gametocytes are elongated or crescent-shaped cells that stretch, but remain within, the erythrocyte. Macrogametocytes are slightly longer than microgametocytes, the two measuring 12–14 μm and 9–11 μm long, respectively. Hemozoin, as well as **Maurer's dots** or **clefts** (cytoplasmic precipitates in the cytoplasm of erythrocytes infected with *P. falciparum*), tend to aggregate around the nuclear region of gametocytes.

## Epidemiology

Endemicity of human malaria is usually determined by the geographic distribution of its arthropod vector, an anopheline mosquito. Areas where the vector is not present are free of the disease. For instance, since there are no anopheline

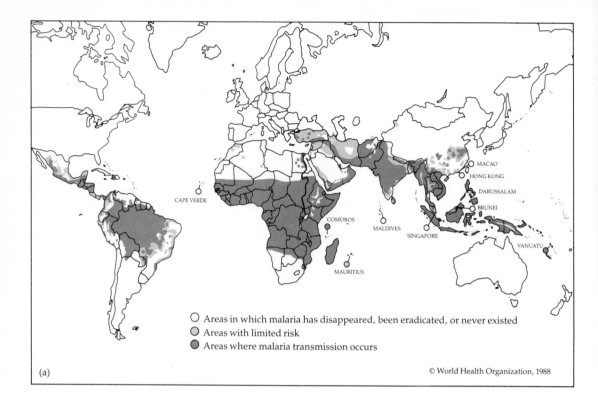

MACAO
HONG KONG
DARUSSALAM
BRUNEI
CAPE VERDE
COMOROS
MALDIVES
SINGAPORE
VANUATU
MAURITIUS

○ Areas in which malaria has disappeared, been eradicated, or never existed
◐ Areas with limited risk
● Areas where malaria transmission occurs

(a)                                                          © World Health Organization, 1988

**Figure 7–5**
**Global distribution of malaria.**
(a) Epidemiological assessment
of the status of malaria.

mosquitoes in Hawaii, many southeastern Pacific islands, and New Zealand, malaria does not occur in these areas (Fig. 7–5a).

Local environmental factors determine which particular species of mosquito transmits malaria in a given area; therefore, local epidemiological surveys are used to assay the prevalent transmitters. Precipitin tests of ingested blood from infected mosquitoes reveal whether the vectors have zoophilic or anthropophilic feeding preferences.

Statistical computation of the average number of bites per person per night yields the **critical density.** A continuously declining critical density indicates that malaria in a survey area is waning and may eventually disappear. An accurate critical density assessment must include not only the number of mosquitoes and their feeding preferences, but also the frequency of feeding and the life expectancy of the mosquito species.

Critical density is influenced by environmental factors that affect breeding and/or sporogony. These functions require temperatures between 16 and 34°C and a relative humidity in excess of 60%. Water dependency for breeding

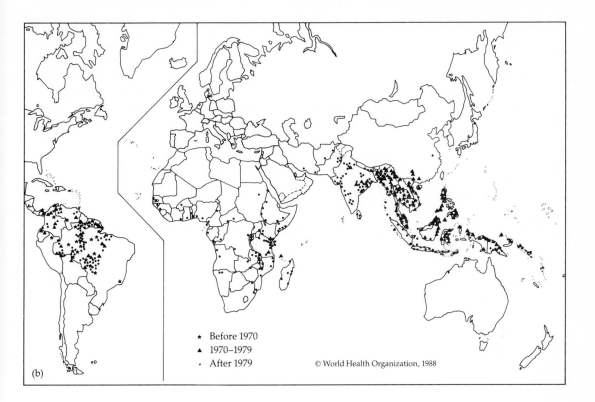

★ Before 1970
▲ 1970–1979
. After 1979

© World Health Organization, 1988

**Figure 7–5 (continued)**
**Global distribution of malaria.**
(b) Areas where chloroquine-resistant *Plasmodium falciparum* has been reported.

varies greatly; some species of *Anopheles* favor small bodies of water, others require large bodies of water such as ponds and even lakes, and still others have intermediate requirements. Females vary also, even as to the preferred feeding locale, that is, indoor **(endophilic)** or outdoor **(exophilic)**. Mosquito populations in areas of low critical density produce a pattern known as **stable malaria,** a universal low-grade infection with little, if any, disease symptoms. The immunity level in the human population is unaffected by environmental and climatic changes. On the other hand, mosquito populations displaying a high critical density are associated with **unstable malaria.** The disease pattern in such areas is noticeably affected by drastic environmental or climatic changes. Incidence is usually transient, alternately producing periods of high mortality and then declining as optimal conditions subside. Since there is insufficient time for immunity to become established under such circumstances, a pattern of recurring epidemics develops.

The control of malaria depends upon a variety of factors, such as availability of antimalarial drugs, use of screens on houses to keep out mosquitoes, proper use of insecticides, elimination of mosquito breeding sites, mosquito eradication, and other environmental controls. Under the auspices of the World Health Organization (WHO), malaria was controlled or drastically diminished in many parts of the world by the 1960's. However, there has been a marked resurgence in the disease since the 1970's. Several factors have contributed to this, most important of which are the development of widespread resistance on the part of anopheline mosquitoes to insecticides and the evolution of chloroquine-resistant *P. falciparum.* Another factor is the reduction in personnel trained to maintain the WHO-established standards for control.

## Relapse and Recrudescence

It has long been known that victims of vivax or ovale malarias, after apparent recovery, may suffer **relapse.** Originally, such relapse was thought to be due to populations of cryptozoites entering the exoerythrocytic cycle. While one population progressed to the usual erythrocytic phase, underwent schizogony, and released merozoites into the circulating blood causing malaria, the other population maintained an ongoing exoerythrocyctic cycle known as a para-erythrocytic cycle. It was thought that parasites in the hepatic stages of the cycle remained protected from host antibodies until activated by some physiological change within the host that allowed them to erupt from the hepatocytes, precipitating another bout of malaria.

A more recent view also recognizes the existence of two different populations of sporozoites. **Short prepatent sporozoites** (SPP's), upon entering the human host, undergo the usual exoerythrocytic and erythrocytic phases of development and cause malaria. **Long prepatent sporozoites** (LPP's), or **hypnozoites,** remain dormant in the hepatocytes for an indefinite period. When a stimulus, such as the physiological fluctuation cited above, activates hypnozoites into the exoerythrocytic and erythrocytic cycles, relapse occurs. The ratio of LPP's to SPP's in *P. vivax* infections in a given human population appears to vary according to strain. For instance, in a North Korean strain found in temperate zones, LPP sporozoites are far more numerous than SPP's. On the other hand, in strains common to tropical regions, the relative proportions are equal or sometimes reversed.

Recurrence of malaria among victims infected by *P. malariae* many years after apparent cure fostered an enduring belief that this species produced relapses like those produced by *P. vivax* and *P. ovale*. However, it has been shown that the periodic increase in numbers of parasites results from a residual population persisting at very low levels in the blood after inadequate or incomplete treatment of the initial infection. The number of parasites is usually so small that infected individuals remain symptomless. This situation may persist for as long as 53 years before something, such as splenic dysfunction, triggers a parasite population explosion with accompanying disease manifestations, a phenomenon termed **recrudescence.** The difference, therefore, between relapse and recrudescence is that the former results from exoerythrocytic stages in the liver as a result of the activation of hypnozoites, while the latter is due to a sudden increase in what was a persistent, low-level parasite population in the blood.

## Symptomatology and Diagnosis

Of the four species of *Plasmodium* responsible for human malaria, *P. falciparum* is the most pathogenic and causes, by far, the highest mortality. For that reason falciparum malaria will be given primary emphasis in the following discussion.

Pathology in human malaria is generally manifested in two basic forms: host inflammatory reactions and anemia. Host inflammatory reactions are initiated by the periodic rupture of infected erythrocytes, which releases malarial pigment such as hemozoin, cellular debris, and parasite metabolic wastes. These ruptures are accompanied by fever paroxysms that are usually synchronous except during the primary attack. As explained earlier, the interval between paroxysms is species specific. However, during the primary attack, since the infection may arise from several populations of liver merozoites at different stages of development, synchrony may not be evident. How the parasites' development gradually assumes a synchronous pattern remains unexplained, but *P. falciparum* tends to be the most persistently erratic. Macrophages, particularly those in the liver, bone marrow, and spleen, phagocytose released pigment. In extreme cases, the amount of pigment is so great that it imparts a dark, reddish-brown hue to visceral organs such as liver, spleen, and brain. With increased erythrocyte destruction, accompanied by the body's inability to recycle iron bound in the insoluble hemozoin, anemia develops.

One pathological element unique to *P. falciparum* is vascular obstruction. Plasma membranes of erythrocytes infected with schizonts, the more mature stages of the organism, develop electron-dense "knobs" by which they adhere to the endothelium of capillaries in visceral organs (Fig. 7–6). Engorged with hordes of infected erythrocytes, the capillaries become obstructed, causing the affected organs to become anoxic. In terminal cases, blocked capillaries (**ischema**) in the brain cause it to become swollen and congested.

A condition known as **blackwater fever** often accompanies falciparum malaria infections. Characterized by massive lysis of erythrocytes, it produces abnormally high levels of hemoglobin in urine and blood. Fever, vomiting with blood, and jaundice also occur, and there is a 20 to 50% mortality rate, usually due to renal failure. The exact cause of this condition is uncertain; it may be a reaction to quinine, or it may result from an autoimmune phenomenon in which hemolytic antibodies are produced.

Diagnosis of malaria usually consists of the microscopical demonstration of the parasites in stained thick and thin blood smears of peripheral blood. Even though synchrony is obvious, diagnostic blood samples can be drawn almost anytime, since a few "stragglers" from the previous episode always remain in the blood. Smears, however, should be made at regular intervals over a period of several days, especially if one smear fails to show parasites. Serological tests

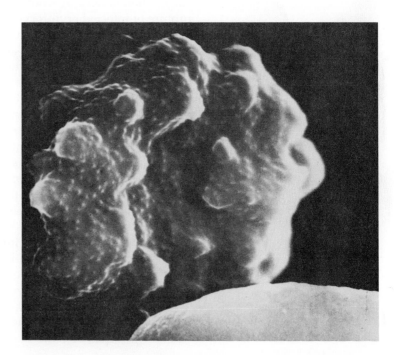

**Figure 7–6**
**Erythrocyte parasitized with**
*Plasmodium falciparum,*
**showing surface knobs.**

are of little clinical value since they make no distinction between present and past infections.

# Chemotherapy

Malaria control requires effective treatment of the disease in humans and continuous efforts to control mosquito populations. The first known effective antimalarial drug was quinine, an extract from the bark of the cinchona tree of South America and other tropical areas. In use since 1640, the drug destroys the schizogonic stages of malaria, but it has little or no effect on exoerythrocytic stages or gametocytes. During World War II, when the Japanese occupied the cinchona plantations in Indonesia, it became necessary for Allied forces to develop alternative drugs. A synthetic drug, Atabrine dihydrochloride (quinacrine hydrochloride), developed in Germany in 1936, proved useful against the erythrocytic stages of all species of *Plasmodium* and in suppressing clinical symptoms. Like quinine, Atabrine is ineffectual against exoerythrocytic stages and, consequently, patients treated with this drug are susceptible to relapse. Also, Atabrine produces a number of undesirable side effects, such as jaundice and gastrointestinal disturbances. Since World War II, research has yielded a number of synthetic drugs, of which the most commonly used are chloroquine, amodiaquin, and primaquine. Each, however, has limited effect upon *Plasmodium* and, for maximum benefit, should be administered in combination with one or more other drugs. For instance, while chloroquine and amodiaquin act to suppress clinical symptoms by destroying the erythrocytic stages, the slow-acting drug primaquine destroys the exoerythrocytic stages. Currently, the optimal chemotherapeutic regimen for treatment of vivax malaria includes a combination of chloroquine and primaquine.

The folic acid cycle provides a suitable metabolic pathway for chemotherapeutic management of malaria. This cycle is vital to the parasite in synthesizing bases for nucleic acid formation. The drug pyrimethamine, used in combination with sulfadoxine, inhibits portions of the cycle and is therefore lethal to the parasites. In 1984, a new antimalarial drug, mefloquine, was tested and approved for use by health authorities. This drug acts against blood schizonts. Currently, mefloquine is being added to the pyrimethamine–sulfadoxine combination in a one-step treatment for human malaria.

An alarming phenomenon in the treatment of malaria is the increasing resistance of the parasites to chemotherapy (Fig. 7–5b), most probably arising from mutagenic changes developed by some strains of *P. falciparum*. Thus, the development of antimalarial drugs must be a continuous process. Similarly, the use of insecticides to eradicate mosquitoes has led to the appearance of resistant mosquito strains in areas that have been sprayed extensively. In Greece, for example, only a few years after apparently successful efforts to control *Anopheles* with DDT, it was necessary to alternate DDT application with dieldrin in order to control the malaria-carrying species.

Ideally, the search for new antimalarial drugs and new insecticides should be directed toward discovery of compounds that block a critical metabolic pathway within the parasite or mosquito. Further, such new compounds should be inexpensive and safe and should produce long-lasting effects. Such an approach, however, must be predicated upon a thorough understanding of the biochemical processes occurring within these parasites, knowledge acquired only after years of intensive research with sophisticated techniques.

## Immunity

In addition to chemotherapy research, development of a protective vaccine against malaria is being vigorously pursued. Indeed, the development of vaccines and immunodiagnostic tests are two of the major priorities of WHO. The basis for development of a successful vaccine is identifying those stages that stimulate protective immune responses in the vertebrate host. Since many of the developmental stages of malarial parasites in the vertebrate host are intracellular and therefore are protected from the host's immune mechanism, the extracellular forms—sporozoites and merozoites—become the targets for a vaccine. A number of approaches using recent technology, such as gene cloning and genetic engineering, are creating a degree of cautious optimism in the quest. Certain singular characteristics of the sporozoite surface coat have already been identified. The coat acts as a renewable "decoy" to the vertebrate host's immune system, stimulating the production of antibodies. When the sporozoite is attacked and its "decoy" coat sloughs off, a replacement coat is synthesized, and the "decoy" effect continues. This system provides ideal protection for the sporozoite, which resides only briefly in the blood before it penetrates a liver cell and is protected from circulating antibodies. This method of protection contrasts with that in trypanosomes (p. 102), which are exposed to the immune system for a long time throughout a lengthy residence in the blood. The surface antigens of African trypanosomes, it will be recalled, undergo continual change, keeping one step ahead of the vertebrate host's immune system.

In endemic areas, premunition is the basis for protective immunity as long as low-level infection persists. With complete cure, however, the victim regains susceptibility. Also, while nursing infants in endemic areas are protected through antibodies in the mother's milk, at the time of weaning the children are at greatest risk, and the highest mortality rate in such regions is among children. Also, *P. falciparum* has been reported to cross the placenta and cause infection of the fetus.

Factors other than immunological ones also may affect susceptibility among humans. Several genetic conditions affect the malarial organism. Susceptibility conferred by the presence of Duffy antigens has already been discussed. Genetic deficiency in glucose-6-phosphate dehydrogenase (G6PDH) activity in erythrocytes **(favism)** creates an inhospitable environment for the parasites. This enzyme is rate-limiting in one of the erythrocyte metabolic pathways that provides pentoses for the malarial organism's synthesis of nucleic acid. Hence, an insufficiency in the enzyme creates a deficiency in the parasite's synthesis of DNA and RNA. Humans heterozygous for **sickle cell anemia** possess a selective advantage over individuals with normal hemoglobin in regions where *P. falciparum* is endemic. The reasons for this advantage are not fully understood, but there is evidence that the sickle cell trait affects the resting potential of the erythrocyte's plasma membrane, causing an excessive leakage of potassium from the cell. Since the malarial parasite requires a higher level of potassium than is available, it dies. In a heterozygous host, up to 40% of the cells are of this type and are, therefore, unsuitable for the parasite's development, thus accounting for the resistance to the disease among such persons. Ironically, the severe pathological effects of falciparum malaria have resulted in the maintenance of this highly deleterious mutation.

## Physiology

Metabolic characteristics of *Plasmodium* provide targets for drug action and immunological attack. Unfortunately, many gaps remain in our understanding of several metabolic aspects of the parasite's intracellular stages—due, in part, to the fact that until very recently there was no satisfactory *in vitro* culture method for these stages. For example, glucose is the main carbohydrate required by the parasite, and most of its energy appears to derive from glycolysis. However, while some intermediates of the Krebs cycle have been demonstrated, there is no evidence of mitochondria in the erythrocytic stages, although the mosquito stages do possess these organelles. The erythrocytic stages are essentially anaerobic, although they use oxygen for synthesis of nucleic acids.

The end-products of carbohydrate metabolism are lactic acid, formic acid, and some acetic acid. The parasite does fix carbon dioxide, and the enzymes that catalyze this reaction are believed to be vulnerable to quinine and chloroquine.

Hemoglobin is essential for the parasite's development, although the precise components required by the parasite are unknown. The parasite digests hemoglobin intracellularly, producing an insoluble by-product, hemozoin. In addition to its effect upon carbon dioxide fixation, chloroquine appears to interfere with the intracellular digestive processes of the parasite. The lysosomotropic agents chloroquine and quinine are weak bases that raise the pH of the lysosomal contents, preventing the parasite from efficiently digesting host hemoglobin.

Although the malarial parasite depends on the host erythrocyte for many essential molecules, it can synthesize folic acid from basic molecules; and folic acid is a key compound in the folic acid cycle for pyrimidine synthesis. Host cells, on the other hand, require outside sources of folic acid. Drugs that block the synthesis of folic acid are, therefore, prime candidates for chemotherapeutic use.

# OTHER APICOMPLEXANS

## *Babesia* species

Although infections of humans by *Babesia* spp. have been known since 1957, human babesiosis has in recent years become sufficiently common on Nantucket Island and Martha's Vineyard in Massachusetts, at Shelter Island on Long Island, New York, and in Wisconsin to attract the attention of medical parasitologists. In each instance, the causative agent has been identified as *Babesia microti*, a natural parasite of the meadow vole and other rodents. The vector in all instances has been identified as the tick *Ixodes scapularis*. Humans acquire the infection when an infected tick accidentally feeds on a human host. Splenectomized persons seem especially vulnerable to babesiosis; indeed, such individuals appear to be susceptible to more than one species of *Babesia*, and most fatalities reported to date have occurred in splenectomized individuals.

**Life Cycle.**   Infection of the vertebrate host begins with the introduction of **vermicles** (= sporozoites) through the bite of the infected tick. The vermicle is approximately 2 μm long and varies in shape from piriform to spiral. There is no exoerythrocytic phase in the life cycle. The vermicle enters the host erythrocyte, where it develops into a trophozoite, rapidly increases in size, and undergoes binary fission, producing numerous merozoites. The merozoites erupt from one host erythrocyte and enter others, where the cycle of growth, division, and re-entry continues, building up an extremely large population in a short time.

The tick acquires the infection initially by ingesting infected vertebrate blood. Parasites are released in the tick's gut and are immediately transformed into motile, polymorphic isogametes. Gametic fusion to form zygotes occurs within 24 hours following the blood meal. The zygotes transform into cigar-shaped ookinetes, 8–10 μm long, that penetrate the tick's intestine and become encysted sporonts, each of which grows to about 16 μm in diameter within 2 days. Each sporont nucleus then undergoes schizogony, and the resulting vermicles, each 9–13 μm long, migrate into the hemocoel, from whence they invade various tissues of the tick, particularly the ovaries. There they undergo several more divisions and invasions within embryonic ticks. Final generations of vermicles eventually migrate to the salivary glands of the newly hatched tick and are injected into the vertebrate host when the young tick takes its blood meal. The passage of *Babesia* from a tick to its progeny in the manner described above is known as **transovarian transmission.**

**Symptomatology   and   Diagnosis.**   Human   babesiosis caused by *Babesia divergens*, reported as a cattle parasite in Ireland, can be fatal. The disease usually mimics relatively mild malaria, and, unless there is reason to suspect babesiosis, the erythrocytic stages in blood smears are often mistaken for malarial organisms. The usual manifestation of the infection is basically hemolytic anemia.

**Treatment.**    Since babesiosis can be mistaken for malaria, it is sometimes treated with chloroquine. In spite of some claims of success, there is no real evidence that the drug is effective in treating this disease. Since most individuals recover spontaneously, treatment of symptoms may be the best way to manage the disease. For patients in whom the number of parasites becomes life-threatening, exchange transfusion may be indicated.

## *Toxoplasma gondii*

Human toxoplasmosis is caused by a coccidian, *Toxoplasma gondii*, originally discovered in 1908 in a desert rodent. This potentially perilous parasite is estimated to infect 50% of the population of the United States. Fortunately, most of the cases are asymptomatic, with clinical toxoplasmosis affecting only scattered individuals. Occasionally, however, minor epidemics do occur. The principal means of acquiring the infection is either ingestion of inadequately cooked meat—including beef, pork, and lamb—or contact with feral or domestic cats. Any cat, no matter how well cared for, may carry and pass the infective stage of *Toxoplasma*. Congenital toxoplasmosis is a very serious disease, and for this reason pregnant women should avoid contact with litter boxes used by cats. Flies and roaches have also been implicated as carriers of the infective stages from cat feces to food.

**Life Cycle** (Fig. 7–7).    *Toxoplasma* can attack a wide variety of tissue cells but seems to favor muscle, lymph nodes, and intestinal epithelium. Infection of intestinal epithelial cells occurs only in felines, probably the "normal" hosts, and this developmental pathway is termed the **enteric** or **enteroepithelial phase.** It is during this stage that sporozoite-containing oocysts are formed that serve as the primary source of human infection. In other hosts, including many species of carnivores, insectivores, and primates, only the **extraintestinal** or **tissue phase** occurs. Ingestion of a sporulated oocyst is the precursor for either developmental phase. Each oocyst measures 10–13 μm by 9–11 μm and contains two sporocysts, each of which, in turn, contains four sporozoites. The sporozoites are released from the oocyst in the lumen of the host's small intestine. In cats, some sporozoites penetrate intestinal epithelial cells to begin the enteric phase, while

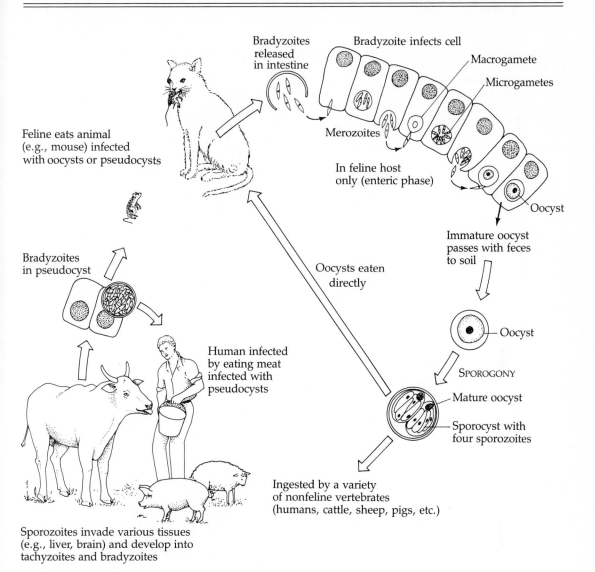

Bradyzoites released in intestine

Bradyzoite infects cell

Macrogamete

Microgametes

Merozoites

In feline host only (enteric phase)

Oocyst

Feline eats animal (e.g., mouse) infected with oocysts or pseudocysts

Immature oocyst passes with feces to soil

Bradyzoites in pseudocyst

Oocysts eaten directly

Oocyst

SPOROGONY

Human infected by eating meat infected with pseudocysts

Mature oocyst

Sporocyst with four sporozoites

Ingested by a variety of nonfeline vertebrates (humans, cattle, sheep, pigs, etc.)

Sporozoites invade various tissues (e.g., liver, brain) and develop into tachyzoites and bradyzoites

**Figure 7–7**
**Life cycle of *Toxoplasma gondii*.**

others penetrate the mucosa and develop in cells of underlying tissues, including lymph nodes and leukocytes.

In the enteric phase, the sporozoites enter the host cell, become trophozoites, and undergo schizogony. The number of schizogonic cycles varies according to the physiological condition of the host, but about 2–40 merozoites (Fig. 7–8) arise from each trophozoite. From 3 to 15 days after infection, some of the merozoites invade new host cells and develop into either microgametocytes (males) or macrogametocytes (females). About 2 to 4% of the gametocytic

**Figure 7–8**
**Apical complex.**
(a) Drawing of merozoite of *Toxoplasma gondii* showing some constituents of the apical complex. (b) Electron micrograph of (a).

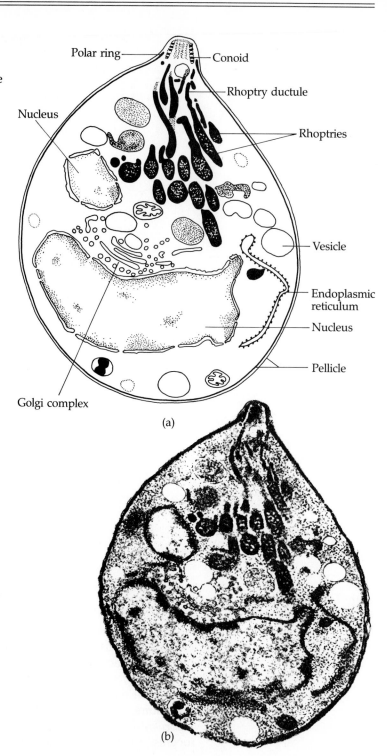

Polar ring

Conoid

Rhoptry ductule

Nucleus

Rhoptries

Vesicle

Endoplasmic reticulum

Nucleus

Pellicle

Golgi complex

(a)

(b)

population are microgametocytes, and each produces about 12 microgametes. Fertilization is intracellular, the microgametes bursting from their host cell to invade other host cells containing the macrogametes. Following fertilization, the resulting zygote develops into an oocyst that breaks out of the cell into the lumen of the feline intestine, to be passed out with feces. Within 1 to 5 days, in the presence of oxygen, the oocyst undergoes sporogony, forming two sporocysts, each containing four sporozoites. The feline enteric phase, therefore, consists of three stages: schizogony with the formation of merozoites, gamogony with the formation of gametes, and sporogony with the formation of oocysts containing the infective sporozoites.

In the cat, extraintestinal development, which follows an entirely different pattern, can occur concomitantly with enteric development. Only the extraintestinal phase occurs in mammals other than cats, including humans.

In extraintestinal development, the sporozoites invade cells other than those of the intestinal epithelium, reproduce, and form rapidly dividing merozoites called **tachyzoites,** which measure 7 by 2 μm. In acute infections, 8 to 16 tachyzoites are produced within a **parasitophorous vacuole** in the host cell, eventually causing the cell to disintegrate, probably by pressure, and releasing the parasites to invade new cells. An accumulation of tachyzoites in a host cell is known as a **group.** As the disease becomes chronic, parasites infecting the cells of the brain, heart, and skeletal muscle reproduce more slowly than during the acute phase. At this time, they are designated **bradyzoites** and accumulate in large numbers within an infected cell. Gradually, thick walls develop around the masses to form **pseudocysts,** which may persist for months or even years, especially in nerve tissue. Therefore, all animals except cats can be considered paratenic hosts, since the parasite never completes its sexual phases in them.

Pseudocyst formation coincides with the development of immunity in the host. This immunity, involving both humoral and cellular reactions, is usually permanent and prevents establishment of a new infection. If immunity wanes, it is restored by release of bradyzoites from cysts to repeat this cycle.

**Epidemiology.**    *Toxoplasma gondii* is cosmopolitan in distribution. All mammals, including humans, are capable of transmitting toxoplasmosis transplacentally. Sporulated oocysts, tachyzoites, and bradyzoites all serve as infective agents. Sources of infections vary, ranging from direct contamination, as from handling cat litter, to ingestion of inadequately cooked food or raw milk.

At least five different strains of *T. gondii* have been identified and studied. They differ primarily in duration of the life cycle and the number and morphology of merozoites produced.

Immunologic surveys reveal that humans throughout the world carry antibodies to *Toxoplasma;* however, clinical toxoplasmosis is rare, and infections are generally asymptomatic. Although all of the influential factors are not yet known, it has been established that the following affect the level of pathology: (1) age of the host, with older hosts being more resistant to the disease; (2) virulence of the strain of *T. gondii* involved; (3) natural susceptibility of the host; and (4) degree of acquired immunity of the host.

**Symptomatology and Diagnosis.**    Symptomatic or clinical toxoplasmosis may be classified as acute, subacute, chronic, or congenital.

Acute toxoplasmosis in humans is characterized by parasitic invasion of the mesenteric lymph nodes and liver parenchyma. The most common symptom is painful, swollen lymph glands in the inguinal, cervical, and subclavicular regions, frequently accompanied by fever, headache, anemia, muscle pain, and sometimes lung complications. The tachyzoites proliferate in many tissues and tend to kill host cells rapidly. When cells from sites such as the retina or brain are involved, serious lesions often develop. Subacute toxoplasmosis is merely a prolongation of the acute stage.

Normally, the duration of the chronic stage is limited by the host's immunological system. However, if immunity develops slowly, the course of clinical toxoplasmosis can be protracted. During this period, tachyzoites continue to destroy cells, producing extensive lesions in lung, heart, liver, brain, and eyes. Damage is usually greater in the central nervous system than in non-nerve tissues because of lower immunocompetence in the former. The onset of chronic toxoplasmosis occurs when immunity in the host becomes sufficient to suppress tachyzoite proliferation, which coincides with the formation of cysts. The cysts may remain intact for years, producing no clinical symptoms. A cyst wall may occasionally rupture, releasing bradyzoites; most of these are killed by host responses, although some may penetrate cells and form new cysts. Death of bradyzoites elicits a hypersensitive reaction. In the brain, nodules of glial cells gradually form at the sites of such reactions. In cases in which there are sufficient numbers of such nodules, the victim may develop symptoms of chronic encephalitis, sometimes accompanied by spastic paralysis. This is especially true for AIDS (autoimmune deficiency syndrome) patients, in whom *Toxoplasma* may cause severe brain damage. The occurrence and rupture of cysts in the retina and choroid may lead to blindness. Chronic toxoplasmosis may also cause myocarditis, leading to permanent heart damage and pneumonia.

Congenital toxoplasmosis results from fetal transplacental infection. Such infection may result in stillbirth, or, if liveborn, the child may exhibit a variety of abnormalities. Approximately 12% of infected infants born alive die shortly after birth, and fewer than 20% of surviving infected infants are normal at 4 years of age. Abnormalities appear in the central nervous system, eyes, and viscera, with symptoms such as jaundice, microcephaly, and hydrocephaly appearing at birth or shortly thereafter.

Diagnosis is based, primarily, on serological tests using killed antigens. Demonstration of organisms in mice following their inoculation with suspected fluid or biopsied tissue (xenodiagnosis) constitutes positive diagnosis.

**Treatment.**    Oral administration of pyrimethamine, usually accompanied by trisulfapyrimidines, is the treatment of choice at this time. Since pyrimethamine may cause folic acid deficiency, supplementary folinic acid may also be added to the regimen.

## Pneumocystis carinii

There has been a dramatic upsurge in the incidence of *Pneumocystis carinii* pneumonia (PCP) coincident with the appearance of AIDS. Of the opportunistic diseases associated with AIDS, PCP is the most common cause of death, affecting an estimated 60% of AIDS patients. In addition to its prevalence among AIDS patients, PCP is common in children and premature infants who are malnourished or debilitated or who suffer from primary immune deficiency disorders. The disease also is found in cancer patients being treated with immunosuppressive drugs.

A universally accepted taxonomic designation for *P. carinii* has yet to be agreed upon. A number of authorities place it provisionally in the kingdom Protista, phylum Apicomplexa. Others classify *Pneumocystis* as a protistan of independent systematic position. Still others place it in the kingdom Fungi. Not only is its taxonomy open to question, but its life cycle, natural reservoirs, and modes of transmission are obscure.

**Life Cycle** (Fig. 7–9).    Little of the life cycle of *P. carinii* has been established. What is known has been derived from morphological studies of forms collected from infected humans and other mammals. No information is available on forms existing outside these hosts. *P. carinii* is an extracellular parasite found in interstitial tissues of the lungs and alveoli.

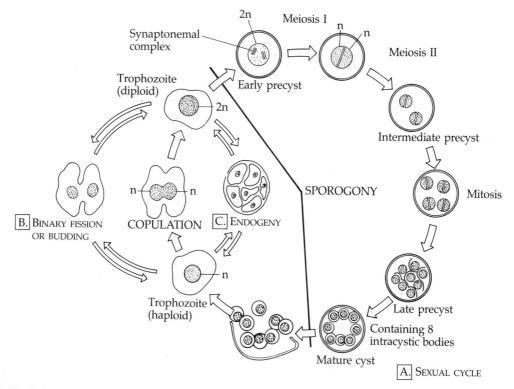

**Figure 7–9**
**Life cycle of *Pneumocystis carinii*.**
Only the intrapulmonary cycle is known. In the sexual cycle A (trophozoite-cyst cycle), the diploid trophozoite meiotically divides through the precyst stages into the mature cyst with eight haploid intracystic bodies. This ruptures, releasing the intracystic bodies that develop into haploid trophozoites. This process is equivalent to sporogony. As well as the sexual cycle, the trophozoites seem to have two modes—B and C—of asexual division: binary fission or budding of the trophozoite (B) and endogeny (C). It is unknown which type of trophozoite (diploid or haploid) is involved in the asexual development. All cycles are extracellular.

**Figure 7–10**
**An irregularly shaped**
**trophozoite (right) and a**
**rounded cyst (left) of**
*Pneumocystis carinii.*
The trophozoite has a thin
pellicle and contains a nucleus,
a few lamellae of rough
endoplasmic reticulum,
mitochondria, and electron
dense bodies. The cyst has a
thicker pellicle and contains
intracystic bodies.

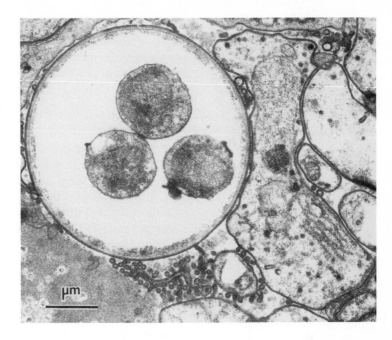

Three morphological stages—**trophic, precystic,** and **cystic**—have been identified. In the pleomorphic trophic stage (Fig. 7–10), the parasite, measuring 2–8 μm, is bounded by a thin pellicle, 20–40 nm thick, consisting of a plasma membrane and an electron-dense outer layer. Associated with the pellicle are small, tubular expansions sometimes regarded as filopodia. Trophic stage forms are usually uninucleate, although binucleate forms occasionally occur.

The precystic stage is a transitional link between the trophic and cystic stages. The precystic organism is oval and 3–5 μm long, with a clump of mitochondria in its cytoplasm. In this stage, the pellicle begins to thicken, varying from 40 to 120 nm, with few tubular expansions. The number of nuclei increases to eight.

The cyst measures 4–6 μm and has a thick pellicle (70–140 μm) consisting of three layers: plasma membrane, electron-lucent middle layer, and electron-dense outer layer. Eight **intracystic bodies,** or sporozoites, arranged in a rosette pattern (Fig. 7–9) form meiotically within the cyst during sporogony. Each intracystic body measures 1–1.5 μm; possesses a nucleus, a mitochondrion, and a rough endoplasmic reticulum; and can be spherical, crescent-shaped, or amoeboid. The intracystic bodies rupture from the cyst, and each develops to the trophic stage. This activity occurs in the alveolar lining layer, and each new form selectively attaches to squamous (type I) alveolar epithelial cells. While the mode of transmission from one human to another has not been established, the most plausible means, based on rat-to-rat transmission studies, appears to be inhalation of cysts from the air.

**Symptomatology and Diagnosis.**    In immunologically normal individuals, *Pneumocystis* infection is asymptomatic; however, immunosuppression is capable of activating such latent infections into virulent ones. *Pneumocystis* is found in the lungs of the host, usually in the lumen of the alveolus. The alveolar septa thicken and become infiltrated with plasma cells, and the organisms fill the alveoli. These events occur in rapid succession and are accompanied by fever, difficulty in breathing, coughing, and cyanosis. In untreated patients, death from pneumonia is the inevitable outcome. Diagnosis is made by identifying the organism from lung biopsies or bronchial lavages.

**Treatment.**    Treatment consists of the administration of trimethoprim–sulfamethoxazole or pentamidine isothionate; however, because the immune system has been compromised, treatment is unsuccessful in a majority of cases.

## SELECTED READINGS

Desowitz, R. S. 1976. How the wise men brought malaria to Africa. *Natural History* 85, 36–44.

Friedman, M. J., and Trager, W. 1981. The biochemistry of resistance to malaria. *Scientific American* 244, 154–165.

Godson, G. N. 1985. Molecular approaches to malaria vaccines. *Scientific American* 248, 52–59.

Hermentin, P. 1987. Malaria invasion of human erythrocytes. *Parasitology Today* 3, 52–55.

Jacobs, L. 1973. New knowledge of toxoplasma and toxoplasmosis. *Advances in Parasitology* 11, 631–669.

Matsumoto, Y., and Yoshida, Y. 1986. Advances in pneumocystis biology. *Parasitology Today* 2, 137–142.

Spielman, A. 1988. Lyme disease and human babesiosis: Evidence incriminating vector and reservoir hosts. In *The Biology of Parasitism* (Englund, P. T., and Sher, A., eds.), pp. 147–65. Alan R. Liss, New York.

# PART TWO
## THE TREMATODA

# CHAPTER EIGHT

## GENERAL CHARACTERISTICS OF THE TREMATODA

The phylum Platyhelminthes includes various dorsoventrally flattened animals commonly known as flatworms (Fig. 8–1). All members are typically bilaterally symmetrical, lack a body cavity, and have a digestive tract that, if present, is incomplete. That is, the caeca end blindly, so the only opening to the exterior, the mouth, serves for both ingestion and egestion. Skeletal, circulatory, and respiratory systems are usually lacking. The space between the body wall and the internal organs is filled with connective tissue fibers, muscle, and unattached and fixed cells of various types. The intercellular spaces are filled with body fluids. The fibers and cells and the spaces between them are referred to collectively as the **parenchyma.**

Four classes make up the phylum. Two of these, Trematoda and Cestoidea, contain flatworms parasitic to humans. One evolutionary scheme for the trematodes proposes that they arose from a stock of free-living flatworms, progenitors of present-day rhabdocoel turbellarians, that apparently became intimately associated with molluscs and ultimately became parasitic. Evolutionary divergence within this endoparasitic population gave rise to two groups that are designated as subclasses Digenea and Aspidogastrea. The ancestral digeneans proliferated asexually in the mollusc, the adult forms later parasitizing vertebrates when they arose. The ancestral, nonproliferative, aspidogastrean forms, on the other hand, remained in molluscs through adulthood. All trematodes parasitic to humans belong to the subclass Digenea.

Digenetic trematodes are one of the largest groups of platyhelminths, parasitizing a wide range of invertebrate and vertebrate hosts, including humans. Within human hosts, these worms are found in numerous organs, including the intestine, lungs, liver, and vascular system.

## STRUCTURE OF ADULT

Despite superficial differences, the morphology of the various groups of digenetic trematodes is basically the same. The following description represents a hypothetical composite exemplifying the various anatomical features (Fig. 8–1).

**Figure 8–1**
**Generalized digenetic**
**trematode.**
(a) Diagram of entire organism.
(b) Detailed diagram of
common genitalia, showing
relationship of male (right) and
female (left) sex organs.

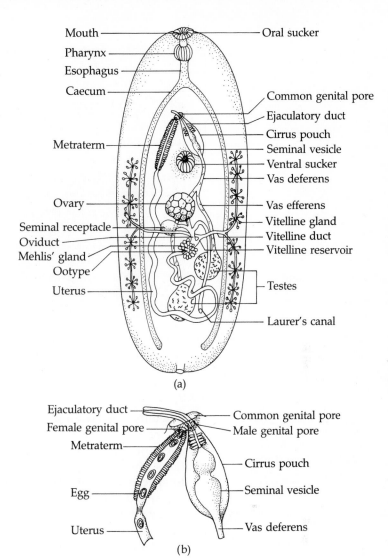

Mouth — Oral sucker
Pharynx
Esophagus
Caecum — Common genital pore
— Ejaculatory duct
Metraterm — Cirrus pouch
— Seminal vesicle
— Ventral sucker
— Vas deferens
Ovary — Vas efferens
Seminal receptacle — Vitelline gland
Oviduct — Vitelline duct
Mehlis' gland — Vitelline reservoir
Ootype
Uterus — Testes
— Laurer's canal

(a)

Ejaculatory duct — Common genital pore
Female genital pore — Male genital pore
Metraterm
— Cirrus pouch
— Seminal vesicle
Egg
— Vas deferens
Uterus

(b)

# Tegument

Once considered a nonliving, protective "cuticle," the tegument is now recognized as a dynamic, cellular structure. Under the light microscope, it appears as a more or less homogeneous layer about 7–16 μm thick (Fig. 8–2). The tegument is a **syncytium:** a multinucleated tissue with no cell boundaries (Fig. 8–3). The outer zone of this syncytium, the **distal cytoplasm,** is delineated at its surface by a plasma

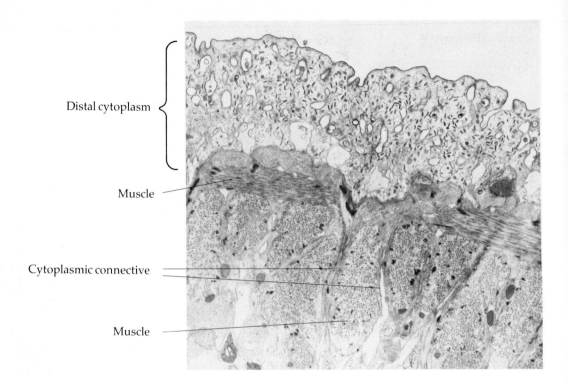

Distal cytoplasm

Muscle

Cytoplasmic connective

Muscle

**Figure 8–2**
**Transmission electron**
**micrograph of the tegument of**
**a digenetic trematode.**

membrane measuring about 10 nm thick. Associated with the plasma membrane is a surface coat, or **glycocalyx,** that varies in thickness according to species. Surface invaginations, the number and extent of which also vary according to species, serve to increase tegumental surface area, much like microvilli on the surface of human intestinal cells. The ability of the tegument to absorb exogenous molecules is generally proportional to the number and extent of invaginations and the number of mitochondria in the distal cytoplasm. Hydrolytic enzymatic activity in the glycocalyx facilitates the uptake of certain molecules from the environment. The glycocalyx is also a protective structure, shielding the worm from hostile environmental influences such as antibodies and host digestive enzymes. For instance, the presence of acid mucopolysaccharides in the glycocalyx is of particular significance since such molecules are known to inhibit a number of digestive enzymes. Their presence on the body surface may account for the ability of intestinal trematodes to resist host digestive enzymes.

Embedded in the distal cytoplasm of some species are tegumental spines, with bases lying just above the basal

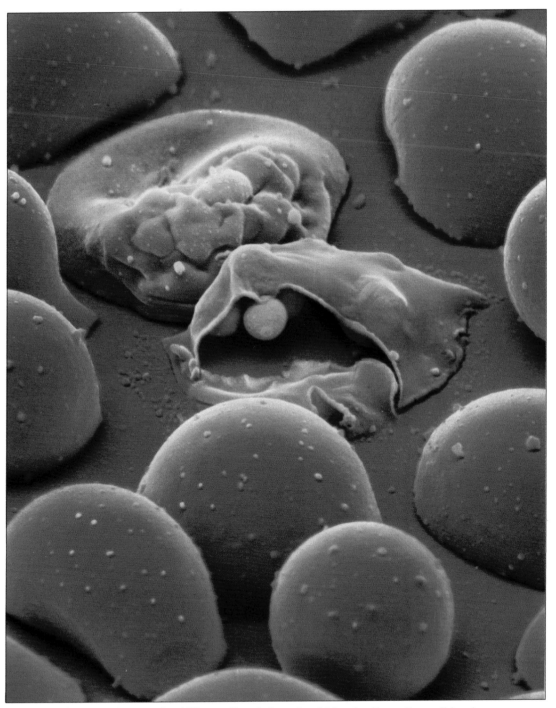

**Scanning electron micrograph of *Plasmodium*-infected red blood cells.** One cell has burst open, releasing malaria merozoites.

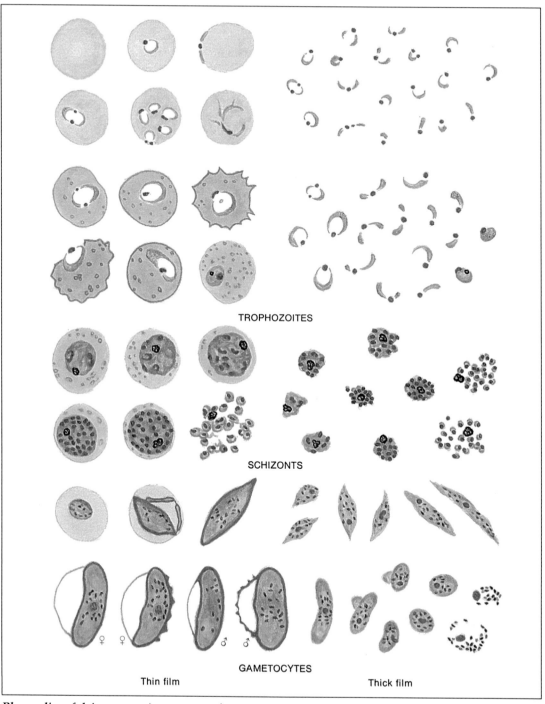

TROPHOZOITES

SCHIZONTS

GAMETOCYTES

Thin film                    Thick film

***Plasmodium falciparum.*** Appearance of parasite stages in Giemsa-stained thin and thick blood films.

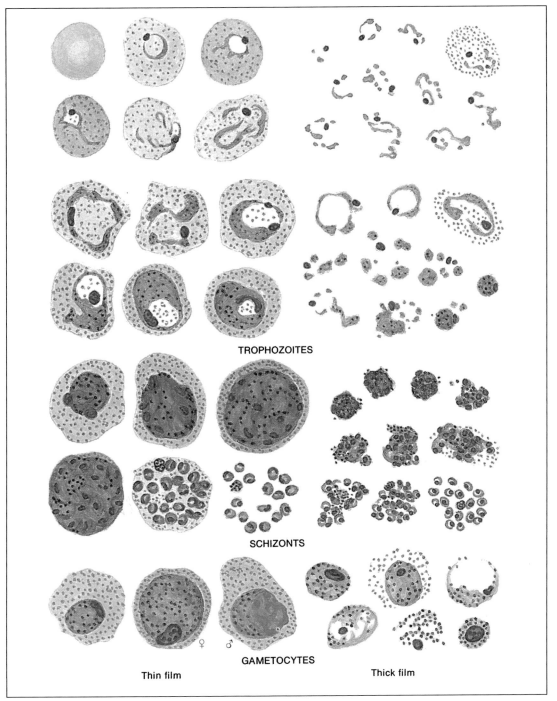

TROPHOZOITES

SCHIZONTS

♀   ♂

GAMETOCYTES

Thin film                              Thick film

*Plasmodium vivax.*   Appearance of parasite stages in Giemsa-stained thin and thick blood films.

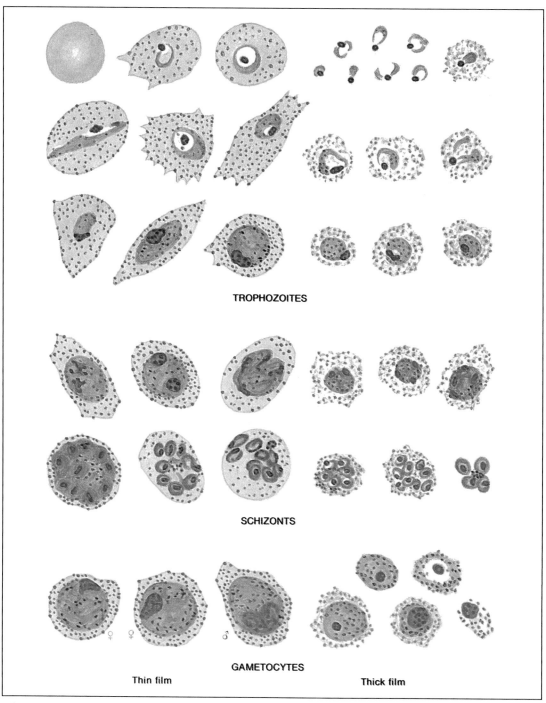

**TROPHOZOITES**

**SCHIZONTS**

**GAMETOCYTES**

Thin film

Thick film

*Plasmodium ovale.* Appearance of parasite stages in Giemsa-stained thin and thick blood films.

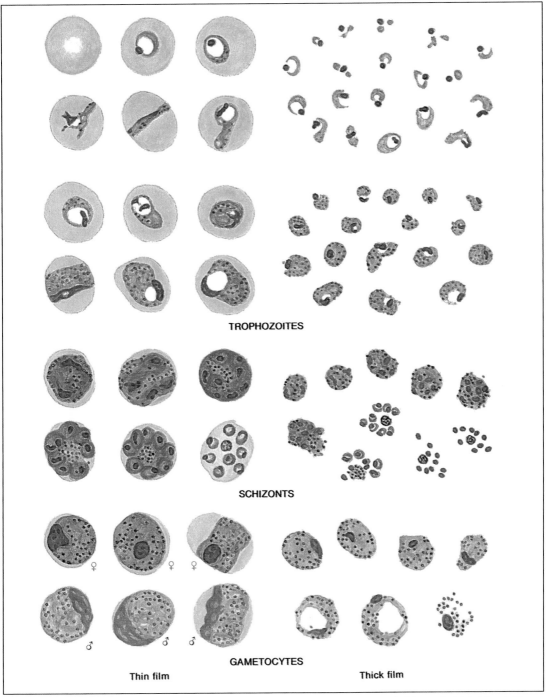

**TROPHOZOITES**

**SCHIZONTS**

**GAMETOCYTES**

Thin film                    Thick film

*Plasmodium malariae.*    Appearance of parasite stages in Giemsa-stained thin and thick blood films.

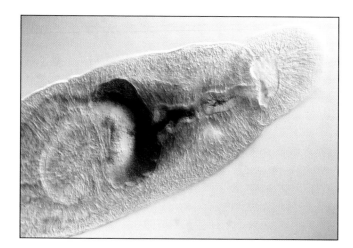

**Anterior end of male *Schistosoma mansoni*.**

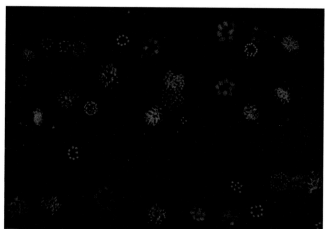

**Fluorescent DNA-stained rosettes of schistosome spermatogenesis.**

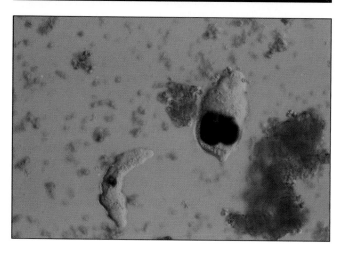

**Schistosomule of *Schistosoma mansoni*.**

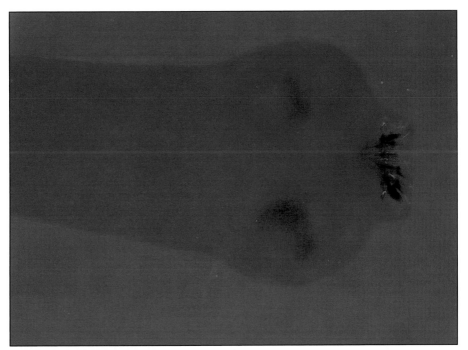

Scolex of adult *Taenia solium*.

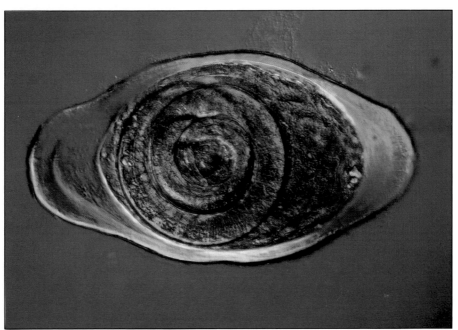

Nurse cell enclosing *Trichinella spiralis* larva.

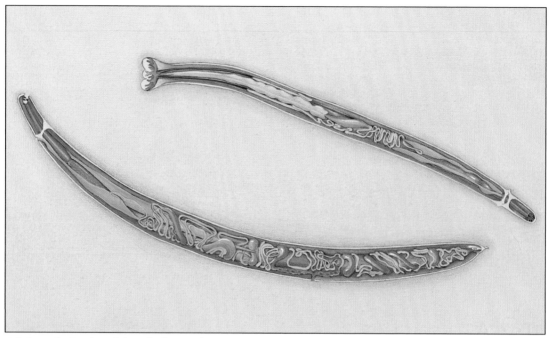

**Adult male (top) and female (bottom)** *Ancylostoma duodenale.*

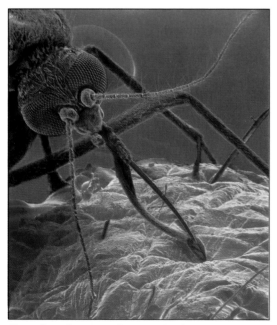

**Scanning electron micrograph of** *Anopheles* mosquito feeding through human skin.

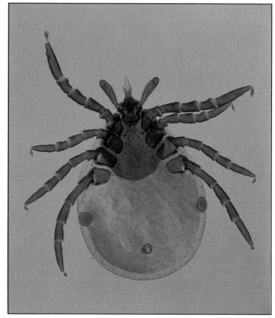

**Light microscope view of an** *Ixodes* tick.

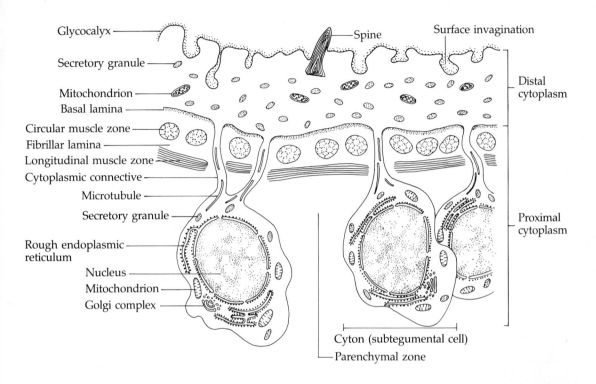

Glycocalyx
Secretory granule
Mitochondrion
Basal lamina
Circular muscle zone
Fibrillar lamina
Longitudinal muscle zone
Cytoplasmic connective
Microtubule
Secretory granule
Rough endoplasmic reticulum
Nucleus
Mitochondrion
Golgi complex

Spine
Surface invagination
Distal cytoplasm
Proximal cytoplasm
Cyton (subtegumental cell)
Parenchymal zone

**Figure 8–3**
**Diagrammatic representation of the tegument of a digenetic trematode.**

plasma membrane of the distal cytoplasm and tips projecting outward but still covered by the surface membrane. Although the function of these spines has not been firmly established, it is speculated that they may serve as ancillary holdfast mechanisms and/or storage sites for certain essential molecules. The matrix of the distal cytoplasm also contains one or two types of secretory vesicles.

The outer, distal cytoplasm is connected to the inner, **proximal cytoplasm** (= **cyton region**) by cytoplasmic bridges. The proximal cytoplasm contains nuclei, endoplasmic reticula, Golgi complexes, glycogen deposits, mitochondria, and various types of vesicles. This region of the tegument is the locus for the synthesis of materials for repair and maintenance of the distal cytoplasm. The vesicles observed in the distal cytoplasm are packets of substances, produced in the proximal cytoplasm, that continually maintain the outer plasma membrane and its glycocalyx and assist in the maintenance of the matrix and the spines. The translocation of these vesicles from proximal to distal cytoplasm is facilitated by microtubules in the cyton region and in the cytoplasmic bridges.

# Digestive Tract

Digenetic trematodes possess incomplete digestive tracts (Fig. 8–1). The anterior mouth, surrounded by a muscular oral sucker, leads into a bulbous, muscular pharynx, in many species via a short prepharynx. The esophagus connects the pharynx and the alimentary tract, the latter bifurcating into two **caeca.** The mouth, pharynx, and esophagus make up the foregut, analogous to that of higher forms. The lining of the foregut is morphologically similar to the general tegument since it is a syncytium consisting of two cytoplasmic zones, distal and proximal. There are, however, no spines associated with this lining. The foregut is the site of ingestion and assimilation of food, and the ability to accomplish these functions is enhanced by specific modifications of the foregut in these organisms. For instance, in many forms, the proximal cytoplasm produces enzymes that are released into the lumen of the foregut, where they partially degrade ingested food. In addition, heavily muscularized regions of the foregut, such as the pharynx or, in some species, the esophagus, break food into smaller particles.

**Figure 8–4**
**Section through tegument–gastrodermis junction.**
Note abrupt transition at desmosome region (arrow).

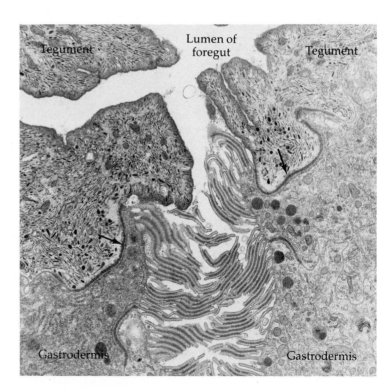

The transition from the tegumentlike structure of the foregut to the simple epithelium, or **gastrodermis,** of the branched caeca is abrupt and marked by a prominent cell junction (Fig. 8–4). The gastrodermis consists of cells either with or without distinct lateral cell boundaries (i.e., a syncytium). There is no discernible physiological basis for this variation. The caeca are two longitudinal, blind tubes of variable length. In many species, they extend almost to the posterior tip of the body; in others, they may extend no further than a third of the body length. In some larger digeneans, the caeca exhibit extensive diverticulation.

The gastrodermal surface is bounded by a plasma membrane amplified in either fingerlike microvilli (Fig. 8–5a) or leaflike lamellae (Fig. 8–5b). Digestion and absorption of food occur in the caeca, and such amplifications increase the absorptive surface. The type of amplification is independent of the type of food ingested. Some blood-feeding digeneans, for example, display a microvillar type, while others display

**Figure 8–5**
**(a) Microvillar amplification of gastrodermis of *Megalodiscus* sp. Bottom left is cross-section through microvilli.**
**(b) Lamellar amplifications of gastrodermis of *Brachycoelium* sp.**

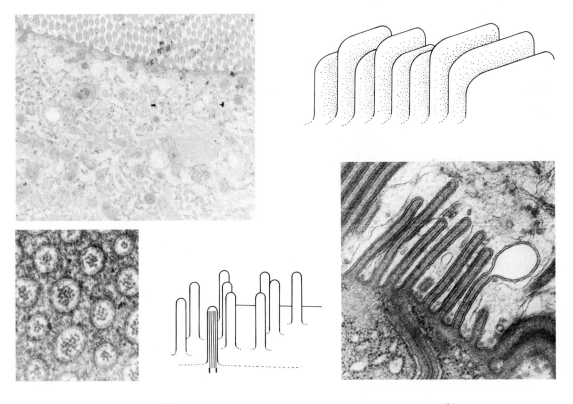

(a)                                    (b)

the lamellar type. Associated with the plasma membrane is a prominent glycocalyx that, similar to the tegumental glycocalyx, appears to afford protection as well as aid in the uptake of certain molecules, the latter function abetted by its enzymatic activity. Digestion is typically extracellular, occurring in the gut lumen.

The gastrodermis is highly active in protein synthesis and secretion, for which it possesses abundant rough endoplasmic reticulum, Golgi complexes, many mitochondria, and vesicles, most of the last originating from the Golgi complex. The vesicles contain either the material for maintaining the glycocalyx or the hydrolytic enzymes that are released into the caecal lumen for digestion of food. The basal plasma membrane of the gastrodermis often displays extensive infoldings that seem to be associated with the organism's ability to transport ions. The basal plasma membrane rests on an extensive **basal lamina** in which are embedded two layers of muscles—one circular, the other longitudinal.

## Muscular and Nervous Systems

There are two muscle zones in adult digenetic trematodes. Underlying the tegument is the **subtegumental zone,** which consists of three layers of muscle—longitudinal, circular, and diagonal. Contractile activity by these muscles is usually minimal, although there are species with more active subtegumental musculature. The muscle layers are typically more distinct in the anterior part of the body. The orientation of contractile fibers allows the organism to elongate, contract, and/or twist its body in almost any given plane. This zone consists of smooth muscles, with the nucleated region, or **myoblast,** connected to the bundles of myofibers. The second zone of musculature, the **gastrodermal zone** described in the previous section, helps move food up and down the caecal lumen. Well-developed contractile fibers also occur in the oral and ventral suckers.

The nervous system of adult digeneans (Fig. 8–6) is of the "ladder" type. Three pairs of longitudinal nerve trunks—a prominent ventral pair, a lateral pair, and a dorsal pair—extend posteriorly and anteriorly from two connected dorsal ganglia (= brain) near the pharynx; all three pairs of trunks are interconnected by transverse commissures. Smaller branches, emanating from the brain and longitudinal trunks, supply motor and sensory innervation to the tegument, suckers, reproductive systems, and other organs.

**Figure 8–6**
**(a) Nervous system of a digenetic trematode.**
**(b) Innervation of the anterior end and sucker of a digenetic trematode.**

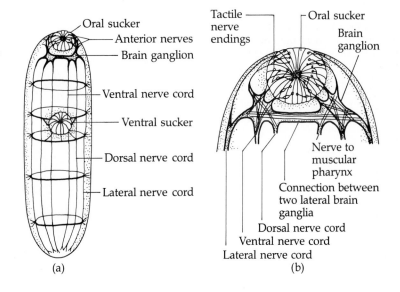

(a)

Oral sucker
Anterior nerves
Brain ganglion
Ventral nerve cord
Ventral sucker
Dorsal nerve cord
Lateral nerve cord

(b)

Tactile nerve endings
Oral sucker
Brain ganglion
Nerve to muscular pharynx
Connection between two lateral brain ganglia
Dorsal nerve cord
Ventral nerve cord
Lateral nerve cord

Sensory organs are evident in some tissues of the digenean body, particularly the tegument and gastrodermis. These usually appear as modified cilia projecting from bulbous nerve endings, and they extend outward from the tegumental surface or from the gastrodermis into the lumen of the digestive tract. They may serve as pressure, touch or rheotactic sensors, or even as chemoreceptors.

In larval stages, types of sensory organs vary widely, including papillae, pigmented eyespots, uniciliated organs, and organs containing up to six ciliary eyespots. Such diversity undoubtedly aids these free-swimming larvae in locating hosts. Nerve end organs act as chemo-, mechano-, and photoreceptors.

## Osmoregulatory System

This system is of the typical protonephridial type: a tubular system closed at one end and open at the other. Currents are produced at the closed ends by **flame cells,** each of which is equipped with a tuft of fused, vigorously beating cilia (Fig. 8–7). The number and arrangement of such cells in digeneans are specific enough to serve as taxonomic indicators of phylogenetic relationships (Fig. 8–8). Each cell opens into a terminal tubule, several of which converge to form larger collecting tubules. The collecting tubules on each

**Figure 8–7**
**Transmission electron micrograph of the ciliary tuft of a trematode flame cell.**

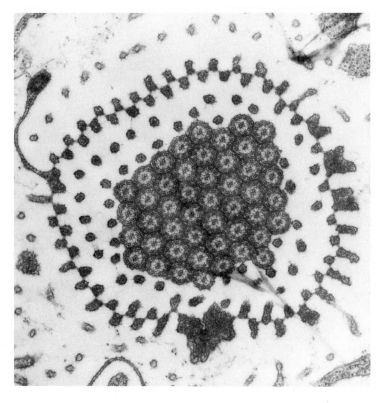

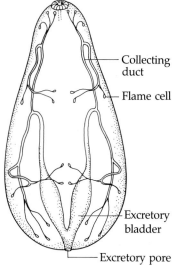

Collecting duct

Flame cell

Excretory bladder

Excretory pore

**Figure 8–8**
**Excretory system of *Heterophyes heterophyes*.**

side of the body lead posteriorly and empty into a common **excretory bladder** (Fig. 8–9), the duct of which opens to the exterior through the excretory pore located at or near the posterior end of the body.

While it seems likely that this system serves in both osmoregulation and/or excretion, not all details of these functions are clearly defined. In some forms, structural and biochemical features suggest reabsorptive functions. For instance, microvilli and alkaline phosphatase activity, both characteristic of absorptive epithelium, occur in the walls of the collecting ducts in such forms.

The major nitrogenous waste product in digeneans is ammonia, although other soluble compounds, such as urea and other nitrogenous compounds, also occur. It is not entirely clear how much of each of these compounds is eliminated through the tegument, digestive tract, or excretory system. In a number of forms, uric acid forms in the excretory bladder and tubules and is eliminated as insoluble crystals via the excretory pore.

**Figure 8–9**
**Shapes of excretory vesicles of digenetic trematodes.**
(a) V-shaped vesicle. (b) Y-shaped vesicle. (c) I-shaped vesicle.

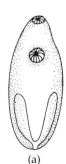 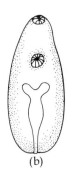 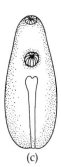

(a)                    (b)                    (c)

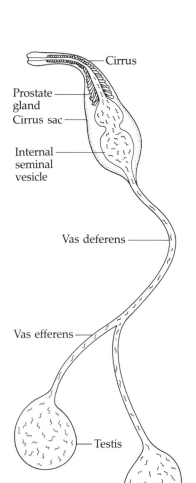

Cirrus

Prostate gland

Cirrus sac

Internal seminal vesicle

Vas deferens

Vas efferens

Testis

**Figure 8–10**
**Diagram of the male reproductive system of a digenetic trematode.**

# Reproductive Systems

With the exception of schistosomes, digenetic trematodes are hermaphroditic. The male reproductive system may mature prior to the female system, reducing the likelihood of self-fertilization.

**Male System.** The male reproductive system (Fig. 8–10) generally includes two testes, although schistosomes are multitesticular. The position of the testes in the parenchyma varies according to species, as do shape and orientation to each other. For instance, testes can be located anywhere from the middle to the posterior portion of the body. They can be ovoid, round, smooth, branched, or lobed. They can be at tandem, side by side, or diagonal to each other. Such characteristics are useful in the identification of species. Spermatogenesis in the testes produces biflagellated sperm.

Leading from each testis is a **vas efferens,** each of which unites with others anteriorly to form the common **vas deferens.** Distally, this duct forms the male copulatory organ, or **cirrus.** The cirrus may be surrounded by a **cirrus sac** into which it can invaginate when it is not everted. Also enclosed by the cirrus sac are the sperm-storing **seminal vesicle** and the **prostate gland.** The eversible cirrus can be protruded to the exterior through a genital pore on the ventral surface of the organism.

Among digeneans, there are certain variations in the components of the vas deferens and their relative positions. One or more of its components may be missing (e.g., the prostate gland and/or the cirrus sac and/or a protusable cirrus), and the seminal vesicle often varies in size and position. The seminal vesicle, usually enclosed within the cirrus

**Figure 8–11**
**Schematic drawing showing formation of constituents of a digenetic trematode egg (see text for description).**

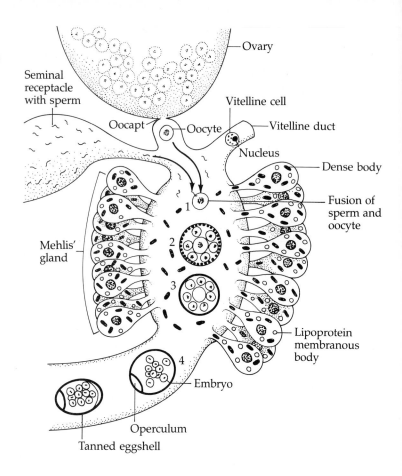

sac, is sometimes located outside the sac, in which case it is designated as an **external seminal vesicle.**

**Female System.**   The female reproductive system consists of a single ovary embedded in the parenchyma, either anterior or posterior to or between the testes, depending upon the species. **Ova** (actually secondary oocytes) formed by the ovary are released via a short **oviduct,** passing through a sequence of events analogous to an assembly line (Fig. 8–11). After leaving the ovary, each ovum passes down the oviduct to a minute chamber, the **ootype.** In this vicinity, the duct of the seminal receptacle, in which sperm deposited earlier are stored, joins the oviduct. Fertilization occurs at this point, whereupon oogenesis is completed and cleavage begins. The ootype is surrounded by **Mehlis' gland** consisting of two groups of unicellular glands, each group characterized by the type of material it secretes into the ootype.

One group secretes a membranous body, while the other secretes a dense body. Among several functions suggested for these secretions, the most likely is that the membranous body provides a template for the deposition of shell material (Fig. 8–12) and the dense body provides lubrication for the passage of the forming shelled egg. Other functions postulated for these secretions include activation of sperm, activation of vitelline glands to release shell material, and enhancement of the hardening process of the eggshell.

Other glands that communicate with the ootype are the **vitelline** (Fig. 8–13). In digeneans, these glands are composed of numerous multicellular clusters. Each cell synthesizes globules, which are then stored in its cytoplasm. As each cell attains a certain level of maturity, it detaches and enters a vitelline ductule. Groups of glands are usually situated bilaterally, although distribution may vary according to species. The smaller vitelline ductules converge to form right and left **vitelline ducts;** they, in turn, merge to form the **common vitelline duct,** which opens into the ootype. In some digeneans, the right and left vitelline ducts merge into

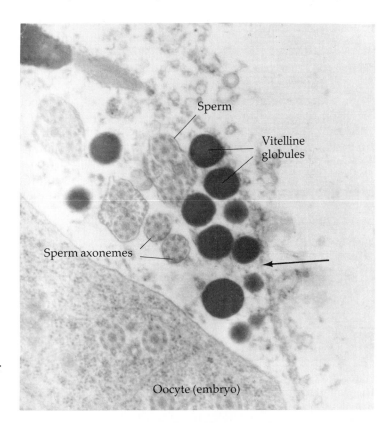

**Figure 8–12**
**Transmission electron micrograph of a forming egg shell of a digenetic trematode.** Vitelline globules line the inner aspect of the lipoprotein membrane (arrow) prior to fusion.

**Figure 8–13**
**Transmission electron**
**micrograph through the**
**vitelline gland of a digenetic**
**trematode.**

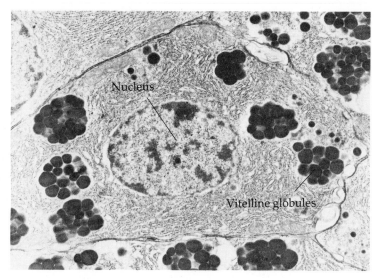

a common chamber, the **vitelline reservoir,** which is connected to the ootype by a short duct.

The vitelline gland cells play an essential role in eggshell formation. They release into the ootype globules that then become aligned against the membranous template derived from Mehlis' gland. These globules then coalesce and eventually toughen to form the shell. This toughening process is accomplished by enzymatic cross-linking of proteins in the coalesced globules. In some species, tyrosine residues of the proteins are oxidized into a "tanned" eggshell. This type of shell is rather hard and brownish in color. In other forms, disulfide links are formed, producing an eggshell more elastic than the tanned form. Cytoplasm of the vitelline cells also serves as nutrient for the developing embryo. According to some authorities, the uterine lining in some digeneans may also supply essential elements for eggshell formation.

The uterus is a long, often convoluted tube through which shelled eggs are transported to the exterior via the genital pore. In some species, a muscular, distal portion of the uterus, a **metraterm,** helps propel the eggs out of the uterus as well as serving in copulation. In addition to transporting eggs to the exterior, the uterus also permits sperm to move in the opposite direction to the seminal receptacle. During copulation, the cirrus is inserted into the distal end of the uterus; sperm, ejaculated into the metraterm or the uterus, then swim to the seminal receptacle where they are stored. In some species, a **Laurer's canal,** originating on the surface of the ootype, passes to the dorsal surface, where it

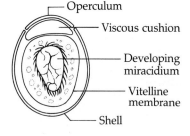

**Figure 8–14**
**Diagram of a typical digenetic**
**trematode egg.**

**Figure 8-15**
**Eggs of some digenetic trematodes parasitic in humans.**
(a) *Clonorchis sinensis* egg, 27–35 by 12–20 μm, flask-shaped with operculum at narrow end. (b) *Paragonimus westermani* egg, 80–118 by 48–60 μm, oval, with operculum at flattened end. (c) *Fasciolopsis buski* egg, 130–140 by 80–85 μm, ellipsoidal, with inconspicuous operculum. (d) *Schistosoma japonicum* egg, 70–100 by 50–65 μm, round to oval, with short lateral spine and no operculum. (e) *Schistosoma mansoni* egg, 114–175 by 45–68 μm, elongate oval, with longer lateral spine and no operculum. (f) *Schistosoma haematobium* egg, 112–170 by 40–70 μm, spindle-shaped, with posterior terminal spine and no operculum.

may or may not open to the exterior. This canal may represent a vestigial vagina, or it may serve as an outlet for excess sperm and extraneous matter formed during egg formation.

**The Egg.** The ovoid, shelled egg contains vitelline substance, the embryo and ancillary membranes, and other materials (Fig. 8–14). The eggshell is typically provided at one end with a lidlike structure, the **operculum,** which allows the larva to hatch. The eggshells of human blood flukes possessing no operculum rupture longitudinally when they hatch. Hatching occurs only under certain conditions of temperature, osmolarity, and light. For instance, in schistosomes infecting humans, hatching of embryonated eggs is inhibited by an osmolarity equivalent to 0.85% saline and a temperature of 37°C, thereby reducing the likelihood that the egg will hatch prematurely within the host's body. Most digenean eggs are unembryonated when they pass out of the human host and are unable to hatch until further development occurs.

Distinctive size and structural characteristics of trematode eggs, especially those of medically important species, are useful in diagnosis (Fig. 8–15).

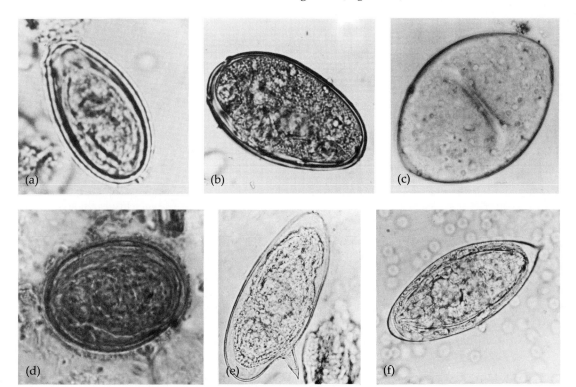

◇

# GENERALIZED LIFE CYCLE PATTERNS

The following brief overview of the life cycles of digeneans that infect humans will provide a clearer picture of the various larval stages and the relationship of each to the one that follows it. (Fig. 8–16)

Eggs are usually released into the lumen of the host's organ occupied by the adult worm (gut, lungs, urinary bladder, etc.) and pass to the exterior through feces, sputum, or urine. After finding its way to water, an egg completes its development and a free-swimming **miracidium** hatches (Fig. 8–17). Within 24 hours, the miracidium must find and penetrate the integument of a suitable freshwater or marine snail host (the first intermediate host), shedding its ciliated epidermis in the process and metamorphosing into a **primary sporocyst** (Fig. 8–18), which may produce numerous secondary sporocysts or **primary rediae** asexually (Fig. 8–19). In some forms, the egg must be ingested by the snail (particularly if the snail is a terrestrial one) before the miracidium hatches.

**Figure 8–16**
**Flowchart showing life cycles of trematodes infecting humans.**

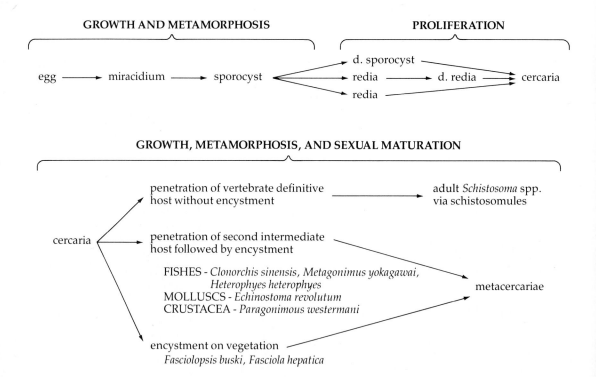

**Figure 8–17**
**Miracidium of *Schistosoma.***

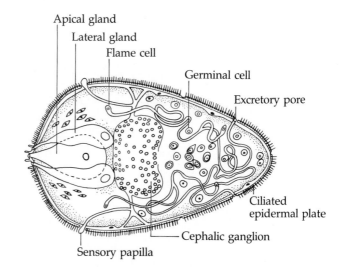

Apical gland
Lateral gland
Flame cell
Germinal cell
Excretory pore
Ciliated
epidermal plate
Cephalic ganglion
Sensory papilla

While the digestive gland is a common site for further development, the gonad, the mantle, and the lymph spaces surrounding the intestine, as well as other organs, may also serve for such development. Once established in a suitable location, the sporocyst or redia grows, matures, and continues further proliferation.

**Figure 8–19**
**Redia of *Fasciola hepatica.***

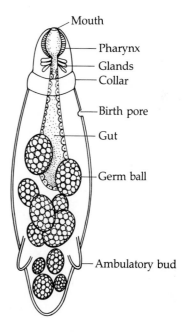

Mouth
Pharynx
Glands
Collar
Birth pore
Gut
Germ ball
Ambulatory bud

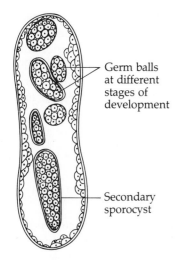

Germ balls
at different
stages of
development

Secondary
sporocyst

**Figure 8–18**
**Primary sporocyst.**

**Figure 8–20**
**Cercaria of *Clonorchis sinensis*.**

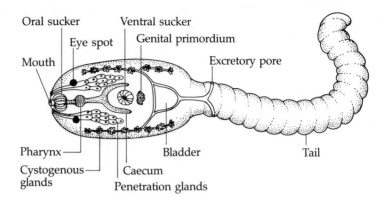

Sporocysts are commonly elongate and hollow and contain germ cells, formed in the miracidium, that multiply by mitosis and develop into **germ balls.** Rediae differ from sporocysts in possessing a functional, sac-like gut and a pharynx.

Rediae or secondary sporocysts (depending on species) eventually give rise to a tailed larva called **cercaria** (Fig. 8–20). Cercariae that escape from the molluscan host experience only a brief (several hours) free-swimming existence since they do not feed outside the host. In some species, the cercariae may actively penetrate or attach to the surface of a second intermediate host or attach to vegetation; they lose their tails and encyst, and they are then known as **metacercariae** (Fig. 8–21). Upon ingestion by a vertebrate definitive host, the encysted metacercaria excysts in the vertebrate small intestine, migrates to the definitive site, and gradually matures into the adult stage. In schistosomes, cercariae penetrate the definitive host directly, thereby foregoing an encysted metacercaria stage.

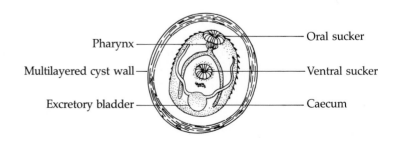

**Figure 8–21**
**Drawing of generalized encysted metacercaria.**

# The Miracidium

The miracidium is a ciliated, nonfeeding larva (Fig. 8–17). Under favorable conditions, it escapes from the eggshell, usually through the operculum, into the environment. The miracidium is elongated and covered with flattened, ciliated epidermal plates. At the junctures of adjacent epidermal plates are **cytoplasmic ridges,** which play a prominent role during the miracidium's metamorphosis into the next larval stage. Beneath the epidermal plates are well-developed circular and longitudinal muscles.

At the anterior tip of the miracidium is a flexible **apical papilla** with sensory organs and three secretory glands—the apical gland and two lateral glands—that secrete materials at the tip of the papilla during host penetration. During penetration, the papilla becomes partially invaginated, and secretions from the glands are captured in the depression. The papilla thus acts as a suction cup, holding the miracidium to the site of penetration and allowing the secretions to exert both adhesive and lytic actions. In addition to the sensory structures in the papilla, there may be two to three anterior **eyespots,** as well as **lateral papillae,** on each side of the body. The "brain" of the miracidium lies in the parenchyma behind the apical region, from which nerve fibers innervate various tissues and organs of the body.

The miracidium also has a simple, protonephridial excretory system. Waste-containing body fluids are collected by two or three pairs of flame cells and excreted through two lateral excretory pores.

During differentiation of the miracidium, germ cells grow and divide to form germ balls. Each germ ball eventually develops into a distinct, membrane-enclosed entity that is the next larval generation.

# The Sporocyst

First-generation sporocysts, having differentiated from miracidia, are usually observed near the site of penetration (mantle and headfoot), but occasionally they can reach the hemocoel in the digestive gland of the molluscan host. Less often, they occur along the digestive tract, depending upon the species. The sporocyst varies in shape from ovoid to elongate to tubular and may even be extensively branched (Fig. 8–18).

The thickness of the sporocyst wall, as seen in cross-section, varies according to age and species. Its outermost layer, as in all subsequent stages in the life cycle of digeneans, is a syncytial tegument derived from the cytoplasmic ridges of the miracidium. Prior to completely penetrating the first intermediate host, or shortly thereafter, the miracidial epidermal plates are shed; as the miracidium transforms into a sporocyst, the cytoplasmic ridges spread to form the tegument (Fig. 8–22). In most sporocysts, microvilli produce extensive amplification of the tegumental surface.

Beneath the tegument lies a thin basal lamina in which is embedded a layer of circular muscles. A thin layer of parenchyma underlies this area. These layers form the lining of the fluid-filled **brood chamber,** a cavity containing the germ balls. Sporocysts possess no digestive tracts, and essential nutrients must diffuse across the absorptive tegument. Carbohydrates derived from body fluids of the infected mollusc are the chief source of energy for this stage. Definitive nervous and reproductive systems also are lacking, although flame cells are generally present.

In some species, germ balls in the brood chamber of mother (or primary) sporocysts differentiate to form secondary (or daughter) sporocysts. In other species, the germ balls differentiate into rediae. Daughter sporocysts usually are morphologically similar to primary sporocysts but can be

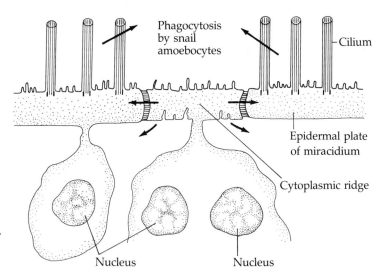

**Figure 8–22**
**Drawing showing changes in the body of a miracidium after its penetration of the snail.**
Epidermal plates are shed and phagocytozed by snail amoebocytes. Cytoplasmic ridges expand to form the outer layer (= tegument) of the sporocyst.

distinguished by their larger size and their common occurrence in deeper body organs, such as the digestive gland and gonads of the molluscan host.

## The Redia

Rediae, if present, develop from germ balls in the brood chamber of the primary sporocyst. They eventually escape from the sporocyst through the molluscan tissue and migrate to the digestive gland.

Each redia is elongate and normally possesses two or four bud-like, antero- and posterolateral projections: the **ambulatory buds** (or **procruscula**) (Fig. 8–19). As their name implies, the ambulatory buds facilitate movement of the larva through the tissues of the molluscan host. This movement is abetted by contractions of the redial body. Unlike the sporocyst, the redia possesses a digestive tract with an anterior mouth, a muscular pharynx, and an unbranched caecum. As the redia moves through the host's tissues, it actively ingests host cells, digesting them in the lumen of the caecum. Some rediae augment these intestinal feedings by secreting hydrolytic enzymes to the exterior and lysing surrounding host cells. The resulting molecules are then absorbed through the tegument. The physical damage inflicted upon the molluscan host by rediae is considerably greater than that caused by sporocysts.

On each side of the pharynx is a cephalic ganglion from which nerve fibers radiate. Flame cells occur in most rediae, terminating at the bladder(s) with either single or multiple excretory pores.

As stated earlier, a tegument identical to that of the sporocyst covers the surface of the redia.

Usually, near the mouth there is a birth pore, leading from the brood chamber. Within the brood chamber of the redia, germ balls differentiate into either secondary (daughter) rediae or the next larval stage, the cercaria.

## The Cercaria

Cercariae differentiate from the germ balls in the brood chambers of secondary, tertiary, or subsequent generations of sporocysts or rediae depending upon the life cycle of the digenean. A cercaria is usually equipped with a tail, enabling it to swim; a few species, such as the human lung fluke, have minute tails, forcing the cercaria to crawl on a substrate rather than swim. After escaping from the brood chamber through the birth pore, cercariae leave the molluscan host and actively seek the next host or suitable vegetation.

The distribution of internal organs in all cercariae, regardless of species, usually resembles that of the adult worm (Fig. 8–20). The mouth, situated at the anterior end of the body and surrounded by the oral sucker, leads into the foregut and paired caeca. There is a variably positioned ventral sucker, its location remaining constant through adulthood. In many cercariae, openings of several types of glands are found anteriorly. The name of a gland indicates its assumed function. For instance, in schistosome cercariae, a pair of **escape glands** lie near the mouth (Fig. 8–23). The contents of

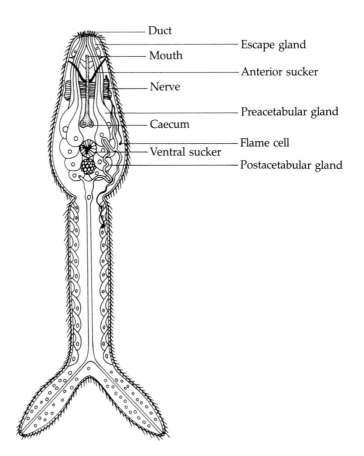

**Figure 8–23**
**Cercaria of *Schistosoma* spp.**

these glands are secreted during the cercaria's emergence from the sporocyst in which it had developed and from the snail host. In liver fluke cercariae, there are **cystogenous glands** that secrete substances to form a cyst wall. Other glands, such as **penetration glands** and **mucoid glands,** may be involved in host penetration; these may be further augmented by cuticular stylets capable of puncturing chitin-covered arthropods.

Embedded in the parenchyma, near the ventral sucker, is a genital primordium, a mass of germinal cells that eventually forms the male and female reproductive systems of the adult.

Cercariae also have protonephridial (flame cell) excretory systems. But, unlike sporocysts and rediae, cercariae have two lateral collecting tubules that empty into a common, posterior, excretory bladder from which a tube may extend posteriorly into the tail. The arrangement of flame cells in cercariae is very similar to the arrangement in the adult. Thus, if the flame cell pattern in a cercaria is known, it can be used to correlate the larval form with its adult stage.

## The Metacercaria

The next larval stage of most digeneans is the metacercaria. When the free-swimming (or crawling) cercaria locates a suitable substrate or penetrates a second intermediate host, it sheds the tail and encysts. Within the cyst wall, the metacercaria may grow and develop into a more mature juvenile pre-adult. Its genital primordium may differentiate into a complete reproductive system that usually is nonfunctional. Many cercarial features, such as various glands and sensory structures, shortly disappear.

Very little is known about the metabolism of metacercariae. It is generally assumed that they subsist primarily, if not exclusively, on stored nutrients. However, while many metacercariae appear metabolically quiescent, some encysted in animal tissues do grow and, in fact, may affect their host's metabolism dynamically. They commonly induce the host's cellular defenses to encapsulate them with fibrous connective tissue. All metacercariae, however, undergo one common developmental change: they become infective to their definitive host.

# GERM CELL CYCLE

Reproduction in the miracidium–sporocyst–redia–cercaria progression is asexual, with the progeny arising through differentiation of germinal cells passed from one generation to the next. This phenomenon is known as the **germ cell cycle.** Only in the adult does sexual reproduction occur. Currently, the most widely accepted concept of intramolluscan reproduction among digeneans is that of **sequential polyembryony,** the production of multiple embryos from the same zygote with no intervening gamete production. Some evidence of parthenogenesis in sporocysts has been reported in several digeneans, in addition to polyembryonic proliferation.

Of particular importance to those interested in gene expression is the observation that all stages in the digenean life cycle carry identical sets of genes. Yet the expression of these genes differs among the several stages. It is apparent, then, that certain genes are activated while others are suppressed at various times during the sequence of larval development. For example, genes responsible for the development of an intramolluscan larva into a redia are suppressed in circumstances in which development into a sporocyst is indicated, and vice versa. What triggers this activation–suppression cycle has yet to be established.

Although the life cycle in a given species almost always follows the same pattern, environmental factors, such as temperature changes, and experimental manipulations, such as transplanting from one mollusc to another, can alter the sequential pattern in some digeneans. These alterations consist primarily of variations in the number and type of intramolluscan generations of larvae.

# PHYSIOLOGY

During the past two decades, considerable information has been complied concerning the biochemistry and physiology of digenetic trematodes. Much of this information has been derived from studies on the adult sheep liver fluke *Fasciola hepatica.* A number of factors are responsible for this emphasis: the adult worms are large and easy to work with; the life cycle can be maintained in the laboratory; and the economic and medical importance of this species attracts interest and funding for experimentation. The physiology of human blood flukes, or schistosomes, also has been studied intensively for similar reasons. Unfortunately, physiological and biochemical information on other genera and on larval forms is meager. Much of the following overview of the physiology of digeneans is the result of studies of the genera *Fasciola* and *Schistosoma*.

Substrate phosphorylation, via glycolysis, is the main source of energy for these forms, with glycogen and glucose as the main carbohydrates metabolized. Even in the presence of oxygen, as in the blood vessel environment of schistosomes, glycolysis provides the primary energy supply. In *Fasciola*, oxygen is used when available, but its contribution toward satisfying the organism's overall energy requirements is difficult to assess. A functional Krebs cycle exists in *Fasciola* and possibly in the schistosomes, but here, too, the overall role in energy production is probably minimal. Some enzymes usually considered Krebs cycle enzymes actually may serve in other metabolic pathways.

The dependence of digeneans on glycolysis for energy has been used to advantage in devising effective drugs for treatment of patients infected with these parasites. For instance, the efficacy of trivalent antimony compounds in treating schistosomiasis derives from their ability to inhibit phosphofructokinase, an important enzyme in the glycolytic pathway. Because it is requisite for any effective drug, the equivalent host enzyme must not be affected by the same level of drug concentration that affects the parasite.

The miracidia and cercariae of all species studied to date are obligate aerobes, relying on oxidative phosphorylation for energy. The metabolism of intramolluscan stages, on the other hand, resembles more closely that of adult forms in their dependency upon substrate phosphorylation to supply energy-rich compounds.

The limited information available on the synthetic abilities of *Fasciola* and the schistosomes shows that these parasites depend upon their hosts for a number of essential compounds, including pyrimidines, arginine, and lipids such as sterols and saturated and unsaturated fatty acids. The worms can probably synthesize complex lipids, provided they are supplied with basic molecules such as fatty acids.

## SELECTED READINGS

Bogitsh, B. J. 1975. Cytochemical observations on the gastrodermis of digenetic trematodes. *Transactions of the American Microscopical Society* 94, 524–528.

Bogitsh, B. J. 1986. An overview of surface specializations in the digenetic trematodes. *Hydrobiologia* 132, 305–310.

Llewellyn, J. 1965. The evolution of parasitic platyhelminths. In *Evolution of Parasites* (Taylor, A., ed.). Blackwell Scientific Publications, Oxford, England.

Schell, S. C. 1970. *How to Know the Trematodes.* William C. Brown, Dubuque, IA.

Smyth, J. D., and Halton, D. W. 1983. *The Physiology of Trematodes,* 2nd ed. Cambridge University Press, New York.

Whitfield, P. J., and Evans, N. A. 1983. Parthenogenesis and asexual multiplication among parasitic platyhelminths. *Parasitology* 86, 121–160.

# CLASSIFICATION OF THE TREMATODA*

## PHYLUM PLATYHELMINTHES

### CLASS TURBELLARIA
Mostly free-living worms in terrestrial, freshwater, and marine environments; some are commensals or parasites of invertebrates, especially of echinoderms and molluscs.

*ORDER ACOELA*

*ORDER NEORHABDOCOELA*

*ORDER ALLOEOCOELA*

*ORDER TRICLADIDA*

*ORDER POLYCLADIDA*

### CLASS MONOGENEA
All are parasitic, mainly on the skin or gills of fish; although most are ectoparasites, a few live within the stomadaeum, proctodaeum, or their diverticula.

### CLASS TREMATODA
All are parasitic, mainly in the digestive tract, of all classes of vertebrates; there are three subclasses.

### Subclass Aspidogastrea
Most have only one host, a mollusc; a few mature in marine turtles or fishes and have a mollusc or lobster intermediate host.

### Subclass Digenea
At least two hosts in life cycle, the first almost always a mollusc; perhaps most diversification in bony marine fish, although many species in all other groups of vertebrates.

*SUPERORDER ANEPITHELIOCYSTIDA*
Embryonic excretory vesicle (bladder) retained in adult, not replaced by mesodermal cells; vesicular wall thin, not epithelial; cercaria with forked or simple, straight tail; cercaria without oral stylet.

*Superfamily Strigeoidea*

*Superfamily Schistosomatoidea*
Dioecious adults in vascular system of definitive host; pharynx absent; no second intermediate host in life cycle; cercaria furcocercous with relatively short rami; oral sucker of cercaria replaced by protractile penetration organ; cercarial eyespots either pigmented or not; parasites of fishes, reptiles, birds, and mammals. (Genus mentioned in text: Family Schistosomatidae[†]—*Schistosoma*.)

---

*Only those taxa that include parasitic species are defined.

[†]For diagnoses of families subordinate to the Digenea, see Yamaguti, S. 1958, *Systema Helminthum*, Vol. 1 (two parts). Interscience, New York.

*Superfamily Bucephaloidea*

*Superfamily Echinostomatoidea*
Adult and cercaria usually with circumoral collar, commonly armed with spines; parasites of reptiles, birds, and mammals. (Genera mentioned in text: Family Fasciolidae[†]—*Fasciola, Fasciolopsis.* Family Echinostomatidae—*Echinostoma*).

*Superfamily Clinostomatoidea*

*Superfamily Brachylaemoidea*

*Superfamily Paramphistomoidea*

*Superfamily Azygioidea*

*Superfamily Cyclocoeloidea*

*Superfamily Fellodistomatoidea*

*Superfamily Transversotrematoidea*

*Superfamily Notocotyloidea*

*SUPERORDER EPITHELIOCYSTIDIA*
Wall of embryonic excretory vesicle (bladder) replaced by epithelial cells of mesodermal origin; cercaria with simple, straight tail; cercarial oral stylet commonly present.

*Superfamily Plagiorchioidea*

*Superfamily Allocreadioidea*
Adult one of several morphologic types; with or without eyespots; oral sucker usually simple, but some with appendages; acetabulum in anterior half of body; testes in posterior half of body; ovary pretesticular; cercaria one of several morphologic types; cercaria usually with eyespots; parasites of fish, amphibians, reptiles, and mammals. (Genus mentioned in text: Family Troglotrematidae—*Paragonimus.*)

*Superfamily Opisthorchioidea*
Cercaria with well-developed penetration glands; cercarial oral sucker protractile; cercarial ventral sucker rudimentary; cercarial tail one of several types; parasites of fish, amphibians, reptiles, birds, and mammals. (Genera mentioned in text: Family Opisthorchiidae[†]—*Opisthorchis, Clonorchis.* Family Heterophyidae—*Heterophyes, Metagonimus.*)

*Superfamily Hemiuroidea*

*Superfamily Isoparorchioidea*

---

[†]For diagnoses of families subordinate to the Digenea, see Yamaguti, S. 1958, *Systema Helminthum*, Vol. 1 (two parts). Interscience, New York.

# CHAPTER NINE

# VISCERAL FLUKES

Species of seven genera, representing five families, commonly infect various visceral organs of humans. Members of the genera *Fasciola, Clonorchis,* and *Opisthorchis* reside in the liver; another four, *Fasciolopsis, Heterophyes, Metagonimus,* and *Echinostoma,* inhabit the small intestine; and several members of the genus *Paragonimus,* especially *P. westermani,* live in the lungs. For the sake of convenience, discussion of the organisms is structured according to site of infection rather than phylogenetic relationships. The classification system at the end of Chapter Eight summarizes phylogenetic affinities.

## LIVER FLUKES

### *Fasciola hepatica*

*Fasciola hepatica* is one of the largest digeneans parasitizing humans, measuring 30 mm long by 13 mm wide (Fig. 9–1). In addition to its size, *F. hepatica* can be distinguished from other digeneans by its highly branched testes and intestinal caeca; the short, convoluted uterus; oral and ventral suckers of equal size, the former situated on an anterior prominence called the **cephalic cone;** and vitellaria that extend along the lateral edges of the body to the posterior end. Adult worms live in the bile passages, liver tissue, and gall bladder of their mammalian hosts.

**Life Cycle** (Fig. 9–2).    *Fasciola hepatica* occupies a prominent place in parasitology because among digenetic trematodes its life cycle was the first to be completely elucidated, and that achievement has been the impetus for all subsequent investigations on life histories.

The ovoid eggs are relatively large (130–150 μm by 63–90 μm), operculate, and yellowish-brown in color. They are expelled while the miracidium is only partially developed, pass into the host's alimentary tract via the common bile duct, and eventually reach the exterior with feces, at which time they must encounter fresh water if the cycle is to continue.

After 4 to 15 days in water at approximately 22°C, the completely developed miracidium escapes when the operculum opens. The miracidium has eyespots and is positively phototropic. Within 8 hours after hatching, the miracidium must seek out and penetrate a suitable snail host or it will

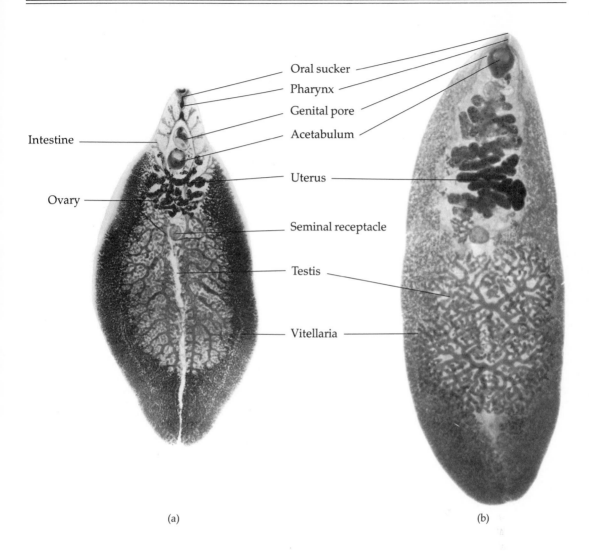

Oral sucker
Pharynx
Genital pore
Acetabulum
Intestine
Uterus
Ovary
Seminal receptacle
Testis
Vitellaria

(a)                                                          (b)

**Figure 9–1**
**Two fasciolid flukes.**
(a) *Fasciola hepatica*, the sheep
liver fluke. (b) *Fasciolopsis buski*.

die. Members of the amphibious snail genera *Lymnaea, Suc-cinea, Fossaria,* and *Practicolella* serve as first intermediate hosts. Upon penetration, each miracidium metamorphoses into a sporocyst that gives rise to mother rediae that, in turn, give rise to daughter rediae. Germ balls in the brood chambers of daughter rediae develop into cercariae, which emerge from the snail and become free-swimming. Upon reaching aquatic, emergent vegetation (e.g., grasses) or even submerged bark, the cercariae shed their tails and encyst as metacercariae on plants upon which sheep and cattle commonly feed. Humans become infected by eating contaminated watercress and other vegetation.

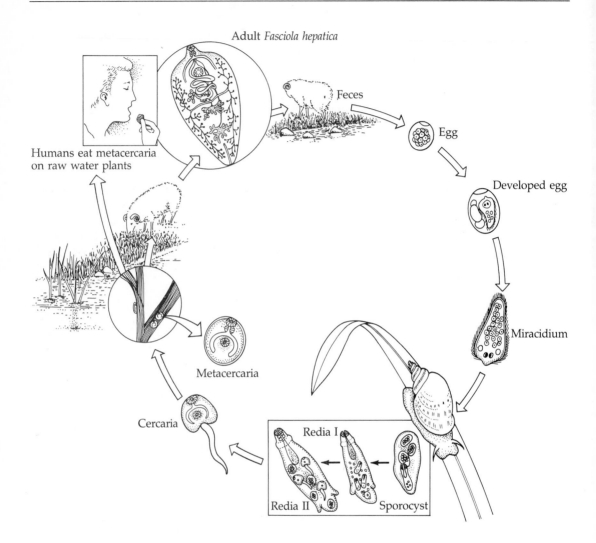

Adult *Fasciola hepatica*

Feces

Egg

Developed egg

Miracidium

Humans eat metacercaria on raw water plants

Metacercaria

Cercaria

Redia I

Redia II    Sporocyst

**Figure 9–2**
**Life cycle of *Fasciola hepatica.***

Metacercariae swallowed by the definitive host excyst in the duodenum, penetrate the intestinal wall, and enter the liver capsule via the body cavity. Migration through the liver parenchyma allows them to consume liver cells and blood before they reach the bile ducts, where they attain sexual maturity in approximately 12 weeks.

**Epidemiology.**    Human infection by *F. hepatica* occurs throughout the world and is of increasing importance in some Caribbean islands and South America, as well as southern France, Great Britain, and Algeria. Ecologically, sheep- and cattle-raising regions are the primary areas for human infection. Infections in cattle and sheep produce serious economic losses in wool production, milk, and meat. In one abattoir, economic losses from infected beef liver were estimated at thousands of dollars per year.

**Symptomatology and Diagnosis.**    Infection with *F. hepatica* in humans, or fascioliasis, is characterized by extensive destruction of liver tissue and bile ducts, hemorrhage, atrophy of portal vessels, and secondary pathological conditions that may be lethal. In addition to causing mechanical damage, the worms also may evoke inflammatory reactions when the host becomes sensitized to the worm's metabolic products. Juvenile worms may get lost in the body cavity, encyst in ectopic tissues, and eventually become calcified.

Initial symptoms frequently include severe headache, backache, chills, and fever. An enlarged, tender, or cirrhotic liver, accompanied by diarrhea and anemia, indicates advanced infection.

Laboratory diagnosis is based on identification of the characteristic eggs from the feces (Fig. 8–15). Complement-fixation tests have also proven diagnostically useful, especially in extrahepatic infections.

It is of interest that, when eaten by humans in the Middle East, raw bovine liver harboring *Fasciola hepatica* causes pain, irritation, hoarseness, and coughing due to young worms becoming attached to buccal or pharyngeal membranes. This condition, known as **halzoun,** is more commonly caused by pentastomids, or tongue worms, acquired in a similar manner.

**Treatment.**    Some patients respond well to treatment with dichlorophen. Dehydroemetine hydrochloride and emetine hydrochloride are also used, but the same caution must apply as when these drugs are used in the treatment of amoebiasis. Since they are cardiotoxins, bed rest is essential during therapy. Globally, praziquantel is currently the drug of choice, although in the United States it has only limited approval for human use.

## *Clonorchis sinensis*

*Clonorchis sinensis*, the Chinese, or Oriental, liver fluke, is distributed widely in Korea, Japan, China, Taiwan, and Vietnam and has been estimated to infect at least 19 million persons. It belongs to the family Opisthorchiidae, whose members possess small suckers and infect the biliary systems of reptiles, birds, and mammals. Prosobranch snails serve as the molluscan hosts, and freshwater fishes such as carp serve as second intermediate hosts.

**Life Cycle** (Fig. 9–3). The adult worm resides in the bile ducts and varies in size from 12 to 20 mm long and from 3 to 5 mm wide. The body is tapered anteriorly, while the posterior end is somewhat blunt (Fig. 9–4). The poorly developed ventral sucker lies about one-fourth the body length from the anterior end, just behind the common genital pore. The caeca extend to the posterior region of the body. A centrally located ovary lies just anterior to the deeply lobed, tandemly arranged testes. The vitellaria are lateral, and a loosely coiled, gravid uterus extends from the region of the

**Figure 9–3**
**Life cycle of *Clonorchis sinensis*.**

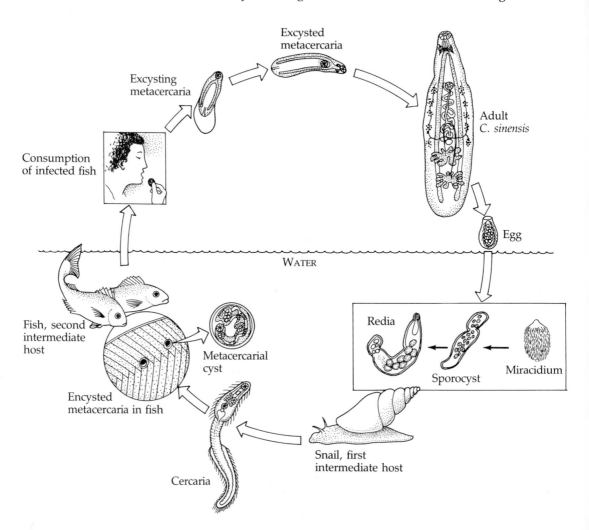

ovary to the genital pore. The tanned eggs, which measure 29 by 16 μm, are operculated, with a ridge or collar at the base of the operculum, giving them an unusual urn shape (Fig. 8–15).

Eggs containing partially developed embryos are deposited in the biliary ducts and pass to the outside with the host's feces. Although the egg contains a fully developed miracidium when it reaches fresh water, it does not hatch immediately. Instead, hatching occurs only when the egg reaches the digestive tract of a suitable snail intermediate host belonging to any of the genera *Parafossarulus*, *Bulimus*, *Semisulcospira*, *Alocinma*, or *Melanoides*. The released miracidium first penetrates the intestinal wall of the snail into the

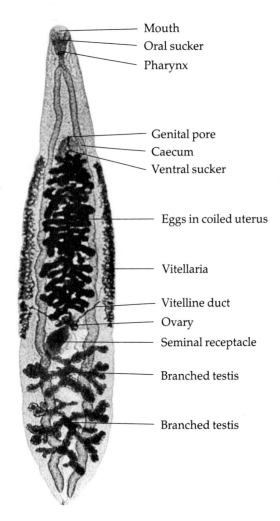

Mouth
Oral sucker
Pharynx

Genital pore
Caecum
Ventral sucker

Eggs in coiled uterus

Vitellaria

Vitelline duct
Ovary
Seminal receptacle

Branched testis

Branched testis

**Figure 9–4**
**The digenetic trematode**
*Clonorchis sinensis.*

hemocoel and then the digestive gland, where it metamorphoses into a sporocyst. The sporocyst gives rise to rediae, which erupt from the sporocyst and, in turn, produce cercariae. The free-swimming cercariae that emerge from the snail must penetrate the skin, gills, fins, or muscles of freshwater fish hosts within 24 to 48 hours. Each burrows into these tissues, loses its tail, and encysts as a metacercaria. A wide variety of fish species belonging to the family Cyprinidae serve as second intermediate hosts. Humans become infected by eating raw or poorly cooked fish (including steamed, smoked, or pickled). The metacercaria excysts in the duodenum, migrates up the common bile duct and into the biliary ducts where it reaches sexual maturity, continually feeding on the contents of the ducts. Following excystation, the worm takes a month to mature sexually. *Clonorchis sinensis* has been known to live up to 25 years in the human host.

**Epidemiology.**    Reservoir hosts—including cats, dogs, tigers, foxes, badgers, and mink—play a significant role in maintaining Oriental liver fluke populations in endemic areas. The high incidence of mammalian infection, the increase in freshwater fish farming in the Orient, and the practice of eating fish raw have made clonorchiasis a serious problem. Oriental aquaculture ponds are commonly fertilized with human excrement to enhance the growth of vegetation on which the fish feed. In Hong Kong, where fish farming is very common, the prevalence of human clonorchiasis is about 14%; in the rural endemic areas, it may reach 80%.

**Symptomatology and Diagnosis.**    Most of the damage to human hosts occurs in the bile ducts, manifested by mechanical and toxic irritation. The amount of damage is proportional to the number of worms present, with some infections running into the thousands; for example, over 6000 adult worms were recovered from one person at autopsy. In such extreme cases, liver enlargement, thickening of the bile ducts, fibrosis, and some destruction of liver parenchyma occur. Unlike *Fasciola*, however, *Clonorchis* does not invade liver tissues and, therefore, does not cause extensive necrosis. Intestinal disturbances also are common, but clonorchiasis is rarely fatal except when patients succumb to secondary infections due to lowered resistance.

Positive diagnosis depends on identification of eggs from either feces or biliary drainage, and these must be differentiated from eggs of heterophyids (see below). Clinical examination is warranted whenever there is liver enlargement coupled with a history of residency in endemic areas.

**Treatment.**    Praziquantel administered over a two-day period is the treatment of choice. In light infections, prognosis is good even without treatment since tissue invasion is not involved.

## *Opisthorchis felineus* and *O. viverrini*

*Opisthorchis felineus* and *O. viverrini* are parasitic in the bile ducts of fish-eating mammals, including humans (Fig. 9–5). *O. felineus* is most common in southern, central, and eastern Europe, Turkey, the southern part of the Soviet Union, Vietnam, India, and Japan. It is also present in Puerto Rico and possibly other Caribbean islands. In Thailand, Laos, and southeast Asia, *O. viverrini* occurs in an estimated 1 to 3 million humans. Patients harboring these worms suffer from diarrhea and thickening and eventual erosion of the bile duct wall.

**Figure 9–5**
**(a)** *Opisthorchis felineus* **adult.**
**(b)** *O. viverrini* **adult.**

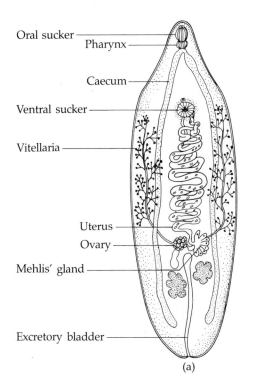

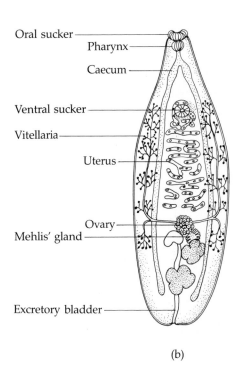

(a)                                    (b)

The life cycle of *O. felineus* and *O. viverrini* is similar to that of *C. sinensis*, employing intermediate hosts belonging to the snail genus *Bithynia* and cyprinid fishes, such as the chub or tench. Although infection by these worms is more common in animals, human infection results from eating raw or improperly cooked fish infected with encysted metacercariae. Felines are important reservoir hosts in endemic areas for both *O. felineus* and *O. viverrini*.

Diagnosis and treatment of both infections are similar to those for clonorchiasis.

## INTESTINAL FLUKES

### *Fasciolopsis buski*

*Fasciolopsis buski* is the largest digenean infecting humans, reaching a size of 75 mm long and 20 mm wide. It is morphologically similar to *Fasciola hepatica* with a few notable differences (Fig. 9–1). The most obvious of these are that, in *F. buski*, the caeca lack side branches, the ventral sucker is much larger than the oral sucker, and there is no cephalic cone. It differs further from all other members of the family Fasciolidae in that the definitive habitat is the small intestine of humans and pigs rather than the liver.

**Life Cycle** (Fig. 9–6).   Adult worms inhabit the duodenal and jejunal regions of the small intestine, either attached by the suckers to the mucosal epithelium or lying buried in the mucus secretions. Daily each deposits about 25,000 eggs that are indistinguishable from *F. hepatica* eggs; they pass out in feces and must reach fresh water in order to continue the cycle. In fresh water, miracidia develop and hatch in about 3 to 7 weeks, depending on temperature. They locate and penetrate a snail of the genus *Segmentina* or *Hippeutis* and metamorphose into sporocysts, followed by two redial generations. Cercariae emerge from the daughter rediae 4 to 7 weeks after miracidial penetration of the snail, re-enter the water, and encyst on freshwater vegetation, most commonly water chestnut, water caltrop, water bamboo, and lotus. Encysted metacercariae are ingested when humans eat contaminated raw plants or peel the pods or stalks with their teeth before eating, thereby freeing and swallowing the encysted metacercaria. Metacercariae excyst in the small intestine, attach to the mucosa, and develop to sexual maturity in 25 to 30 days.

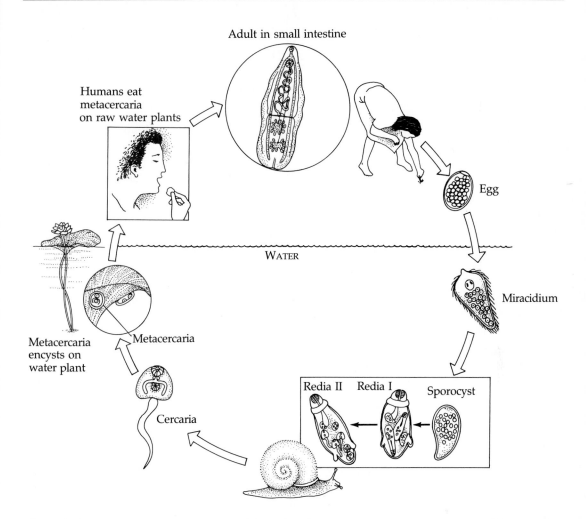

**Figure 9–6**
**Life cycle of *Fasciolopsis buski.***

**Epidemiology.** Human infection by *F. buski* occurs throughout central and south China, Taiwan, Thailand, Laos, Vietnam, Cambodia, India, Korea, and Indonesia. The infection is usually acquired by ingestion of encysted metacercariae from fresh plants grown in ponds fertilized with human or pig excrement. Drying or cooking the plants before eating kills metacercariae. Hogs are the most important animal reservoirs for *F. buski.*

**Symptomatology and Diagnosis.** The worm feeds actively not only on the intestinal contents but also on the superficial mucosa, causing inflammation, ulceration, and abcesses at sites of attachment. Diarrhea, nausea, and intestinal pain are common, especially in the morning hours. Intestinal edema occurs in heavier infections. Ingestion of food may relieve the abdominal distress unless it happens to consist of infested aquatic plants, in which case symptoms will eventually exacerbate. Due to the large size of the worms, intestinal obstruction may also occur. Reaction to the worms' metabolites can produce such clinical symptoms as leukocytosis, anemia, and eosinophilia. Patients purged of the worms usually recover completely, although advanced, heavy infections can be fatal.

When clinical symptoms develop in an endemic area, diagnosis must be confirmed by fecal examination for eggs, or, occasionally, by examination of whole worms vomited or passed in feces.

**Treatment.**    Praziquantel is the drug of choice where available; dichlorophen or tetrachloroethylene are the usual alternatives.

## *Echinostoma revolutum*

Several members of the genus *Echinostoma* and related genera occasionally infect humans as well as other mammals. Adult echinostomes, while varying greatly in size, are easily identified by the collar of spines along the dorsal and lateral sides of the head. In general appearance (Fig. 9–7), the adult worm is elongated, with a massive ventral sucker situated immediately behind the head. The testes lie in tandem in the posterior portion of the body; the ovary is anterior to the testes, and the short uterus consists only of an ascending limb terminating at the genital pore anterior to the ventral sucker. Large, operculate eggs measure 90–126 μm long by 54–71 μm wide, with only a few in the uterus at any given time. *Echinostoma revolutum* is the prototype for echinostome species infecting humans, essential differences consisting primarily of the number and arrangement of collar spines.

**Life Cycle.**    The life cycle of *E. revolutum* is typical of most echinostomes. Operculated eggs are passed from the definitive host with feces and must reach fresh water for the cycle to continue. The enclosed miracidium is at a very early stage of development when the egg is deposited and requires 2 to 5 weeks to develop to maturity, after which it hatches and penetrates a snail of the genus *Lymnaea*, *Physa*, or *Bithynia*. Various freshwater pelecypods and gastropods serve as hosts for other echinostomes. A single sporocyst generation and two redial generations develop in the molluscan host. Free-swimming cercariae escape from daughter rediae, enter

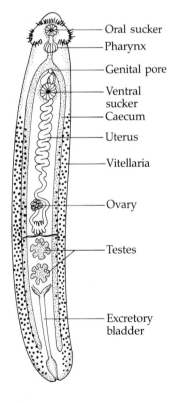

Oral sucker
Pharynx
Genital pore
Ventral sucker
Caecum
Uterus
Vitellaria
Ovary
Testes
Excretory bladder

**Figure 9–7**
*Echinostoma revolutum* **adult.**

the water, and penetrate and encyst in molluscs—including species that serve as first intermediate hosts—and a variety of other aquatic animals and, at times, on aquatic vegetation. The life cycle is completed when the definitive host ingests encysted metacercariae, which excyst and develop to sexual maturity in the small intestine.

**Epidemiology.**    While as many as 15 species of *Echinostoma* have been reported in humans, most are incidental parasites. *E. revolutum*, for instance, is a common parasite of birds and mammals in the United States. Human infections of *E. ilocanum* are most frequently reported from such Oriental countries as the Philippines, China, Taiwan, and Indonesia. Infection occurs when the infected second intermediate host is eaten either raw or improperly cooked. Because of the variety and number of potential intermediate and definitive hosts, it is impossible to control the parasite, but human infections can be prevented if food is cooked adequately.

**Symptomatology and Diagnosis.**    Echinostomiasis in humans is usually a minor affliction, often causing nothing more serious than diarrhea. In heavy infections, the spinose collar may cause ulceration of the intestinal mucosa. Children sometimes experience abdominal pain, diarrhea, anemia, and/or edema.

Diagnosis of eggs from feces depends on features that distinguish echinostome eggs from those of other intestinal helminths, namely their dark brownish color and the very immature larvae, even uncleaved zygotes.

**Treatment.**    As with most intestinal flukes, best results are achieved with praziquantel, with tetrachloroethylene as an alternative.

## *Heterophyes heterophyes* and *Metagonimus yokagawai*

*Heterophyes heterophyes* and *Metagonimus yokagawai* belong to the family Heterophyidae. Measuring 1.4 mm long and 0.5 mm wide, they are among the smallest digeneans infecting humans (Fig. 9–8). These pyriform flukes are covered by a tegument containing scalelike spines. In *H. heterophyes*, the genital pore, situated postero-lateral to the prominent ventral sucker, is surrounded by a genital sucker or **gonotyl**. In *M. yokagawai*, the ventral sucker and gonotyl are fused, and the

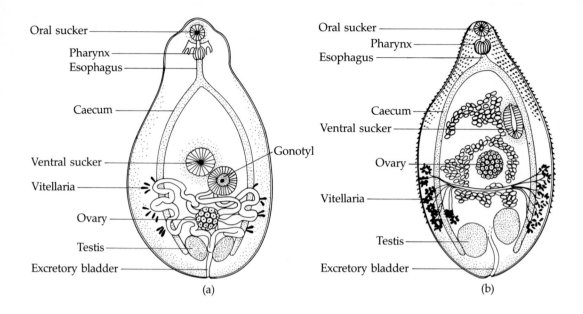

Oral sucker
Pharynx
Esophagus
Caecum
Ventral sucker
Vitellaria
Ovary
Testis
Excretory bladder
Gonotyl

(a)

Oral sucker
Pharynx
Esophagus
Caecum
Ventral sucker
Ovary
Vitellaria
Testis
Excretory bladder

(b)

**Figure 9–8**
**(a)** *Heterophyes heterophyes*
**adult. (b)** *Metagonimus*
*yokogawai* **adult.**

complex is displaced to the left side of the body. The reproductive system is located in the posterior half of the body, with the testes lying side by side. The ovary is medial, just anterior to the testes, with lateral, follicular vitelline glands restricted to the posterior third of the body. The gravid uterus loops between the long intestinal caeca, terminating at the gonotyl. The eggs of both these species resemble those of *Clonorchis sinensis* except for their indistinct opercular shoulders and the presence of an abopercular knob.

**Life Cycle.**    *Heterophyes heterophyes* and *Metagonimus yokagawai* commonly inhabit the middle of the small intestine, and their life cycles are almost identical. Human infection by *H. heterophyes* occurs in Asia, Egypt, and Hawaii, while *M. yokagawai* is the most common intestinal fluke of humans in the Far East, Spain, and the Balkan countries. Eggs with fully developed miracidia pass out of the body in feces and hatch only when ingested by a suitable molluscan first intermediate host. In *H. heterophyes*, this is a freshwater or brackish water snail of the genera *Pirenella* (in Egypt), *Cerithidia* (in Japan), and *Tarebia* (in Hawaii); *M. yokagawai* infects members of the snail genus *Semisulcospira*. The hatched miracidium penetrates the intestine of the snail and transforms into a sporocyst in the digestive gland. Two generations of rediae follow the sporocyst, with daughter rediae giving rise to cercariae that escape to the external environment, penetrate the musculature of a suitable fish, and encyst as metacercariae. One of the principal fishes used by *H. heterophyes* as the second intermediate host is the mullet, which can harbor several thousand metacercariae. Salmonoid fishes commonly serve as second intermediate hosts for *M. yokagawai* metacercariae. Human infection results from consumption of raw or improperly cooked fish. The metacercariae excyst in the duodenum, migrate to the jejunum, and become sexually mature in about a week.

**Epidemiology.**    There is an unusually high incidence of infection with *H. heterophyes* in Egypt, especially in parts of the lower Nile valley. Poor sanitation practices by local fishermen, boatmen, and other residents continually pollute the water with eggs. One of the principal food fishes is the mullet, and parasitic infection results from eating fresh mullet, either incompletely cooked or poorly pickled. Human infection with *H. heterophyes* is also common in Japan, central and south China, Korea, Taiwan, Greece, Israel, and Hawaii. Infection with *M. yokagawai* occurs when the infected second intermediate host, such as a salmonoid fish, is consumed raw or improperly processed. A variety of fish-eating mammals, including cats and dogs, serve as reservoirs of infection for both of these zoonotic parasites.

**Symptomatology and Diagnosis.**    The pathology, symptomatology, and diagnosis of infection by these two digeneans are very similar. Adult worms often produce little distress to the patient, but heavy infections may elicit inflammatory reactions at sites of contact as well as diarrhea and abdominal pain. Eosinophilia is also common, but without anemia. Adult worms sometimes erode the mucosa and deposit eggs, which infiltrate the lymphatics or venules. The eggs are then carried to various parts of the body where they may cause granulomatous responses in such organs as the heart or brain. Heterophyid myocarditis sometimes precipitates fatal heart attacks, and neurological complications also have been reported.

Diagnosis depends on positive identification of eggs from feces. Because of the great degree of similarity, care must be exercised to differentiate the eggs from those of other heterophyids and of opisthorchids.

**Treatment.**    Treatment is the same for both parasites, i.e., praziquantel or tetrachloroethylene.

# LUNG FLUKES

## *Paragonimus westermani*

*Paragonimus westermani,* the Oriental lung fluke, belongs to the family Troglotrematidae and is one of several digeneans belonging to the same genus that infect the human respiratory tract. The first report of human infection was from Formosa (Taiwan) during the latter part of the nineteenth century. Following that initial account, numerous other infections were quickly diagnosed in the Orient, where the condition remains prevalent today.

The thick-bodied, reddish-brown adult worm measures 7.5–12 mm long and 4–6 mm wide (Fig. 9–9). The male reproductive system consists of two irregularly lobed testes situated side by side about two-thirds down the length of the body. The lobed ovary, anterior to the right testis, is connected via the oviduct to the uterus, a tightly coiled rosette that lies anterior to the left testis at the same level as the ovary. Vitellaria extend bilaterally along the length of the body, lateral to and paralleling the caeca. A medially located ventral sucker lies between the ovary and the uterus. Brownish, operculated eggs (Fig. 8–15), smaller than but similar to those of *Fasciola hepatica,* are released through the genital pore situated in the center of the uterine rosette.

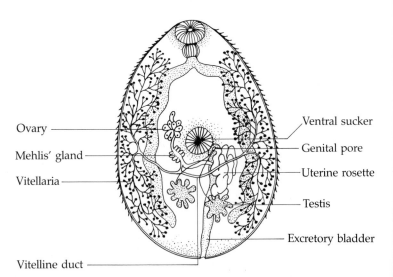

Ovary

Mehlis' gland

Vitellaria

Ventral sucker

Genital pore

Uterine rosette

Testis

Excretory bladder

Vitelline duct

**Figure 9–9**
*Paragonimus westermani* **adult.**

**Life Cycle** (Fig. 9–10).   Paired adult *P. westermani* are usually found encapsulated in the bronchioles of the victim's lungs. Commonly, eggs containing uncleared embryos or zygotes are coughed up and expelled with sputum when the capsules enclosing the adult worms rupture. However, some eggs may be swallowed with sputum, pass through the digestive system, and be expelled with feces, while others get trapped in the surrounding lung tissue and produce bronchial abcesses. Once the egg reaches water, several weeks are required for the miracidium to develop. When the miracidium is fully developed, hatching is spontaneous, and the miracidium must then locate and penetrate a suitable

**Figure 9–10**
**Life cycle of *Paragonimus westermani*.**

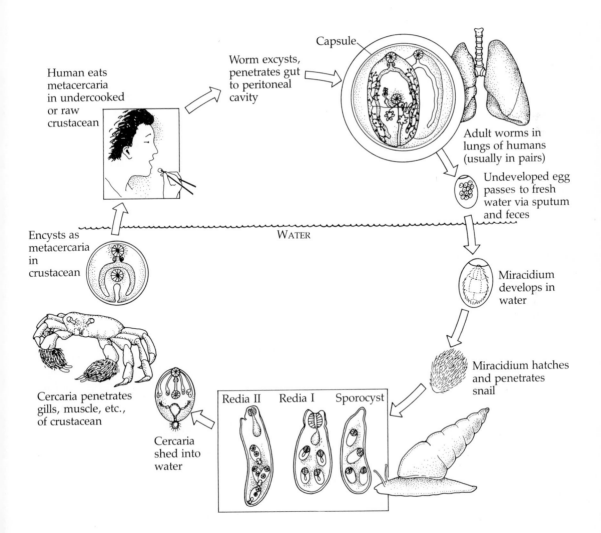

Human eats metacercaria in undercooked or raw crustacean

Worm excysts, penetrates gut to peritoneal cavity

Capsule

Adult worms in lungs of humans (usually in pairs)

Undeveloped egg passes to fresh water via sputum and feces

Encysts as metacercaria in crustacean

WATER

Miracidium develops in water

Cercaria penetrates gills, muscle, etc., of crustacean

Cercaria shed into water

Redia II    Redia I    Sporocyst

Miracidium hatches and penetrates snail

snail host of the genus *Semisulcospira, Tarebia,* or *Brotia* within 24 hours or perish. Following penetration of the snail host and metamorphosis into a sporocyst, two redial generations are produced in the digestive gland. Cercariae, formed within the brood chambers of the daughter rediae, emerge from the snail tissue into the surrounding water approximately 11 weeks after the snail is infected. The cercariae possess knoblike tails useless for swimming; instead, the cercariae crawl over solid surfaces until they encounter suitable crustaceans, such as freshwater crabs and crayfish. Using a sharply pointed, cuticular stylet, they can penetrate the crustacean's exoskeleton at various vulnerable sites. There is evidence that the crustacean second intermediate host may also acquire infection by eating infected snails. Once inside the host, they encyst in the muscles, gills, and viscera (Fig. 9–11), where they develop into metacercariae. The encysted metacercaria is not folded over ventrally, as are most encysted metacercariae, but lies in an extended position within the cyst wall.

Humans acquire infection by eating infected freshwater crustaceans raw, inadequately pickled, or incompletely cooked. The metacercaria excysts in the small intestine and partially penetrates the intestinal wall. Young adults remain at this site for several days before entering the coelom. Then, traversing the diaphragm and pleura, they enter the peribronchiolar tissues of the lungs, where they become encapsulated in pairs by host connective tissue and develop to sexual maturity within 8 to 12 weeks. During migration, young adult worms often become lodged in other organs, producing ectopic lesions before succumbing to host reactions.

**Figure 9–11**
**(a) Encysted metacercaria of *P. westermani.***
**(b) Several metacercariae encysted in gill filament of crab host.**

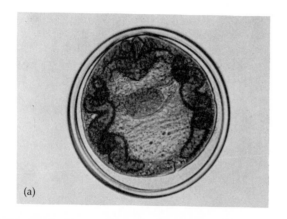

(a)

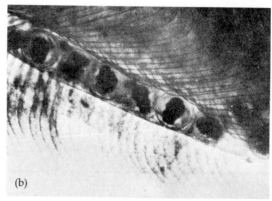

(b)

**Epidemiology.**    While *P. westermani* is worldwide in distribution, human infections are confined mainly to such Oriental countries as Japan, South Korea, Thailand, Taiwan, China, and the Philippines. As noted previously, human infection results from consumption of infected freshwater crustaceans that are raw or improperly pickled or cooked. The pickling process coagulates muscle protein, giving the meat the appearance of being cooked and therefore harmless, while actually it has no effect upon the encysted metacercariae. Metacercariae dislodged from the crustacean during the cleaning process may also adhere to utensils, which then become a source of infection to food handlers. Humans may also become infected by consuming the juices obtained from crushed crabs, a practice common in parts of the Orient.

**Symptomatology and Diagnosis.**    *Paragonimus westermani* adults and eggs stimulate formation of connective tissue capsules in the host, both in the lungs and at ectopic sites. In addition to adult worms, the capsules contain eggs and infiltrated host cells in a hemorrhagic, semifluid mass. The capsules often ulcerate, giving the lungs a peppered appearance. Early symptoms include a cough producing blood-tinged sputum, pulmonary pain, and even pleurisy. A low-grade fever usually accompanies these symptoms. At present, paragonimiasis is difficult to distinguish from other pulmonary disorders such as pneumonia and tuberculosis.

Encysted worms may be found at such ectopic sites as the abdominal wall, lymph nodes, heart, and portions of the nervous system. Infection of the abdominal wall may produce abdominal pain, diarrhea, and bleeding. In the brain, infection may produce a variety of neurological symptoms such as epilepsy and paralysis. Fatalities have been recorded from cardiac involvement as well as from heavy pulmonary infections.

Identification of eggs from sputum or feces is the most reliable diagnostic procedure. Patients from endemic areas who show such symptoms as pulmonary distress, blood-tinged sputum, and eosinophilia should be examined carefully. For ectopic infections, immunological tests such as complement-fixation and intradermal tests with *Paragonimus* as antigen have proven useful.

**Treatment.**    A 24-hour course of treatment with praziquantel is recommended in countries that permit its use. In the United States, oral administration of bithionol for 10 to 15 days is recommended.

# ◇
# SELECTED READINGS

Boray, J. C. 1969. Experimental fascioliasis in Australia. *Advances in Parasitology* 7, 96–210.

Koniya, Y. 1966. *Clonorchis* and clonorchiasis. *Advances in Parasitology* 4, 53–106.

Yokagawa, M. 1969. *Paragonimus* and paragonimiasis. *Advances in Parasitology* 7, 375–387.

# CHAPTER TEN

## BLOOD FLUKES

The human disease complex known as schistosomiasis is also referred to as bilharziasis or snail fever. It is caused primarily by three members of the genus *Schistosoma* (family Schistosomatidae): *S. haematobium, S. mansoni,* and *S. japonicum.* There are several other species that infect humans, but they are much less common or even rare. Human infections by these flukes number in excess of 250 million worldwide, and in spite of efforts to control this disease, the level of incidence has shown no significant decrease. In the People's Republic of China alone, a recent estimate indicated at least 15 million cases of schistosomiasis japonica, representing the single most serious disease in that country. As a result of concerted control measures, incidence in China has been somewhat reduced. Egypt has one of the most heavily infected populations in the world, since not only is *S. haematobium* endemic to that country, but *S. mansoni* also occurs with great frequency. In the population of some endemic areas of the Nile valley, the infection rate exceeds 80%. Other areas of high incidence include tropical and subtropical Africa, parts of South America, and several of the Caribbean islands (Fig. 10–1).

While it was not until 1852 that the young German parasitologist Theodor Bilharz, working in Egypt, discovered

**Figure 10–1**
**(a)** Global distribution of schistosomiasis due to *Schistosoma mansoni* and *S. intercalatum.*
**(b)** Global distribution of schistosomiasis due to *Schistosoma haematobium, S. japonicum,* and *S. mekongi.*

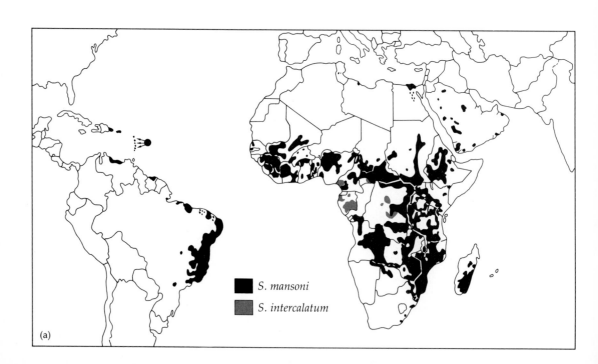

■ *S. mansoni*

▨ *S. intercalatum*

(a)

one of the parasites (*S. haematobium*) responsible for urinary schistosomiasis, there are recorded accounts of the disease dating from pharaonic times. In the Ebers papyrus from 1500 B.C., there is a reference to treatment of hematuria (bloody urine), and calcified eggs of *S. haematobium* have been found in the viscera of Egyptian mummies dating from 1200 B.C.

Fossilized bulinid snails that serve as intermediate hosts for *S. haematobium* have been uncovered in the ancient biblical city of Jericho. An interesting hypothesis, based on this discovery, is that the city's well was infested with infected snails, producing a high incidence of schistosomiasis among the citizenry. Too debilitated by the disease to defend their city or repair its decaying walls, they were easily defeated by Joshua's army. Without knowing the cause of this heinous disease, Joshua, in order to prevent its spread, destroyed Jericho and proclaimed a curse upon any who would rebuild it, thus precluding subsequent repopulation. The city remained deserted for more than 500 years. Centuries of recurring drought apparently destroyed the snails, and the city became, and still remains, free of the parasite.

The French invasion of Egypt during the early part of the nineteenth century was probably one of the first large-

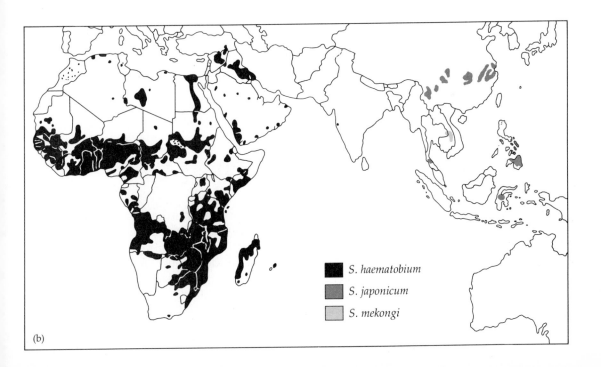

(b)

scale contacts people of the Western world had with schistosomiasis. Besides amoebic dysentery, the French had to contend with two other diseases previously unknown to them—hematuria and the eye disease known as trachoma. The former, as we now know, is caused by *S. haematobium*, while the latter is caused by a fly-transmitted microorganism (see p. 372). Both diseases remain firmly entrenched in Egypt.

## MORPHOLOGY

Figure 10–2 depicts adult male and female worms. The mouth of the adult schistosome is surrounded by an oral sucker, and a ventral sucker is located immediately posterior to the level of bifurcation of the gut. While no pharynx is present, there is an esophagus with prominent **esophageal glands.** The paired caeca reunite posteriorly, forming a single caecum that extends along the remaining length of the body. Schistosomes are unique among digeneans in being dioecious and sexually dimorphic. The adult male is larger in circumference than the female, with a ventral fold or groove called the **gynaecophoral canal.** The female, longer and more slender than the male, is held in this canal, permitting almost continuous mating.

The male possesses from 5 to 9 testes, and the male genital pore opens ventrally, immediately posterior to the ventral sucker. There is no cirrus. In the female, the position of the single ovary varies according to species, and the uterus may be long or short, depending on the position of the ovary relative to the female genital pore.

## LIFE CYCLE

The life cycles (Fig. 10-3) of the three species are virtually identical and will be so treated. Individual differences will be noted in the section following description of the life cycle.

Adult schistosomes reside in mesenteric veins that drain the intestine (*S. mansoni* and *S. japonicum*) or in vesicular veins serving the urinary bladder (*S. haematobium*). In single-sex infections, the sexual organs of female worms are underdeveloped, leading to the hypothesis that one or more male factors are essential for complete maturation of the female.

The female usually migrates to smaller venules before depositing eggs. The morphology of the egg is distinctive in each species and serves as a criterion for diagnosis (Fig. 8–15). The enclosed miracidium is poorly developed at the time of oviposition, but is well formed before it reaches the lumen of the infected organ. The egg must penetrate the venule endothelium and then traverse the intervening tissues and the mucosal lining before entering the lumen of the gut or the bladder to escape to the outside. The method by which the egg passes through the tissues remains speculative but probably involves hydrolytic secretions emitted through the porous shell. The process is obviously in-

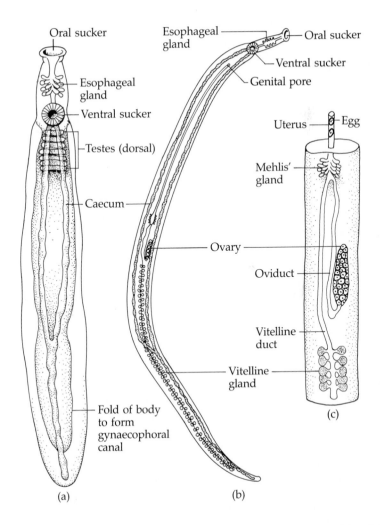

**Figure 10–2**
**Diagram of generalized adult schistosomes.**
(a) Male. (b) Female.
(c) Enlargement of female reproductive system.

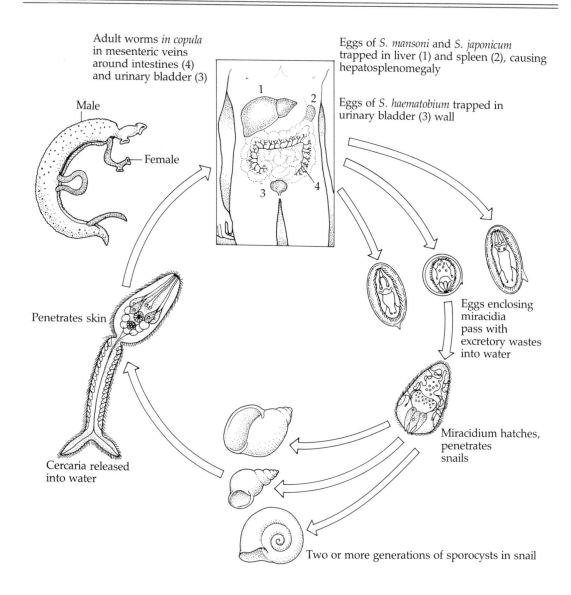

Adult worms *in copula* in mesenteric veins around intestines (4) and urinary bladder (3)

Male

Female

Eggs of *S. mansoni* and *S. japonicum* trapped in liver (1) and spleen (2), causing hepatosplenomegaly

Eggs of *S. haematobium* trapped in urinary bladder (3) wall

Eggs enclosing miracidia pass with excretory wastes into water

Penetrates skin

Miracidium hatches, penetrates snails

Cercaria released into water

Two or more generations of sporocysts in snail

**Figure 10–3**
**Life cycle of a blood fluke.**

efficient since only about one-third of the eggs produced reach the exterior; the remaining eggs are either trapped in the urinary bladder or intestinal walls or are swept back by the blood flow to become lodged in ectopic sites such as the liver (Fig. 10–4) and, occasionally, the spleen and other tissues. After reaching the lumen, the egg passes out in either feces or urine.

Upon reaching fresh water, the egg escapes the inhibitory osmolarity of the host's body fluids, thereby activating the miracidium to hatch. Since schistosome eggs have no

**Figure 10–4**
*Schistosoma mansoni* egg in liver.

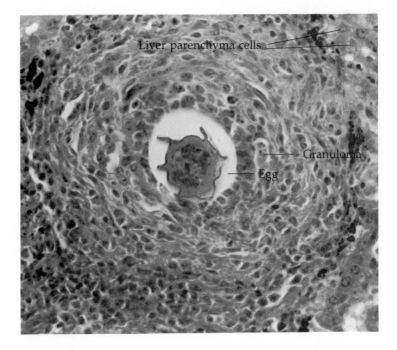

operculum, hatching occurs through a rupture of the egg-shell along a line known as the **stigma.**

The free-swimming miracidium (Fig. 10–5) must penetrate a suitable snail intermediate host within a few hours after hatching or it dies. After transforming into a sporocyst stage in the headfoot of the snail (Fig. 10–6), it produces a second generation of migratory sporocysts, which move to the digestive gland or gonads where they produce either additional generations of sporocysts or the cercarial generation. The cercariae leave the sporocyst in which they have developed via a birth pore and pass through the tissues of the snail to the exterior. This passage is facilitated by secretions from a pair of **escape glands** located in the cephalic region of the cercaria (Fig. 10–7a).

Actively swimming cercariae possess distinctive forked tails and move in a figure-eight pattern characteristic of schistosomes. They may swim upward to the surface of the water and then sink slowly toward the bottom, or they may adhere to the surface film and come to rest, awaiting contact with their next host. The cercariae are stimulated to attach and penetrate by the secretions of mammalian skin. In fresh water, a mucoid surface coat protects the free-swimming cercariae from the hypo-osmolarity of the environment. Cercariae have five pairs of unicellular penetration glands. Two

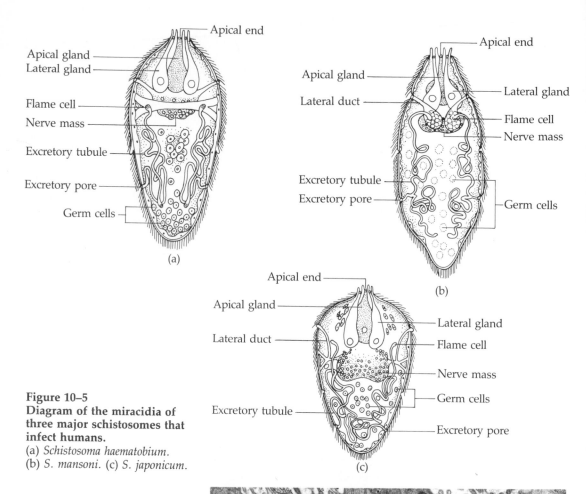

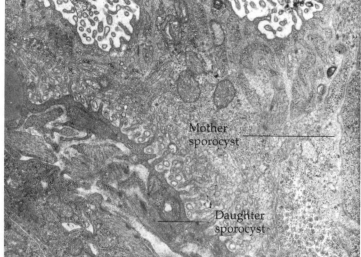

**Figure 10–5**
**Diagram of the miracidia of three major schistosomes that infect humans.**
(a) *Schistosoma haematobium.*
(b) *S. mansoni.* (c) *S. japonicum.*

**Figure 10–6**
**Transmission electron micrograph of the tegument of a mother and daughter sporocyst of *Schistosoma mansoni* with daughter sporocyst developed within.**

**Figure 10–7**
**Cercaria of a schistosome.**
(a) Diagram of entire cercaria.
(b) Diagram of head gland.

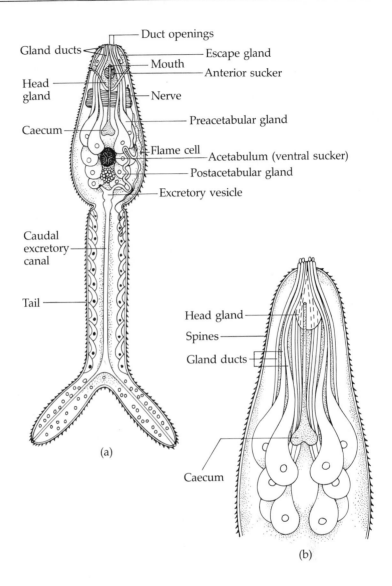

Duct openings
Gland ducts
Escape gland
Mouth
Anterior sucker
Head gland
Nerve
Caecum
Preacetabular gland
Flame cell
Acetabulum (ventral sucker)
Postacetabular gland
Excretory vesicle
Caudal excretory canal
Tail

(a)

Head gland
Spines
Gland ducts
Caecum

(b)

of these—the **preacetabular glands**—are anterior to the ventral sucker, while the other three pairs—the **postacetabular glands**—lie behind the ventral sucker. Each gland cell has a duct that empties separately at the anterior margin of the oral sucker (Fig. 10–7b).

The cercaria adheres its body to the skin of the definitive host using both its muscular suckers and the mucoid secretions of the postacetabular glands. Secretions from the preacetabular glands are more highly enzymatic, facilitating lysis of host skin during the penetration process.

Once the cercaria enters the skin, it burrows to the peripheral capillary bed or enters the lymphatic system; in either case, the worm reaches the right side of the heart and then enters the lungs. During the penetration process, three significant morphological changes occur in the cercaria: the tail is lost, the surface coat is lost, and the contents of the penetration glands are spent. Following these changes, the transformed cercaria is called a **schistosomule.**

Schistosomules appear in pulmonary capillaries by the third day post-penetration. On day 4, these juveniles begin feeding on host erythrocytes, initiating a period of rapid growth and development. The period spent in the host's lungs varies even within the same schistosome species. After a week to 10 days, the schistosomules move through the pulmonary vein to the right side of the heart and then into the systemic circulation. Approximately 3 weeks post-penetration, the worms reach the hepatic portal veins, where they reach sexual maturity and mate after 40 days. Worm pairs then migrate against the portal flow to venules at the definitive sites. The sex of the worms is genetically determined at the time of fertilization.

## Variations

While the morphology and life cycles of the three major schistosomes are basically similar, certain clinical differences exist, which aid in diagnosis.

*Schistosoma haematobium* (Fig. 10–8a).  Except in India and Portugal where intermediate hosts for *S. haematobium* belong to the snail genera *Ferrissia* and *Planorbarius*, respectively, in all major endemic areas—from north to south Africa (particularly the Nile valley), central and west Africa, and a number of countries in the Middle East—several species of the snail genus *Bulinus* serve as intermediate hosts. The male worm may attain a length of 15 mm, while females may reach 20 mm. There are 4 or 5 testes in the male; in the female, the single ovary is situated at about the midpoint of the body. The tegument of the male has many knoblike tubercles on the dorsal surface, while the tegument of the female is smooth. In both sexes, the caeca reunite posteriorly at about two-thirds of the body length.

Females deposit about 30 eggs daily, each egg measuring 112–170 mm long by 40–70 mm wide. The *S. haematobium* egg is readily identifiable by its small, distinct terminal

**Figure 10–8**
**Diagrams of the adults of three major schistosomes that infect humans.**
In each pair, male is on left, female on right. (a) *Schistosoma haematobium*. (b) *S. mansoni*. (c) *S. japonicum*.

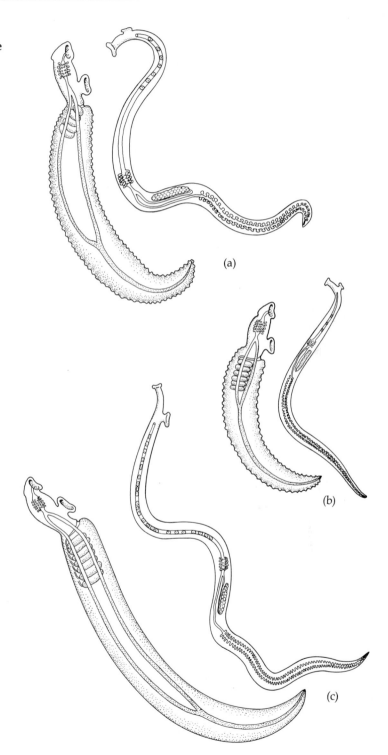

spine (Fig. 8–15). Intramolluscan development requires approximately 4 to 6 weeks after penetration by the miracidium. The prepatent period for *S. haematobium* in the human host is 10 to 12 weeks.

*Schistosoma mansoni* (Fig. 10–8b). This species occurs widely throughout Africa and South America, especially in Brazil, Venezuela, Surinam, and Guyana, and in several Caribbean islands, including Puerto Rico, the Dominican Republic, St. Lucia, Martinique, and Guadeloupe. Introduction into the Western Hemisphere may have occurred during the time of the African slave trade when a number of susceptible snail hosts was introduced, possibly in casks of drinking water brought with the infected slaves.

The male worm measures up to 10 mm in length; the female up to 14 mm. As in *S. haematobium*, the tegument of the male has tubercles on the dorsal surface, while that of the female is smooth. The male has 6 to 9 testes, while in the female a single ovary is situated in the anterior half of the body. Female worms deposit 190 to 300 eggs daily, each measuring 114–175 μm long by 45–68 μm wide. The egg bears a prominent, lateral spine (Fig. 8–15). Many species of the genus *Biomphalaria* are suitable snail hosts. Intramolluscan development requires 3 to 4 weeks, and the prepatent period in humans is 7 to 8 weeks.

*Schistosoma japonicum* (Fig. 10–8c). This schistosome occurs in the Far Eastern countries of China, Japan, and Philippines, Taiwan, and Indonesia. The snail hosts belong to the genus *Oncomelania*. Adult worms are the largest schistosomes infecting humans, with males attaining a length of 20 mm and females 26 mm. The tegumental surface of both sexes is smooth. The male has 7 testes, while the female has a single ovary lying in the posterior half of the body. The relatively long uterus may contain as many as 300 eggs at any given time. The female is a prodigious egg-producer, capable of depositing 3500 eggs per day, and, unlike those of *S. haematobium* and *S. mansoni*, the eggs are deposited in clusters, rather than singly. The eggs of *S. japonicum* are the smallest of the three species, measuring 70–100 μm long by 50–65 μm wide, and may bear a minute, lateral spine (Fig. 8–15). Intramolluscan development requires 4 to 9 weeks, while the prepatent period in the human is 5 to 6 weeks.

# SYMPTOMATOLOGY AND DIAGNOSIS

The first symptom is a localized dermatitis, often observed following cercarial penetration of the skin. It is characterized by itching and local edema, which usually disappear after 4 days. Following skin penetration, the symptoms of human schistosomiasis appear in three phases. The first is the migration phase, characterized by toxic reactions and pulmonary congestion accompanied by fever. This phase may last 4 to 10 weeks, during which the worms migrate from the lungs to the liver where they reach sexual maturity and mate. Mated pairs of *S. mansoni* and *S. japonicum* then move via the hepatic portal system back into the mesenteric veins. The second phase is considerably longer, lasting 2 months to several years. Characteristic symptoms, such as bloody stools (schistosomiasis mansoni and japonica) and hematuria (schistosomiasis haematobium), are caused by the passage of eggs through the intestinal and urinary bladder walls. Pathological alteration of these organs accompanies these incursions. The last phase, the most serious, is characterized by severe intestinal, renal, and hepatic pathology, caused primarily by the reaction of the host to the schistosome eggs.

Hepatosplenomegaly (enlargement of the liver and spleen) is a common symptom of advanced schistosomiasis. Eggs trapped in the walls of the intestine and urinary bladder as well as in ectopic regions, notably the liver and spleen, elicit inflammatory reactions resulting from leucocytic and fibroblastic infiltration and producing cirrhosis, anemia, etc. Eventually, a **granuloma** (pseudotubercle) forms around each egg or cluster of eggs (Fig. 10–4). Small abcesses, accompanied by occlusion of small blood vessels, lead to necrosis and ulceration.

In endemic areas, where reinfection is common, repeated penetration of the intestinal and urinary bladder walls by migrating eggs results in extensive scar tissue formation, which impedes the normal functioning of these organs. For instance, *S. haematobium* infections alter absorptive properties of the urinary bladder wall, predisposing it to malignancy. As a result, in Egypt, for example, *S. haematobium* infection is commonly associated with bladder cancer among male agricultural workers. Because formation of scar tissue also blocks the migration of the eggs through these infected organs, more eggs are swept back to other sites, producing organ enlargement, i.e., hepatosplenomegaly.

The surest means of diagnosis is finding and identifying characteristic eggs in excreta or in tissue biopsies—particularly rectal biopsies. In chronic cases in which very few, if any, eggs are passed, biopsies can be used advantageously, but these are expensive and require the services of trained specialists. Current research efforts are directed toward the development of inexpensive, reliable diagnostic procedures adaptable to primitive conditions. Currently, the most promising utilize immunodiagnostic techniques; however, positive results from these tests should be confirmed by identification of eggs, since false positives sometimes result from concomitant infections with other parasites or exposure to various animal schistosome cercariae. The latter sometimes produces a severe dermatitis reaction called **swimmer's itch** (see pp. 208–10).

## TREATMENT

Treatment varies according to species. No reliable prophylactic regimen is presently available other than the observance of proper sanitation procedures, avoidance of cercariae-infested waters, and prevention of water contamination by human excreta. Any of four chemotherapeutic agents is recommended for treatment of *S. haematobium* infections: metrifonate, niridazole, praziquantel, or antimony sodium dimercaptosuccinate. Unfortunately, all have potentially toxic side effects, although metrifonate and praziquantel are the least toxic. The most effective drug against *S. mansoni* is oxamniquine. The drugs recommended for *S. haematobium* infections can also be used to treat *S. mansoni* infections; however, they are more toxic than oxamniquine. *S. japonicum* infection is the most difficult form of human schistosomiasis to manage chemotherapeutically. Praziquantel is the only effective drug against this parasite and has been approved by the U.S. Food and Drug Administration for human use against schistosomiasis. The biochemical mechanism by which praziquantel is effective is not clear; however, vacuolization of the adult worm's tegument and rapid paralytic contractions of its musculature result from exposure to the drug.

According to the World Health Organization, the key to future schistosomiasis control lies in a four-pronged attack: population-based chemotherapy, with repeated drug administration to infected individuals; use of molluscicides; introduction of biological controls, such as carnivorous snails and fish; and education of the population. Evidence has surfaced, not only of differences in the susceptibility of the parasites to drugs, but of the development of drug resistance as well. Therefore, research efforts to improve existing drugs and to synthesize new, more effective ones must continue, at least until a vaccine becomes available.

## IMMUNITY

Immunity to human schistosomiasis is not totally understood. It is known that animals experimentally infected with schistosomes that normally infect humans develop immunity and that infected humans develop at least partial immunity. The life span of adult schistosomes in the human host can be longer than 30 years. As pointed out earlier, during much of this time the worms are prolific egg producers, and this ability—augmented by their longevity—elicits a wide range of immune responses, both humoral and cell-mediated. Actually, such responses can be correlated with several parasitic stages in the human host. The first, or skin penetration, stage is characterized by a response to the penetrating cercaria's glycocalyx and penetration gland secretions, both released into the host's tissues. The second, or early development, stage produces two responses. One is caused by the tegumental changes of the migrating schistosomule; the other is a response to immunogens released from either migrating or trapped eggs. The immunogens are macromolecules that diffuse through micropores in the eggshell. Some of these macromolecules facilitate migration of eggs through the tissues. They also elicit a granulomatous response to eggs trapped in the tissues, causing pronounced pathological changes. The third, or adult worm, stage is a response to immunogens released from the adult worm's intestine, tegument, and excretory system.

The question may well be asked, "If worms produce immunogens to which the host responds, how do the worms evade this response?" While a complete answer to this question is not yet available, several factors are known. Perhaps the most remarkable of these is the ability of the adult worm to acquire protective host antigens on its surface. The antigens afford protection by disguising the worm's surface so that it escapes detection by the host immune mediators. Antigen acquisition apparently begins during the early schistosomule stage. Logically, therefore, the target for an effective vaccine must be the larval stage before such acquisition has occurred.

## OTHER SCHISTOSOMES

In this age, new discoveries of metazoan parasites pathogenic to humans occur only rarely. There were, for many years, pockets of what were thought to be *S. japonicum* infections in southeast Asia, especially in parts of Laos and Cambodia. However, American involvement in southeast Asia during the Vietnam War prompted a reevaluation of the causative organism for schistosomiasis in that region; as a result, that parasite is now considered to be a separate species, *Schistosoma mekongi*. While it closely resembles *S. japonicum* in pathology and morphology, there are differences. For instance, the molluscan intermediate host is *Tricula aperta*, its eggs are smaller, and the prepatent period is a week longer than for *S. japonicum*.

Another schistosome species, *Schistosoma intercalatum*, is known to cause human schistosomiasis in the Camaroons and Zaire in Africa. In the Camaroons, this parasite utilizes *Bulinus foskalii* as the molluscan intermediate host, while in Zaire, it uses *B. globosus*. Although *S. intercalatum*, normally a parasite of cattle, is generally thought to be more closely related to *S. haematobium* because of the presence of a terminal spine on its eggs, the eggs, like those of *S. mansoni*, are voided in feces rather than in urine. *S. intercalatum* is also less pathogenic to humans than *S. haematobium*.

## SWIMMER'S ITCH

An interesting aspect of schistosome biology concerns cercarial dermatitis, or "swimmer's itch." While the condition is not life-threatening, it can have a negative im-

**Figure 10–9**
**Swimmer's itch.**
Note the localized
inflammatory reaction on the
thigh.

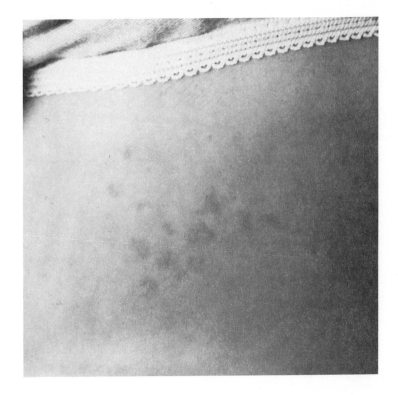

pact on the economy of regions where outbreaks occur, especially those popular with tourists. A number of lake and seashore resorts in Michigan, Minnesota, New Jersey, New England, Wisconsin, and Canada have suffered economic losses when outbreaks have driven vacationers away. The condition is caused when cercariae of blood flukes that normally parasitize aquatic birds and mammals penetrate the human skin, sensitizing the areas of attack and causing pustules and an itchy rash. Since humans are not suitable definitive hosts for these flukes, the cercariae do not normally enter the blood stream and mature. Instead, after penetrating the skin, they are destroyed by the victim's immune responses. Allergenic material released from dead and dying cercariae produces a localized inflammatory reaction (Fig. 10–9). In freshwater lakes of North America, cercariae of the genera *Trichobilharzia*, *Gigantobilharzia*, and *Bilharziella*, which normally infect birds, are the most common dermatitis-producing schistosomes, while the mammal parasite *Heterobilharzia* is prevalent in the Gulf Coast states. One of the most common causative agents of marine swimmer's itch on both the east and west coasts of North America is *Microbilharzia variglandis*, a blood fluke of sea gulls, the cercariae of which develop in the mudflat snail *Ilyanassa obsoleta*. However, the condition is by no means confined to North America; outbreaks have also been reported in Asia, Africa, Europe, and the Middle East.

## SELECTED READINGS

Butterworth, A. E., and Hagan, P. 1987. Immunity in human schistosomiasis. *Parasitology Today* 3, 11–15.

Jordan, P., and Webbe, G. 1982. *Schistosomiasis: Epidemiology, Treatment, and Control*. Wm. Heinemann Medical Books Ltd., London.

Loker, E. S. 1983. A comparative study of the life-histories of mammalian schistosomes. *Parasitology* 87, 343–369.

Stirewalt, M. A. 1974. *Schistosoma mansoni:* Cercaria to schistosomule. *Advances in Parasitology* 12, 115–182.

# PART THREE

# THE CESTOIDEA

# CHAPTER ELEVEN

## GENERAL CHARACTERISTICS OF THE CESTOIDEA

The Cestoidea, or tapeworms, being a class of parasitic flatworms, possess all the characteristics of the phylum Platyhelminthes presented in Chapter 8. The most striking difference between members of this class and the class Trematoda is that tapeworms lack a mouth and a digestive tract. All tapeworms belong to one of two subclasses: the Eucestoda, or true tapeworms (= cestodes), to which those that infect humans belong, and the Cestodaria, a smaller, less well-known group.

The Eucestoda are the most highly specialized flatworm parasites known. Adults of this subclass are endoparasitic in the alimentary tract and associated ducts of various vertebrates, including humans; the larvae, on the other hand, infect both vertebrates and invertebrates. The life cycle requires one or two intermediate hosts, in each of which the tapeworm undergoes a specific phase of its development.

There is much speculation about the origin and phylogeny of tapeworms. One evolutionary scheme proposes that they arose from a stock of aquatic, free-living, bottom-dwelling protomonogeneans that, in turn, evolved from a rhabdocoel-like ancestor similar to the ancestral form suggested for digenetic trematodes. The immediate ancestors of modern tapeworms evolved adhesive organs that enabled them to become attached to, and subsequently ectoparasitic upon, bottom-swelling vertebrates. Some representatives of this population migrated internally to the gut of these vertebrates and became endoparasitic. To survive in that hostile environment, these organisms evolved protective modifications, such as a glycocalyx on the body surface and resistant, quinone-tanned eggshells. Such modifications enabled them to resist the actions of the hosts' digestive enzymes. They also underwent physiological adaptations that allowed them to survive in an environment with reduced oxygen tension. At least one branch of these essentially monozoic animals evolved additional modifications, such as the loss of a gut, development of anterior attachment organs, and duplication of reproductive systems, the last feature leading eventually to segmentation of the body. Later modifications, as the group became increasingly diverse, included adoption of intermediate hosts and the appearance of **apolysis,** the release of gravid (egg-filled) body segments from the chain to the exterior. A cause and effect relationship between the development of apolysis and the loss of capacity to form resistant eggshells by tanning—hence, loss of protection from host digestive enzymes—appears certain, although there is a "chicken or egg" kind of question as to which occurred first.

## MORPHOLOGY

The body of the typical adult eucestode consists of three distinct regions: **scolex, neck,** and **strobila** (Fig. 11–1). The scolex, located at the anterior end, is the attachment portion, the morphology and dimensions of which are key features in identification of these worms. The neck, an unsegmented, poorly differentiated region immediately posterior to the scolex, is generally the narrowest part of the worm. It is from the neck region that new segments, or **proglottids,** differentiate. As new proglottids are formed in the neck region,

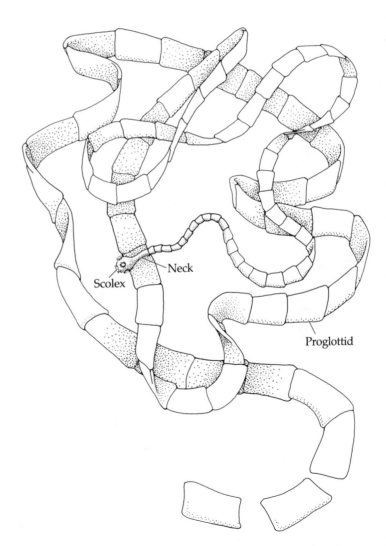

**Figure 11–1**
Diagram showing the three major regions of a generalized eucestode. Note the scolex and neck regions. The remaining region, made up of many proglottids, is the strobila.

they push the older ones progressively posteriad, creating a chain of proglottids, the strobila, that constitutes the third body region. The asexual process of forming segments is termed **strobilation** (Fig. 11–2). As each proglottid is shifted posteriad, its sexual reproductive system matures progressively; hence, the anteriormost proglottids have the least developed reproductive systems, while the more posteriorly the proglottids are located, the greater their level of development. This progressive maturity of the reproductive systems permits a loose subdivision of the strobila into regions of **immature, mature,** and **gravid** proglottids (Fig. 11–2). The reproductive organs in immature proglottids are visible but nonfunctional, while those in mature proglottids are fully functional. At the posterior end of the strobila are the gravid (egg-filled) proglottids. Often, the reproductive organs in gravid proglottids have atrophied. In apolytic species, gravid proglottids detach from the strobila and exit the body of the host with fecal wastes. In **anapolytic** species, eggs are released through a uterine (or genital) pore directly into the host's intestine and, subsequently, also are discharged to the exterior in feces. Most anapolytic tapeworms produce protective, tanned eggshells.

**Figure 11–2**
**Regions along the length of a cestode, *Taenia solium.***
(a) Scolex and neck region.
(b) Immature proglottids.
(c) Mature proglottids.
(d) Gravid proglottid.

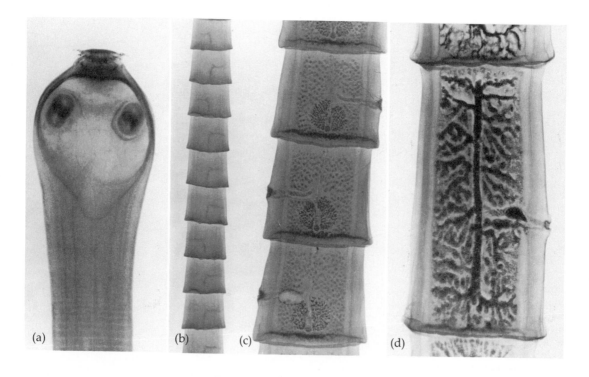

(a)          (b)     (c)                    (d)

# Tegument

### Figure 11–3
**Diagrammatic representation of the tegument of a cestode.** The surface is covered with microthrices, each ending in a thickened, spinelike cap. As is usual, the cell bodies are secretory and produce, among other things, surface coat material.

The tegument of tapeworms (Fig. 11–3) is essentially similar to that of digeneans but with a few notable differences. The surface of the tapeworm tegument bears specialized microvilli, known as **microthrices** (singular, **microthrix**), that project from the outer, limiting membrane of the tegument. The dimensions of these projections vary according to species and location on the strobila. Unlike typical microvilli, each microthrix includes an electron-dense, apical tip separated

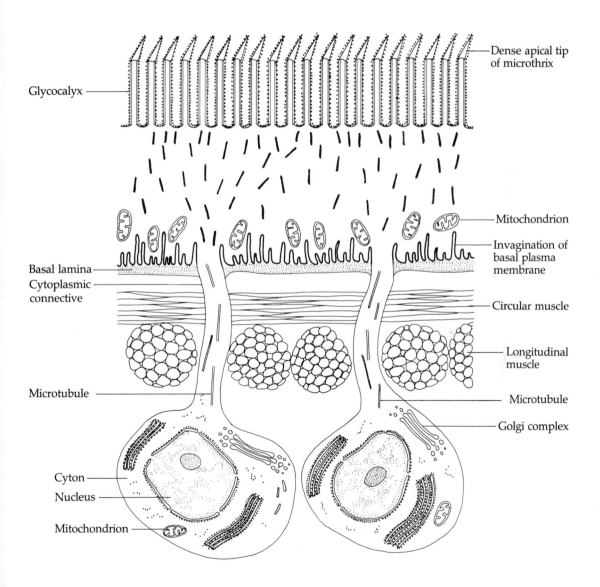

### Figure 11–3
**Diagrammatic representation of the tegument of a cestode.** The surface is covered with microthrices, each ending in a thickened, spinelike cap. As is usual, the cell bodies are secretory and produce, among other things, surface coat material.

Glycocalyx

Dense apical tip of microthrix

Mitochondrion

Invagination of basal plasma membrane

Basal lamina

Cytoplasmic connective

Circular muscle

Longitudinal muscle

Microtubule

Microtubule

Golgi complex

Cyton

Nucleus

Mitochondrion

from the more basal region by a multilaminar plate. These tips, applied to the host's intestinal epithelium, not only provide resistance to the peristaltic movement of the intestine but, with each movement of the worm, agitate intestinal fluids in the immediate microhabitat, thus increasing accessibility of nutrient materials as well as flushing away waste products. Covering the entire surface of the tegument is a layer of carbohydrate-containing macromolecules, the **glycocalyx,** that serves several important purposes, such as protecting the parasite from host digestive enzymes, enhancing nutrient absorption, and maintaining the parasite's surface membrane.

As in digeneans, the tegumental syncytium consists of two cytoplasmic regions, **distal** and **proximal.** The distal cytoplasm is replete with mitochondria, usually aligned in a broad, basal band, as well as several types of vesicles and scattered membranes. Glycogen granules are also present in this region in some species. The vesicles arise in the nucleated, proximal cytoplasm, or **cyton,** sunk deep in the parenchyma. The cyton region contains Golgi complexes, mitochondria, rough endoplasmic reticulum, and other organelles involved in protein synthesis and packaging. The mechanisms involved in protein synthesis and packaging maintain the distal cytoplasmic components; that is, materials so synthesized are translocated, via cytoplasmic connectives abetted by microtubules, to the distal cytoplasm where they maintain the glycocalyx, the membranes, the microthrices, etc.

Underlying the distal cytoplasm are two layers of muscles, collectively known as the **tegumental musculature,** consisting of an outer layer with its contractile fibrils oriented in a circular pattern and an inner layer with contractile fibrils oriented longitudinally.

## Parenchyma

The space enclosed by the tegument—except for the portion occupied by reproductive organs, osmoregulatory structures, muscle fibers, and nervous tissue—is filled with a spongy tissue known as the **parenchyma.** In live tapeworms, fluid fills the spaces between the parenchymal cells. Parenchymal cells are the primary sites for synthesis and storage of glycogen. There is speculation that a single population of cells, the myoblasts, gives rise to both the parenchyma and the musculature of most tapeworms.

# Parenchymal Muscles

**Parenchymal musculature,** as distinguished from tegumental musculature, is unique to eucestodes. Bipolar muscle cells and fibers embedded in the parenchyma form a broad band that encircles each proglottid about midway between the outer surface and the central axis and divides the parenchyma into an outer **cortical** region and an inner **medullary** region. In addition to the dominant, longitudinally aligned, contractile myofibers that help stabilize the strobila against peristalsis in the host intestine, circular myofibers are also present.

# Scolex

To facilitate attachment to the host's intestinal wall, tapeworms utilize several types of structures on their scolices, the most common of which are suckers. Muscles in the scolex make possible the holdfast action of this organ. The musculature of the scolex consists of sets of criss-crossing fibers attached to the inner surfaces of the suckers, enabling them to contract. Scolices of tapeworms that infect humans are categorized as either **acetabulate** or **bothriate,** depending on the type of sucker present (Fig. 11–4). An acetabulate scolex is characterized by the presence of four muscular cups sunk into the equatorial surface of the scolex (Fig. 11–4a). These cups are radially arranged equidistant from each other. While the rim of each cup is usually round, it may be oval or even slitlike in some species, and it may be flush with the surface or project beyond it. Each cup is covered by a thin layer of tegument continual with that covering the entire body of the worm. In addition to the muscular cups, there may be accessory holdfast structures, such as hooks, to help anchor the scolex to the host's intestinal wall—in which case the scolex is called an **armed scolex.** These hooks usually are grouped at the apical end of the scolex on a protrusible **rostellum.** The presence, number, size, and shape of the hooks are of taxonomic importance.

A bothriate scolex is characterized by the presence of two, or rarely four or six, longitudinally arranged, shallow depressions called **bothria** (singular, **bothrium**) (Fig. 11–4b).

Various types of glandular secretions are associated with the scolex of many tapeworms. The function of these secretions has not been established with certainty, although

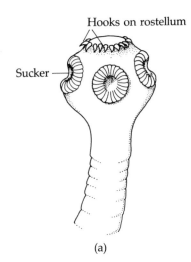

Hooks on rostellum

Sucker

(a)

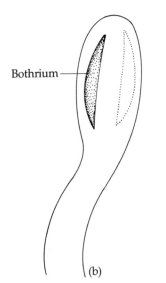

Bothrium

(b)

**Figure 11–4**
**Types of scolices found on tapeworms that infect humans.** (a) Acetabulate, showing three of the four suckers and an armed rostellum. (b) Bothriate, showing one of the two bothridial grooves.

it has been speculated that they are proteolytic, adhesive, and/or stimulatory, depending upon the species.

## Calcareous Corpuscles

Large numbers of concretions, known as **calcareous corpuscles**, occur in the parenchyma of numerous cestode species as well as some trematodes. These spherical bodies, most noticeable in larval forms, consist of organic and inorganic components. The organic portion consists of DNA, RNA, proteins, glycogen, mucopolysaccharides, and alkaline phosphatase; the inorganic portion consists primarily of calcium, magnesium, phosphorus, and traces of metals. While the function(s) of these inclusions remains unclear, it has been suggested that they may act as buffers against anaerobically produced acids, serve as reservoirs for inorganic ions required during development, act as enzyme activators, or be a form of excretory product of metabolism.

## Osmoregulatory System

The cestode osmoregulatory–excretory system is essentially the same as the flame-cell, protonephritic type found in digeneans. In most cases, it serves to maintain within the worm an optimal hydrostatic pressure for extensory movements of the strobila and scolex. Some tapeworms, however, such as *Hymenolepis diminuta*, are known conformers, that is, not being able to regulate osmotic pressure. In these species, the system probably is strictly excretory. The morphology of the system varies somewhat among the different taxa, but sufficient similarity exists to justify the following generalized description.

The osmoregulatory–excretory system consists of two components: the **collecting canals** and the **flame cells.** Four laterally aligned collecting canals—two dorsal and two ventral—extend the entire length of the strobila (Fig. 11–5). All four canals lie just inside the medullary margin of the parenchyma, and a single transverse canal connects the ventral canals at the posterior end of each proglottid. The ventral canals carry fluid away from the scolex, the dorsal canals toward it. In some tapeworms, the four longitudinal canals are linked within the scolex by either a network of canals or a single ring vessel; in others, the dorsal and ventral canals on each side are linked by a simple connection in the region

**Figure 11-5
Morphology of the
osmoregulatory (excretory)
system of cestodes.**
(a) Scolex of *Proteocephalus* sp.
showing single ring type of
connection of the
osmoregulatory canals.
(b) Scolex of *Taenia* sp. showing
network type of
osmoregulatory plexus.
(c) Proglottids showing
longitudinal collecting canals.
Arrows show direction of flow.

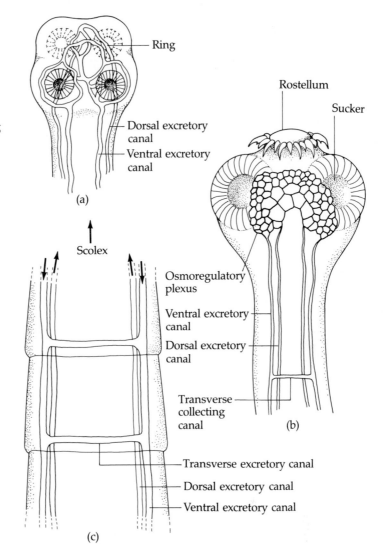

(a)

Ring

Dorsal excretory canal

Ventral excretory canal

Rostellum

Sucker

Scolex

Osmoregulatory plexus

Ventral excretory canal

Dorsal excretory canal

Transverse collecting canal

(b)

Transverse excretory canal

Dorsal excretory canal

Ventral excretory canal

(c)

of the scolex, with no apparent exchange between the two sides.

In the terminal proglottid of young worms, there is an excretory vesicle into which the ventral canals empty. However, in older tapeworms that have sloughed the original posteriormost proglottid, the posterior ends of the ventral canals open independently to the exterior.

Flame cells, usually arranged in groups of four, are associated with the ventral canals. Fluid collected by the flame cells passes through secondary tubules into the main canals. Analysis of fluid within the osmoregulatory system of certain species of tapeworm has revealed that it consists primarily of glucose, soluble proteins, lactic acid, urea, and ammonia. Reabsorption of essential molecules in this system has not been verified.

## Nervous System

The cestode nervous system is relatively complex. The "brain," located in the scolex, is a rectangle or circle of nervous tissue varying in complexity from a simple ganglion to a combination of several ganglia and commissures (Fig. 11–6). It gives rise to short anterior and posterior nerves that richly supply various portions of the scolex with motor fibers and receive sensory fibers from rostellum, suckers, and tegument. Several pairs of longitudinal nerve cords extend posteriorly from this "brain" along the length of the strobila, lateral to the osmoregulatory canals. The cords are connected in each proglottid by cross-connectives, producing a ladderlike appearance. Small motor nerves emanating from the cords and cross-connectives innervate the reproductive organs and musculature, while small sensory nerves supply-

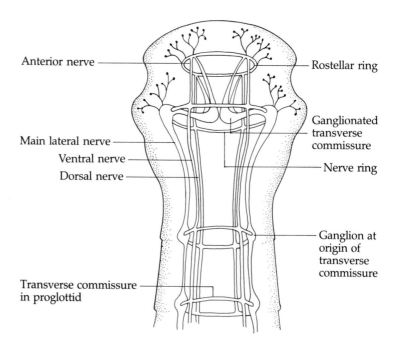

Anterior nerve

Main lateral nerve

Ventral nerve

Dorsal nerve

Rostellar ring

Ganglionated transverse commissure

Nerve ring

Ganglion at origin of transverse commissure

Transverse commissure in proglottid

**Figure 11–6**
**Cestode brain.**

ing the tegument merge with the cords and connectives. Certain organs of both the scolex and the proglottids, such as parts of the reproductive system and suckers, are more extensively innervated than others.

## Reproductive Systems

The general pattern of the reproductive system of cestodes resembles that of digenetic trematodes except for the **cul-de-sac uterus** in some forms (cyclophyllideans), the presence of a separate vaginal canal, and often a laterally situated genital pore. A generalized description of the cestode reproductive system follows, with specific variations noted.

**Male System.**    The male reproductive system consists of one to many testes embedded in the medullary parenchyma of each proglottid (Fig. 11–7). Emanating from each testis is a single vas efferens; in cases of multiple testes, the vasa efferentia unite to form a common vas deferens, which is usually coiled. The distal portion of the vas deferens is modified as a muscular **cirrus**, usually enclosed within a **cirrus sac**. In some species, the cirrus is equipped with spines that hold the organ in place during copulation. The cirrus everts

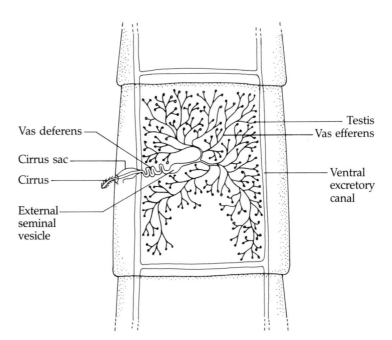

Testis
Vas efferens

Vas deferens

Cirrus sac

Cirrus

Ventral excretory canal

External seminal vesicle

**Figure 11–7**
**Diagrammatic representation of the male reproductive system of a typical eucestode.**

though the male genital pore, which, in turn, opens into the common **genital atrium.**

In most species there is an enlarged area of the vas deferens, the **seminal vesicle**, for storage of sperm. When located within the cirrus sac, it is designated an **internal seminal vesicle**; located outside the sac, it is termed an **external seminal vesicle**. Some species possess both.

**Female System.**   Ova are produced in a single, sometimes bilobed ovary (Fig. 11–8). Following fertilization in the proximal portion of the oviduct, the resulting zygote passes into a region of the oviduct, the **ootype**, equipped with structures involved in eggshell formation similar to those found in digeneans. A **Mehlis' gland** surrounds the ootype and secretes into it material essential to formation of the eggshell; a single, common **vitelline duct** enters the oviduct in the vicinity of the ootype. As in digeneans, the common vitelline duct is formed by the union of many **primary vitelline ducts** arising from vitelline glands, which vary in size and location according to species. Vitelline glands (collectively designated as the **vitellaria**) may form a compact body or consist of numerous follicles scattered throughout the

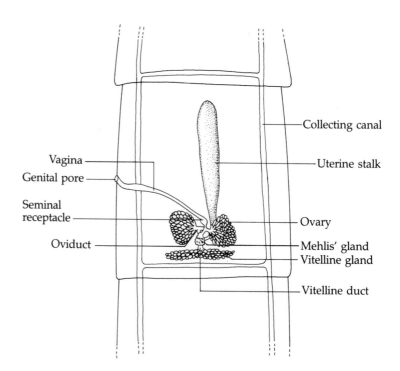

Vagina
Genital pore

Seminal
receptacle

Oviduct

Collecting canal

Uterine stalk

Ovary

Mehlis' gland
Vitelline gland

Vitelline duct

**Figure 11–8**
**Diagrammatic representation of the female reproductive system of a typical eucestode.**

medullary region parenchyma. With few exceptions, secretions of the vitelline glands contain shell precursors as well as provide nourishment for the developing larva. The uterine wall may also contribute materially to extraembryonic membranes and capsules.

The **vagina**, a tubular organ that joins the oviduct at the level of Mehlis' gland, carries sperm from the genital atrium to the oviduct, and fertilization occurs in the region where the vagina and oviduct join. Sperm are stored in an enlargement of the vagina known as the **seminal receptacle**. The oviduct continues as the uterus, which, in some tapeworms—such as the anapolytic members of the order Pseudophyllidea—opens to the outside of the proglottid through a **uterine pore**. Eggs, produced continuously, are expelled through this opening. In other species, including members of the order Cyclophyllidea, the uterus is a blind sac in which developing eggs accumulate. The uterus becomes distended with eggs, filling the medullary region of the proglottid. The gravid proglottid eventually becomes detached from the strobila and is discharged from the host. In some tapeworms (*Dipylidium*, etc.), a modification of uterus–egg interaction occurs in which a much reduced uterus, upon receiving a specific number of eggs, begins pinching off **egg capsules**. The capsules eventually fill the medullary region of the gravid proglottid.

During copulation, the cirrus of one proglottid may be inserted in the vagina of another proglottid of the same worm or another worm. Cross-fertilization between two worms is desirable, at least periodically, to insure vitality and prevent the development of deleterious features due to excessive selfing.

**The Egg.**    The morphology of tapeworm eggs is important for species identification. The following is a brief general description of the basic parts of a typical egg (Fig. 11–9).

The **oncosphere**, containing three pairs of hooks, is encased in an **inner envelope** that, in turn, is surrounded by another membranous structure, the **embryophore**. A cellular zone known as the **outer envelope** lies between the embryophore and the **shell** (or **capsule**), usually the outermost covering of the egg. Tapeworm eggs exhibit certain variations within this basic pattern and are classified into four types: pseudophyllidean, *Dipylidium*, taenioid, and stilesian. Of these, all but the last are represented among tapeworms infecting humans.

**Figure 11–9**
**Diagrammatic representation of the general structure of a cestode egg and oncosphere.**

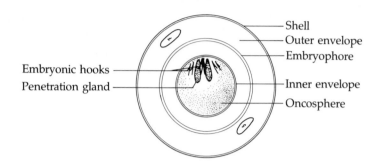

Shell
Outer envelope
Embryophore
Embryonic hooks
Penetration gland
Inner envelope
Oncosphere

The pseudophyllidean egg (Fig. 11–10a), of which the eggs of *Diphyllobothrium latum* are representative, is most similar morphologically and developmentally to those of digenetic trematodes. The fully developed egg has a thick, quinone-tanned shell, usually with a lidlike operculum at one end. Numerous vitelline cells are associated with the zygote, providing stored food for subsequent development. The zygote develops into an oncosphere, which is covered by a ciliated embryophore that enables it to swim upon hatching. This form of the organism is called a **coracidium** (plural, **coracidia**).

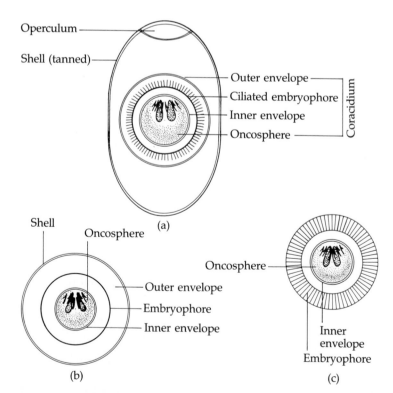

Operculum
Shell (tanned)
Outer envelope
Ciliated embryophore
Inner envelope
Oncosphere
Coracidium
(a)

Shell
Oncosphere
Outer envelope
Embryophore
Inner envelope
(b)

Oncosphere
Inner envelope
Embryophore
(c)

**Figure 11–10**
**Variations in cestode egg structure.**
(a) Pseudophyllidean.
(b) Dipylidean. (c) Taenioid.

**Figure 11–11**
**The three types of egg-forming systems among tapeworms that infect humans.**
(a) Pseudophyllidean, e.g., *Diphyllobothrium latum*. (b) Dipylidean, e.g., *Hymenolepis nana*. (c) Taenioid, e.g., *Taenia solium*.

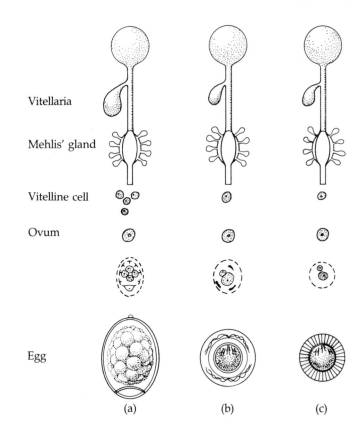

Vitellaria

Mehlis' gland

Vitelline cell

Ovum

Egg

(a)          (b)          (c)

The dipylidean egg, seen in the genera *Dipylidium* and *Hymenolepis*, possesses a thin shell, a thin, nonciliated embryophore, and a relatively thick outer envelope (Fig. 11–10b). In the taenioid egg, characteristic of members of the genera *Taenia* and *Echinococcus*, the shell and outer envelope are lacking, and the thick, nonciliated embryophore constitutes the outermost covering (Fig. 11–10c). In *Dipylidium* and taenioid eggs, in contrast to pseudophyllidean eggs, only one or very few vitelline cells are associated with the zygote (Fig. 11–11).

## LIFE CYCLE PATTERNS

Tapeworms that infect humans display two basic life cycle patterns, one typical of members of the order Pseudophyllidea, the other of members of the order Cyclophyllidea (Fig. 11–12).

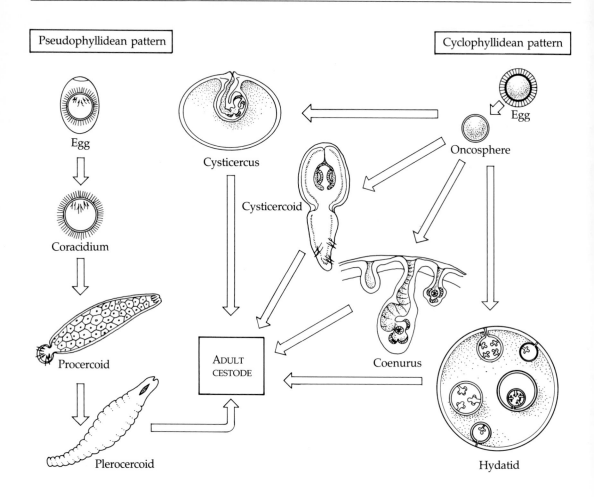

**Figure 11–12**
**Life cycle patterns of**
**tapeworms that infect humans.**

## Pseudophyllidean Pattern

In the order Pseudophyllidea, eggs, containing coracidia, leave the host with feces to water. The coracidium escapes from the eggshell through the operculum and swims for a brief time by means of its ciliated embryophore. Survival of the organism depends upon the coracidium being ingested by the first intermediate host, an aquatic arthropod, within which the embryo sheds its ciliated embryophore and metamorphoses into a globular **procercoid** in the hemocoel. During this development, the oncosphere hooks are retained, albeit nonfunctionally, in a tail-like structure called the **cercomer**. When the first intermediate host is ingested by a second intermediate host, usually a fish, the procercoid migrates via the peritoneal cavity to various parts of the body, principally the musculature, where it grows and develops into a solid, vermiform **plerocercoid** that shows the beginning of strobilation and a self-formed adult scolex. The plerocercoid is infective to humans; when ingested, it attaches to the wall of the small intestine, where strobilation occurs. All the aforementioned stages possess penetration glands that secrete lytic enzymes to aid in penetration of and migration among the various host tissues and organs.

## Cyclophyllidean Pattern

Adapted as it is to terrestrial hosts, the cyclophyllidean hexacanth embryo, or oncosphere, lacks a ciliated embryophore and must remain passive until the egg is ingested by a vertebrate or invertebrate intermediate host. In species that normally utilize an invertebrate intermediate host, usually an arthropod, the oncosphere, upon hatching in the digestive tract, employs its six hooks and its penetration glands to enter the hemocoel, where it metamorphoses into a **cysticercoid**. This form is solid-bodied and possesses a fully developed acetabulate scolex. It is surrounded by several layers of cystic tissue and has a prominent cercomer containing hooks. The cystic layers and the cercomer are digested away in the digestive tract of a definitive host, freeing the scolex and neck to begin strobilation.

In species that utilize a vertebrate intermediate host, the oncosphere, after ingestion, penetrates the intestinal lining and enters a venule. It is carried by the circulating blood to any of several areas of the body, where it develops into a **cysticercus** with an acetabulate scolex invaginated into a fluid-filled vesicle or bladder; hence the common name **bladderworm**. Two other forms that follow this developmental pattern are the **coenurus** and the **hydatid** cysts. In the former, the wall of the bladder develops several invaginated scolices; in the latter, secondary cysts are formed as invaginations on the walls. These second-generation cysts are called **brood capsules** since they, in turn, give rise to scolices, each of which, when ingested by a suitable definitive host, can develop into an adult worm.

In some tapeworms, certain immature stages—including the cysticercus, coenurus, and hydatid cyst of some cyclophyllideans and the plerocercoid of several pseudophyllidean tapeworms—are capable of developing in extraintestinal tissues of humans (see Chapter 13).

# PHYSIOLOGY

The adaptive morphology of adult tapeworms and the environment in which they occur are probably the most significant factors influencing their physiology. Lacking a digestive tract, these worms must derive all nutrient molecules from the host or its microhabitat, and such molecules must cross the tegument. The environment in which tapeworms reside, the small intestine, is one of very low oxygen tension, necessitating anaerobic metabolism. The methods by which nutrients cross the tegument include active transport, facilitated diffusion, and simple diffusion. The most important nutrient molecule is glucose, which, after polymerization within the parasite, is stored as glycogen usually in the parenchyma and interstitial fluid. The only other major, transported carbohydrate is galactose. Considering the intestinal environment, it is not surprising that most energy is derived by substrate phosphorylation via glycolysis. Some tapeworms possess a mammalian-type electron transport system, but its role in energy production is minor. The sites on the tegument over which various molecules are transported vary according to which of the three major types of molecules is being transported. For instance, sites, or loci, differ for the transport of carbohydrates, amino acids, and purines and pyrimidines, the last two molecules being required for synthesis of nucleic acids. Most adult tapeworms also absorb lipids, probably by simple diffusion.

Metabolic rates differ in different parts of the strobila. The neck and immature proglottids have a much higher rate of metabolism than the mature and gravid proglottids, reflecting the high energy requirements for new proglottid formation and organ development. Most of the energy requirement in mature proglottids is for egg production.

# TREATMENT

In most instances, adult tapeworms have little visible effect upon their hosts except in heavy infections, which may result in anemia, weight loss, and various secondary manifestations. The treatment of choice for all tapeworms infecting the small intestine of humans is essentially the same and consists of oral administration of the drug niclosamide, which disrupts proglottids and interferes with the worm's substrate phosphorylation processes, depriving it of required ATP. Two other drugs, quinacrine hydrochloride and aminocrine, have also proven effective in treating tapeworm infections. Praziquantel is an excellent broad-spectrum anthelmintic and, like niclosamide, causes disruption of proglottids. As in the case of schistosomes, additional effects of praziquantel are vacuolization of the tegument and rapid paralysis of the worm's musculature. These drugs should be used cautiously in the treatment of *Taenia solium* infections, since cysticercosis can result from autoinfection by eggs released from disrupted proglottids (see Chapter 13). Five to six weeks after treatment, the patient's feces should be reexamined for the reappearance of eggs—in case the scolex was retained and developed into a "new" worm (Fig. 11–13).

**Figure 11–13**
**Cestode eggs.**
(a) *Hymenolepis nana:* the dwarf tapeworm of humans, rats, and mice. (b) *Hymenolepis diminuta:* the rat tapeworm. (c) *Taenia* sp. (d) *Taenia pisiformis:* the dog tapeworm. (e) *Diphyllobothrium latum.*

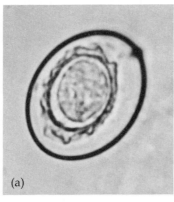
(a)

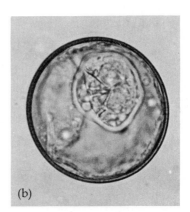
(b)

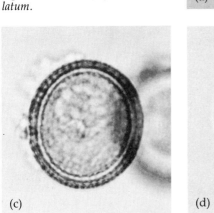
(c)

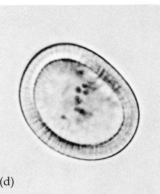
(d)

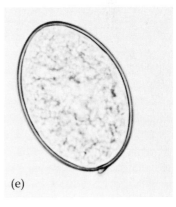
(e)

## SELECTED READINGS

Arai, H. P. (ed.) 1980. *Biology of the Rat Tapeworm, Hymenolepis diminuta*. Academic Press, New York.

Arme, C., and Pappas, P. W. (eds.) 1983. *The Biology of the Eucestoda*. Academic Press, New York.

Kuperman, B. I., and Davydov, V. G. 1982. The fine structure of glands in oncospheres, procercoids and plerocercoids of Pseudophyllidea (Cestoda). *International Journal of Parasitology* 12, 135–144.

Lumsden, R. D. 1975. Surface ultrastructure and cytochemistry of parasitic helminths. *Experimental Parasitology* 37, 267–339.

Pappas, P. W., and Read, C. P. 1975. Membrane transport in helminth parasites: A review. *Experimental Parasitology* 37, 469–530.

Schmidt, G. D. 1985. *Handbook of Tapeworm Identification*. CRC Press, Boca Raton, FL.

Smyth, J. D. 1969. *The Physiology of Cestodes*. W. H. Freeman, San Francisco.

# CLASSIFICATION OF THE CESTOIDEA*

## CLASS CESTOIDEA

All parasites, being common in all classes of vertebrates except Cyclostomata; an intermediate host is required for almost all species.

### Subclass Eucestoda

Polyzoic flatworms (except orders Caryophyllidea and Spathebothriidea); with one or more sets of reproductive organs per proglottid; scolex usually present; shelled embryo with six hooks; parasites of fish, amphibians, reptiles, birds, and mammals.

#### ORDER CYCLOPHYLLIDEA

Scolex usually with four suckers; rostellum present or absent, armed or not; neck present or absent; strobila usually with distinct segmentation; monoecious (or rarely dioecious); genital pores lateral (ventral in Mesocestoididae); vitelline gland compact, single (double in Mesocestoididae), posterior to ovary (anterior or beneath ovary in Tetrabothriidae); uterine pore absent; parasites of amphibians, reptiles, birds, and mammals. (Genera mentioned in text: Family Hymenolepidae*—*Hymenolepis*, Family Taeniidae—*Echinococcus, Taenia*. Family Dilepididae—*Dipylidium*.)

#### ORDER PSEUDOPHYLLIDEA

Scolex with two bothria, with or without hooks; neck present or absent; strobila variable; proglottids anapolytic (senile proglottid detached after it has shed enclosed eggs); genital pores lateral, dorsal, or ventral; testes numerous; ovary posterior; vitellaria follicular as in Trypanorhyncha, occasionally in lateral fields but not interrupted by interproglottidal boundaries; uterine pore present, dorsal or ventral; egg usually operculate, containing coracidium; parasites of fish, amphibians, reptiles, birds, and mammals. (Genus mentioned in text: Family Diphyllobothriidae*—*Diphyllobothrium*.)

#### ORDER PROTEOCEPHALATA

Scolex with four suckers, often with prominent apical organ, occasionally with armed rostellum; neck usually present; genital pores lateral; testes numerous; ovary posterior; vitelline glands follicular, usually lateral, either cortical or medullary; uterine pore present or absent; parasites of fish, amphibians, and reptiles.

#### ORDER TETRAPHYLLIDEA

Scolex with highly variable bothridia, sometimes also with hooks, spines, or sucker; myzorhynchus present or absent; proglottids commonly hyperapolytic (immature proglottid detached before eggs are formed); hermaphroditic, rarely dioe-

*Only those taxa that include parasitic species are defined.

cious; genital pores lateral, rarely posterior; testes numerous; ovary posterior, vitellaria follicular (condensed in *Dioecotaenia* sp.), usually medullary in lateral fields; uterine pore present or not; vagina crosses vas deferens; parasites of elasmobranchs.

## ORDER TRYPANORHYNCHA
Scolex elongate, with two or four bothridia and four eversible (rarely atrophied) tentacles armed with hooks; each tentacle invaginates into internal sheath provided with muscular bulb; neck present or absent; strobila apolytic (gravid proglottids disintegrate or become detached), anapolytic, or hyperapolytic; genital pores lateral, rarely ventral; testes numerous; ovary posterior; vitellaria follicular, cortical, and encircling other reproductive organs; uterine pore present or absent; parasites of elasmobranchs.

## ORDER LECANICEPHALIDEA
Scolex divided into anterior and posterior regions by horizontal groove; anterior portion of scolex cushionlike or with unarmed tentacles, capable of being withdrawn into posterior portion, forming a large suckerlike organ; posterior of scolex usually with four suckers; neck present or absent; testes numerous; ovary posterior; vitellaria follicular, lateral or encircling proglottid; uterine pore usually present; parasites of elasmobranchs.

## ORDER CARYOPHYLLIDEA
Scolex unspecialized or with shallow grooves or loculi or shallow bothria, monozoic; genital pores midventral; testes numerous; ovary posterior; vitellaria follicular, scattered or lateral; uterus as a coiled median tube, opening, often together with vagina, near male pore; parasites of teleost fish and aquatic annelids.

## ORDER APORIDEA
Scolex with simple suckers or grooves and armed rostellum; proglottids distinguished internally or separate proglottids not evident; genital ducts and pores, cirrus, ootype, and Mehlis' gland absent; hermaphroditic, rarely dioecious; vitelline cells mixed with ovarian cells; parasites of anseriform birds.

## ORDER SPATHEBOTHRIIDEA
Scolex feebly developed, undifferentiated or with funnel-shaped apical organ or one or two hollow, cuplike organs; genital pores and uterine pore ventral or alternating dorsal and ventral; testes in two lateral bands; ovary dendritic; vitellaria follicular, lateral or scattered; uterus coiled; parasites of teleost fish.

## ORDER DIPHYLLIDEA
Scolex with armed or unarmed peduncle; two spoon-shaped bothridia present, lined with minute spines, sometimes divided by median, longitudinal ridge; apex of scolex with insignificant apical organ or with large rostellum bearing dorsal and ventral groups of T-shaped hooks; genital pores posterior, midventral; testes numerous, anterior; ovary posterior; vitel-

laria follicular, lateral, or surrounding segment; uterine pore absent; uterus tubular or saccular; parasites of elasmobranchs.

## ORDER NIPPOTAENIIDEA

Strobila small; scolex with single sucker at apex, otherwise simple; neck short or absent; proglottids each with single set of reproductive organs; genital pores lateral; testes anterior; ovary posterior; vitelline gland compact, single, between testes and ovary; osmoregulatory canals reticular; parasites of teleost fish.

## ORDER LITOBOTHRIDEA

Strobila dorsoventrally flattened, with numerous proglottids; scolex a single, well-developed apical sucker; anterior proglottids modified, cruciform in cross section; neck absent; each proglottid with single set of medullary reproductive organs; apolytic or anapolytic; testes numerous, preovarial; genital pores lateral; ovary two or four lobed, posterior; vitellaria follicular, encircling medullary parenchyma; parasites of elasmobranchs.

# CHAPTER TWELVE

# INTESTINAL TAPEWORMS

Adult tapeworms of six genera, representing two orders, infect the human intestinal tract. A single representative of the order Pseudophyllidea, *Diphyllobothrium latum*, is included in this group, while the remaining genera, representing three families, belong to the order Cyclophyllidea. The family Taeniidae is represented by *Taenia solium* and *T. saginata*, Hymenolepididae by *Hymenolepis nana* and *H. diminuta*, and Dilepididae by *Dipylidium caninum*. At least two other members of the family Taeniidae, *Echinococcus granulosus* and *E. multilocularis*, are of medical importance to humans; however, since only the larvae infect humans, they are discussed in Chapter 13.

## *Diphyllobothrium latum*

*Diphyllobothrium latum*, the broadfish tapeworm, parasitizes several larger mammals, including humans, throughout the world. It is most common in Scandinavia, the USSR, and parts of temperate South America.

The adult *D. latum* reproductive system possesses a common genital atrium into which male and female genital pores open on the midventral surface of each proglottid (Fig. 12–1). Sperm enter the female pore and pass down the va-

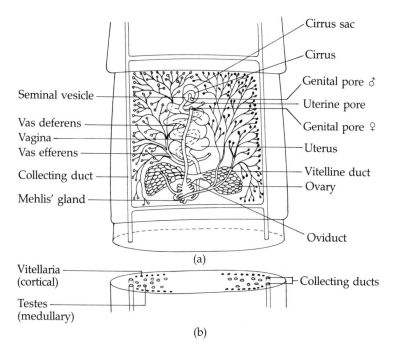

Seminal vesicle

Vas deferens
Vagina
Vas efferens

Collecting duct

Mehlis' gland

Cirrus sac

Cirrus

Genital pore ♂
Uterine pore
Genital pore ♀

Uterus

Vitelline duct
Ovary

Oviduct

(a)

Vitellaria (cortical)

Testes (medullary)

Collecting ducts

(b)

**Figure 12–1**
**Mature proglottid of**
***Diphyllobothrium latum.***
(a) Ventral view. (b) Cross-section.

gina to the oviduct, where fertilization occurs. The bilobed ovary lies in the posterior portion of the proglottid. The oviduct, arising from the ovary, continues anteriad as a coiled uterus, opening to the exterior through the midventral **uterine pore.** Eggs enclosed in tanned eggshells are expelled via the uterine pore. The follicular cells constituting the vitellaria are scattered throughout the cortical fields of the proglottid, and numerous testes are medullary in their distribution except for an area along the midline of each proglottid.

Adult worms may attain a length of 10 meters, may be 10–20 mm wide, and may consist of more than 3,000 proglottids, making *D. latum* the largest tapeworm found in humans. The extraordinary size in this tapeworm is partially due to anapolysis, the retention of terminal proglottids. Approximately 80% of the proglottids are either mature or nearly so. The size of the vertebrate host may also influence the size of the parasite. For example, one of the largest recorded *D. latum,* 12 meters long, was recovered at autopsy from a bear from Yellowstone National Park.

**Life Cycle (Fig. 12–2).**    The adult worm is attached to the mucosal lining of the ileum, and sometimes the jejunum, by both bothria. Ovoid, operculated eggs are released from the uterine pore on the ventral surface of the proglottid. At the time of oviposition, the hexacanth embryo is undeveloped; the eggs must, therefore, lie dormant in the water for approximately 8 to 12 days or longer to complete embryonic development. Typical of the Pseudophyllidea, the hexacanth embryo is covered by a ciliated embryophore and is called a **coracidium**.

Within 24 hours after hatching, the motile coracidium must be ingested by a freshwater copepod belonging to the genera *Diaptomus, Cyclops,* etc., or it will perish. In the digestive tract of the copepod, the ciliated embryophore is shed and the naked hexacanth larva, by means of its hooks and secretions, bores through the intestinal wall into the hemocoel. In 14 to 18 days, the hexacanth embryo, usually one or two per infected copepod, metamorphoses into an elongated, globular **procercoid** larva measuring about 500 μm in length. The prominent cercomer, containing the six larval hooks, projects posteriorly.

When the infected copepod is ingested by a suitable plankton-feeding, freshwater fish, the procercoid penetrates the intestinal wall and migrates to the body muscles. In 7 to

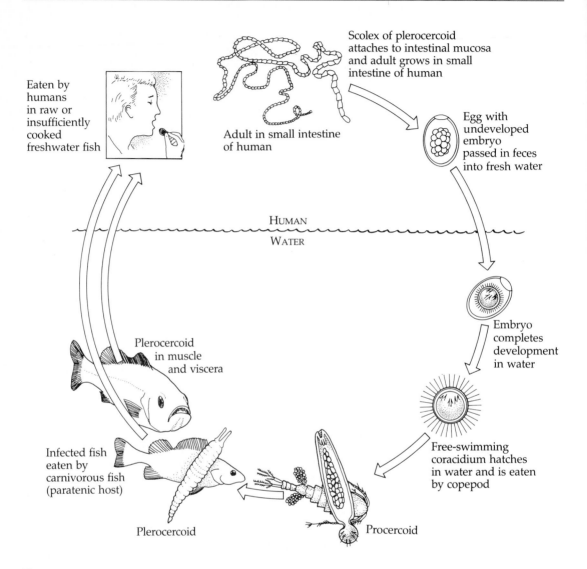

Scolex of plerocercoid attaches to intestinal mucosa and adult grows in small intestine of human

Adult in small intestine of human

Eaten by humans in raw or insufficiently cooked freshwater fish

Egg with undeveloped embryo passed in feces into fresh water

HUMAN

WATER

Embryo completes development in water

Plerocercoid in muscle and viscera

Infected fish eaten by carnivorous fish (paratenic host)

Free-swimming coracidium hatches in water and is eaten by copepod

Plerocercoid

Procercoid

**Figure 12–2**
**Life cycle of *Diphyllobothrium latum*.**

30 days it develops into a long (2 to 4 cm), solid, pseudo-segmented **plerocercoid** larva with an adult scolex at one end. Numerous plerocercoids may be found in a single fish host.

Unlike most pseudophyllidean plerocercoids, the plerocercoid of *D. latum* is coiled and, at times, encapsulated or, more commonly, lying free in muscle tissue. Host reaction, such as encapsulation, depends upon the site the plerocercoid chooses. When the plerocercoid invades the muscles of the body wall, encapsulation rarely occurs; however, when it settles in or on the viscera, encapsulation is common. Infection of the definitive host, including humans, results from ingestion of plerocercoids in poorly cooked, steamed, smoked, pickled, or raw fish. Upon entering the small intestine of the definitive host, the plerocercoid attaches to the mucosa and grows at the rate of about 30 proglottids a day, reaching full maturity in 3 to 5 weeks.

**Epidemiology.**   Human infection with *D. latum* is primarily, although not exclusively, limited to areas where fresh fishes are commonly eaten or where the cleaning and handling of fish is done. A number of coldwater, freshwater fishes—including some of the most prized food fishes, such as pike, salmon, trout, and whitefish—can serve as second intermediate hosts. In addition to being ingested with raw or improperly cooked fish, plerocercoids may be accidentally ingested when they cling to the hands of fish cleaners. In Finland and in some Baltic communities, humans display a relatively high incidence. In North America, 50 to 70% of northern and wall-eyed pike found in some small lakes in the northern United States and Canada harbor plerocercoids of *D. latum*. The parasite is also found in Swiss lakes, the basin of the Danube River, the Middle East, Japan, Chile, Argentina, Peru, and Australia.

Although a number of fish-eating mammals harbor the tapeworm, at worst they are responsible for the spread of the parasite in areas devoid of human inhabitants. Humans, on the other hand, through inadequate sanitation coupled with the presence of suitable intermediate hosts and the practice of eating fish raw or improperly cooked, are responsible for establishing and maintaining its endemicity in the human population. The increased incidence of infected fishes in the United States can be traced directly to the practice of dumping untreated sewage into lakes and streams.

**Symptomatology and Diagnosis.**   Rarely is more than a single worm found in an infected human, and many victims display few, if any, symptoms. Others complain of abdominal pain, weight loss, weakness, and nervous disorders. Many of these vague symptoms are attributable to the patient's reaction to the parasite's metabolic wastes, to degenerating proglottids, or to irritation of the intestinal mucosa, or they are a psychosomatic reaction after the patient learns of the presence of the worm.

Occasionally, the worm is found in the upper portions of the jejunum, in which case it can compete successfully with the host for ingested vitamin $B_{12}$. Since this vitamin is important in the synthesis of hemoglobin, deprivation causes an anemia in the human host similar to pernicious anemia. In endemic areas such as Finland, 5 to 10 of every 10,000 individuals infected with *D. latum* suffer from this type of anemia. If the worm is forced to retreat further down the intestine—by chemotherapy, for instance—the anemia ceases.

Laboratory diagnosis consists of identifying eggs (Fig. 11–15) or the characteristic broad-shaped proglottids from feces or vomitus.

## Taenia solium

This parasite, commonly referred to as the "human pork tapeworm," is common to humans in areas where raw or improperly cooked pork is a regular element of the diet. The adult worm usually measures from 180 to 400 cm (sometimes up to 800 cm) long and comprises 800 to 900 proglottids. The small scolex (Fig. 12–3a), measuring about 1 mm in diameter, is armed with two circles of 22 to 32 rostellar hooks. These hooks are of two sizes—long (180 μm) and short (130 μm)—that alternate in the two circular rows.

The mature proglottid (Fig. 12–4) is squarish in outline, with the common genital pore situated on the lateral edge

**Figure 12–3**
**(a) Armed scolex of** *Taenia solium* **(left) and unarmed scolex of** *T. saginata* **(right). (b) Gravid proglottids of** *Taenia solium* **(left) and** *T. saginata* **(right).**

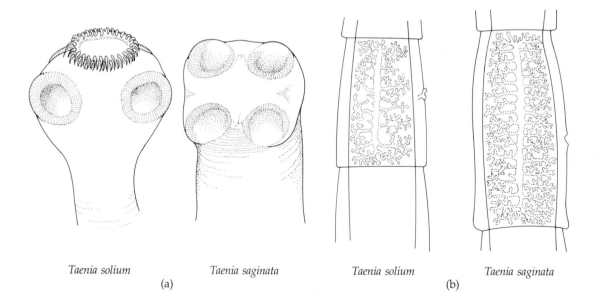

| Taenia solium | Taenia saginata | Taenia solium | Taenia saginata |
| :---: | :---: | :---: | :---: |
| (a) | | (b) | |

**Figure 12–4**
**Diagram of mature proglottid**
**of *Taenia solium*.**

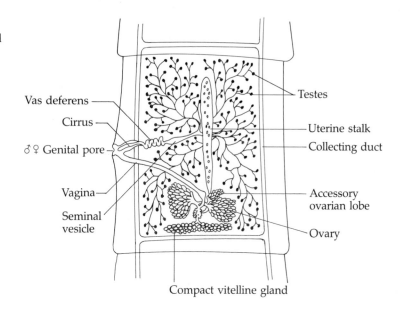

Vas deferens

Cirrus

♂♀ Genital pore

Vagina

Seminal
vesicle

Testes

Uterine stalk

Collecting duct

Accessory
ovarian lobe

Ovary

Compact vitelline gland

about halfway down. The pores on successive proglottids may be on alternate sides or may be positioned unilaterally. The testes are scattered in the medullary region of the proglottid. The ovary consists of two prominent lobes and one small, central lobe. The vitellaria are compact, a feature characteristic of the cyclophyllideans, and are located in the basal part of the proglottid just posterior to the ovary. The oviduct arises at the junction of the three ovarial lobes and continues anteriad as a *cul-de-sac* **uterine stalk**. As eggs are produced, they are "pushed up" into the stalk, which forms lateral branches as the number of eggs increases. The number of lateral branches serves as a tool for distinguishing *T. solium* from *T. saginata; T. solium* has 7 to 12 lateral branches, while *T. saginata* has more than 12 (Fig. 12–3b).

**Life Cycle (Fig. 12–5).**    Groups of 5 or 6 gravid proglottids, each containing thousands of eggs, exit the host daily. Eggs of *T. solium* are indistinguishable from those of *T. saginata.* The outer egg covering is radially striated and covers the oncosphere. The proglottid may rupture either in the host intestine or after it leaves the host. When eggs are ingested by pigs, the liberated oncospheres, using their hooks and penetration glands, penetrate the intestinal wall, gain access to the circulatory system, and are carried by blood or lymph to muscles, viscera, and other organs, where they develop into cysticerci. Each white, ovoid, fluid-filled cysticercus,

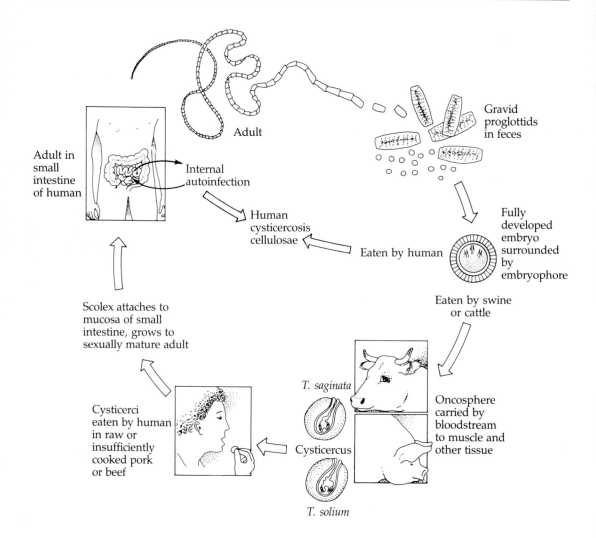

**Figure 12–5**
**Life cycle of *Taenia solium* and *T. saginata*.**

formerly termed *Cysticercus cellulosae*, measures 6–18 mm in length and contains a single, invaginated scolex. When infected, or measly, pork is consumed by a human, the scolex evaginates and attaches to the jejunal wall; there the parasite develops to maturity in 2 to 3 months. Humans are the only known natural, definitive hosts.

**Epidemiology.** The prevalence of pork tapeworm infection in humans varies by region. The very low incidence in the United States can be attributed to the isolation of pigs from human feces. Religious dietary proscriptions forbidding pork consumption by adherents of Islam and Judaism render human infection very rare in Moslem countries and in Israel. It is, however, common in other parts of Africa, India, China, several countries in South and Central America, and Mexico. Conversely, the beef tapeworm is rather rare in Hindu (India) populations, where cows are regarded with reverence and rarely eaten by humans.

**Symptomatology and Diagnosis.** Usually, only a single adult tapeworm infects a human. The armed scolex may cause irritation of the mucosal lining, and there have been cases in which the scolex perforated the intestine, leading to peritonitis. However, the greatest hazard to human health associated with this parasite is infection with the cysticercus, causing the sometimes dangerous disease known as **human cysticercosis** (see Chapter 13).

Identification of proglottids in feces is the most reliable method of diagnosis. Since most taenioid eggs are morphologically indistinguishable (Fig. 11–15), positive diagnosis is established by examination of gravid proglottids to determine the number of main lateral uterine branches (7 to 12 in *T. solium*) (Fig. 12–3b). The morphology of the scolex, particularly the rostellum, is also useful in diagnosis; *T. saginatus* has no rostellum and its scolex bears no hooks, making it easily distinguishable from *T. solium*, which has an armed rostellum.

## *Taenia saginata*

*Taenia saginata* is the most common of the large tapeworms of humans. Morphologically, the adult worm resembles *T. solium*. Usually 35–60 cm long, specimens as long as 225 cm have been reported. The strobila comprises approximately 1000 proglottids. The scolex is unarmed, having neither hooks nor a rostellum (Fig. 12–3a). The morphology of mature proglottids in the two species differs primarily in that *T. saginata* has a bilobed ovary and about twice as many testes as *T. solium* (Table 12–1). As stated above, the gravid uterus of *T. saginata* has in excess of 12 main lateral branches.

**Life Cycle (Fig. 12–5).** The life cycle of *T. saginata* strongly resembles that of *T. solium*. Adults of both species reside in the jejunum of humans, and gravid proglottids detach singly from the strobila and pass to the outside with feces. The eggs of *T. saginata*, indistinguishable from those of *T. solium*, are ingested by a suitable intermediate host, such as cattle or other ungulates. The liberated oncosphere penetrates the intestinal wall and is carried by the lymphatic or blood circulatory system to intramuscular connective tissue, where it develops into a cysticercus known as *Cysticercus bovis*. Humans become infected by ingesting cysticerci in beef, particularly the muscles of the head and heart. Following evagination of the scolex and subsequent attachment to the jejunal wall, the worm develops to maturity in 8 to 10 weeks.

**Epidemiology.**  *Taenia saginata* is distributed throughout the world. Humans acquire infection by eating raw or improperly cooked beef infected with the cysticerci, as in dishes such as steak tartare. Cattle acquire *Cysticercus bovis* by grazing in fields upon which human excrement has been deposited either through fertilization with "night soil" or from poor sanitation. Pastures flooded by rivers and creeks contaminated with human excrement are another source of infection among cattle. Under such conditions, eggs may remain viable for 2 months or longer. Thorough cooking of beef at 57°C until the reddish color disappears or freezing at −10°C for 5 days effectively destroys infective cysticerci.

**Symptomatology  and  Diagnosis.**  Saginatus taeniasis (= taeniosis) in humans is often characterized by such symptoms as abdominal pain, greatly diminished appetite, and weight loss. These symptoms are especially common in patients already debilitated by malnutrition or some other illness. Unlike victims of *T. solium* infection, *T. saginata* victims rarely develop cysticercosis, and the prognosis is generally good.

Diagnostic procedures are the same as those for *T. solium*.

## Hymenolepis nana

Known as the dwarf tapeworm of mice and humans, the adult of this species is the smallest of the tapeworms infecting humans. It ranges from 7 to 50 mm in length and may consist of as many as 200 proglottids. The acetabulate scolex has a retractable rostellum armed with a single circle of small hooks. The mature proglottid (Fig. 12–6), approximately four times as broad as it is long, has a single, common genital atrium on the left margin. The male reproductive system consists of three spherical

**Figure 12–6**
**Diagram of mature proglottid of *Hymenolepis nana*.**

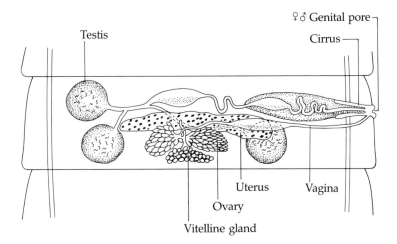

Testis

♀♂ Genital pore

Cirrus

Uterus

Vagina

Ovary

Vitelline gland

testes, one situated near the genital pore and separated from the other two by the bilobed ovary. The medullary region of the gravid proglottid is entirely occupied by a sacculate uterus containing up to 200 eggs.

It is noted that because *H. nana*, unlike *H. diminuta* (see below), possesses an armed rostellum—among other, less conspicuous differences—some consider it to represent a different genus, *Vampirolepis*, hence, *V. nana*.

**Life Cycle (Fig. 12–7).**    The life cycle of *H. nana* is of particular biological significance: it represents a modification of the typical cyclophyllidean life cycle pattern in that the parasite requires only one host to complete its development. Natural definitive hosts, in addition to humans, are rodents, particularly mice and rats. Gravid proglottids from adult worms rupture, releasing oncosphere-containing eggs into the host intestine to be eliminated with feces. The morphology of the egg, infective upon release, is characteristic of hymenolepid eggs. There is a thin shell and an inner membrane with two polar thickenings, from each of which extend four to eight filaments. Upon being ingested by a new host, the oncosphere, freed in the small intestine from its encapsulating membranes, penetrates a villus. There it sheds its six hooklets and, about 4 days later, becomes a modified cysticercoid larva known as a **cercocystis**. The cercocystis erupts from the villus into the lumen of the small intestine, attaches itself to the mucosal lining, and develops into a sexually mature adult in about 30 days. In the case of rodents, an insect, such as the flour beetle, may serve as an

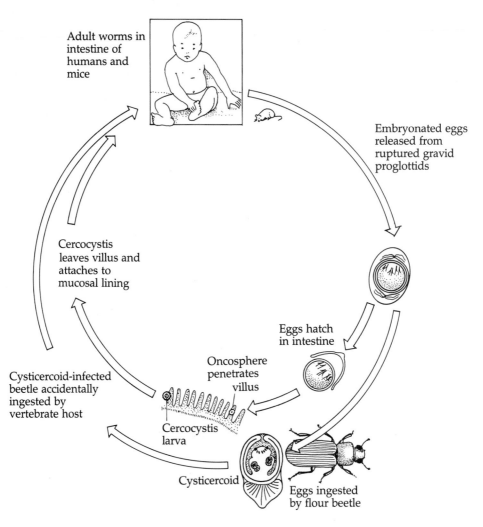

Adult worms in intestine of humans and mice

Embryonated eggs released from ruptured gravid proglottids

Cercocystis leaves villus and attaches to mucosal lining

Eggs hatch in intestine

Oncosphere penetrates villus

Cysticercoid-infected beetle accidentally ingested by vertebrate host

Cercocystis larva

Cysticercoid

Eggs ingested by flour beetle

**Figure 12–7**
**Life cycle of *Hymenolepis nana*.**

intermediate host. In this case, when the insect host is ingested by a rodent, or even accidentally by a human, the cysticercoid attaches to the intestinal wall and develops to sexual maturity. Autoinfection can exacerbate the condition by increasing the number of worms; eggs released from gravid proglottids, instead of passing to the exterior to infect new hosts, hatch in the small intestine and reinfect the same host. The freed oncosphere penetrates a villus and repeats the cycle.

Due to certain physiological variations, many authorities recognize two subspecies of *H. nana*: *H. nana nana*, which infects humans, and *H. nana fraterna*, which infects rodents. The life cycle of the rodent variety includes fleas and beetles as intermediate hosts in which the infective cysticercoid larvae develop. Limited host cross-infectivity does occur.

**Epidemiology.**   *Hymenolepis nana* is cosmopolitan in distribution and is possibly the most common cestode parasite of humans in the world, especially among children. Worldwide prevalence ranges from less than 1% in the United States to about 9% in Argentina, with an average worldwide prevalence of 4%. The usual mode of transmission in humans is hand-to-mouth, although infection may also be acquired through ingestion of contaminated food. However, since infective eggs are very susceptible to such environmental conditions as heat and dessication, the latter occurs infrequently. Infection may also be acquired by accidental ingestion of cysticerci-infected insects. The nature of the life cycle—no essential intermediate host and a high likelihood of autoinfection—makes prevention difficult. Teaching proper personal hygiene to children is perhaps the best preventive measure.

**Symptomatology and Diagnosis.**   Since it is possible for a human victim to harbor massive numbers of these parasites, damage to the intestinal mucosa may be sufficient to produce enteritis. Most infections, however, are light and virtually symptomless—although autoinfection can lead to heavy worm burdens, particularly in children and immunosuppressed patients. In children with a moderate parasite burden, there may be loss of appetite, diarrhea, some abdominal pain, and dizziness.

Diagnosis is by identification of eggs in feces (Fig. 11–15).

## *Hymenolepis diminuta*

*Hymenolepis diminuta*, a common parasite of rats throughout the world, occasionally parasitizes humans. *H. diminuta* exhibits a typical two-host life cycle, utilizing a grain-ingesting insect, such as a flour beetle, as intermediate host. A single worm may reach a length of 90 cm. The scolex in this species is unarmed, and the width of each proglottid is greater than its length. The morphology of proglottids is markedly similar to that of *H. nana* (Fig. 12–6). Of diagnostic relevance, the eggs are usually yellowish-brown and spherical. Unlike that of *H. nana*, the inner membrane in these eggs does not bear conspicuous knobs and filaments at the poles. Insects are infected when they consume rodent feces containing either gravid proglottids or eggs. The oncosphere penetrates the intestinal wall of the insect and enters the hemocoel, where it develops to the cysticercoid stage. The most common intermediate hosts are grain beetles belonging to the genera *Tribolium* and *Tenebrio,* although cockroaches are also known to harbor infective cysticercoid larvae. Humans acquire infection by eating cereals, dried fruits, and other similar foods contaminated with infected insects.

When human infection occurs, children are the most common victims and may suffer abdominal pain, diarrhea, insomnia, and convulsions.

With a life cycle easily maintainable in the laboratory, *H. diminuta* has been a choice parasite for experimental studies for decades. It is perhaps the most studied of all tapeworms.

## *Dipylidium caninum*

*Dipylidium caninum* is a common tapeworm of dogs, cats, and humans, especially children, throughout the world. The parasite can attain a length of 30 cm and possesses on its scolex a conical, retractable rostellum with one to eight (commonly four to six) rows of hooks (Fig. 12–8). It is easily recognizable because each proglottid has two sets of reproductive organs with a genital atrium on each lateral edge. The short, inconspicuous uterus atrophies early, and, as eggs are produced, they are encapsulated in **egg capsules**. Each capsule contains 8 to 25 eggs, and the medullary region of a gravid proglottid is packed with hundreds of egg capsules.

**Life Cycle.**   The adult tapeworm lives in the small intestine of the definitive host, where large, gravid proglottids, 12 mm long by 3 mm wide, separate from the strobila in groups of 2 or 3. The proglottids are capable of moving upon a substrate and can either creep out of the anus or be passed with feces. Eggs and capsules are ingested by larvae of fleas belonging to the genera *Pulex* and *Ctenocephalides* or by the dog louse *Trichodectes canis*. The oncosphere hatches in the gut of the arthropod, burrows through the wall, and develops into a cysticercoid in the hemocoel when the flea or louse ma-

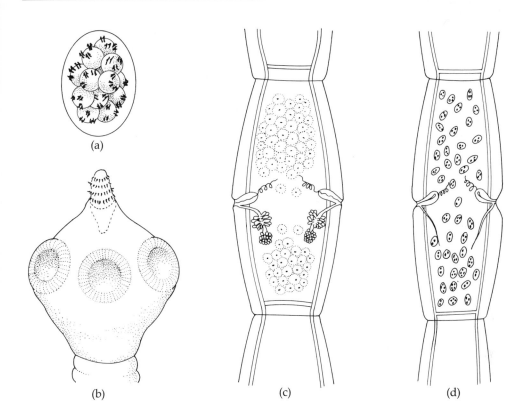

(a)

(b)

(c)

(d)

**Figure 12–8**
*Dipylidium caninum.*
(a) Cluster of eggs in a uterine ball. (b) Scolex with armed rostellum. (c) Mature proglottid with two sets of reproductive organs. (d) Gravid proglottid filled with uterine balls.

tures. When the infected insect is ingested by a suitable definitive host, the cysticercoid is liberated in the small intestine and develops into an adult in about 20 days.

**Epidemiology.** Most human infections are in children younger than 8 years old, with a high percentage falling in the under-6-months age group. This probably is attributable to the fact that a high percentage of dogs are infected, many of which undoubtedly are pets. Transmission to humans usually results from accidental ingestion of infected fleas or lice or from allowing dogs and cats to lick ("kiss") the mouths of children immediately after the pet has bitten an infected arthropod.

**Symptomatology and Diagnosis.** It is rare for humans to harbor more than a single parasite, and symptoms are seldom apparent. Diagnosis is confirmed by discovery of characteristic proglottids or eggs in the feces.

◇
## SELECTED READINGS

Pawlowski, Z., and Schultz, M. G. 1972. Taeniasis and cysticercosis (*Taenia saginata*). *Advances in Parasitology* 10, 269–343.

von Bonsdorff, B. 1956. *Diphyllobothrium latum* as a cause of pernicious anemia. *Experimental Parasitology* 5, 201–230.

# CHAPTER THIRTEEN

# EXTRAINTESTINAL LARVAL TAPEWORMS

This chapter deals with tapeworms having larvae that can be highly pathogenic to humans. Included in this category are several species of *Diphyllobothrium* and related pseudophyllidean cestodes, *Taenia solium*, and at least two members of the genus *Echinococcus*, namely, *E. granulosus* and *E. multilocularis*. The larvae of two other species, *Hymenolepis nana* and *Taenia multiceps*, sometimes infect humans. However, since such accidental human infections are relatively rare (*T. multiceps*) or, when the parasite is in the larval stage, do not produce serious symptoms (*H. nana*) (see p. 249), these species will not be considered in this section.

The human disease known as sparganosis is caused by plerocercoids of any of several pseudophyllideans, human cysticercosis is caused by the cysticercus of *T. solium*, and human hydatidosis results from infection with hydatid cysts of *E. granulosus* or multilocular cysts of *E. multilocularis*.

## HUMAN SPARGANOSIS

The plerocercoid larvae of several pseudophyllidean tapeworms are capable of infecting tissues of humans and other vertebrates (Fig. 13–1). One of the more common of these belongs to the genus *Spirometra*. The plerocercoid larva of

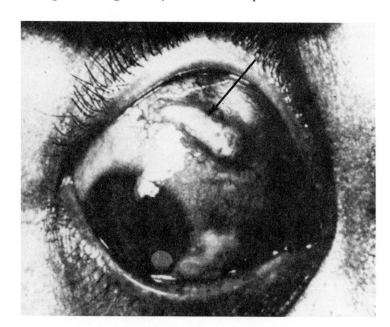

**Figure 13–1**
**Human patient with plerocercoid in conjunctiva.**

*Spirometra* was placed in the genus *Sparganum* before the association between larva and adult worm was established. The term **sparganosis**, signifying an infection with the plerocercoid larva, stems, therefore, from the generic name that has since been dropped.

## Life Cycle

Among various pseudophyllidean tapeworms with plerocercoids that can produce sparganosis in humans, the life cycle of *D. latum* is typical (Fig. 12–2). However, it should be emphasized that human ingestion of *D. latum* plerocercoids will result in the development of the adult worm.

## Epidemiology

Humans become infected in several ways. A common mode is by drinking water contaminated with copepods harboring procercoids. Procercoids released in the gut of the human penetrate the intestinal wall and migrate to various tissues, where they develop into plerocercoids. Backpackers drinking from stagnant pools or lakes are vulnerable to infection in this manner, especially in temperate regions of the world where these parasites are prevalent.

Another way in which humans become infected is by ingesting insufficiently cooked flesh of fishes, amphibians, reptiles, birds, and such mammals as bears, wild boars, and pigs. Plerocercoids of pseudophyllideans other than *D. latum*, ingested when infected muscle is eaten, are freed in the intestine of the human and migrate to various tissues, most commonly the areas in and around the eyes, muscles, viscera of the thorax, and subcutaneous regions of the thorax, abdomen, and thighs.

Humans also acquire infection through the use of poultices, specifically through the practice of placing raw meat over a black eye. Active plerocercoids from infected meat crawl into the orbit and become established. Similar cases of human ocular sparganosis have been reported from the Orient following treatment of skin ulcers or eye inflammations with poultices made from various infected animals, particularly snakes. In Oriental countries the most common plerocercoid causing human sparganosis is that of *Diphyllobothrium erinacei*, a tapeworm of carnivores, while in North America the most common causative plerocercoid is that of *Spirometra mansonoides*, a tapeworm of cats. Another species is capable of asexual proliferation of the scolex in the plero-cercoid stage; hence its species name *Spirometra proliferatum*.

Because practices such as those described above are widespread in the Orient, human sparganosis is common there. However, the disease also occurs, albeit less frequently, in Europe, Australia, Africa, and North and South America.

## Symptomatology and Diagnosis

As noted above, plerocercoids may be found in many parts of the body. The movements and secretions of living plerocercoids can induce localized inflammatory reactions; dead and degenerating larvae sometimes cause edema of the surrounding tissue. Chills and fever may accompany infections. Eye infections, particularly common in the Orient, result in conjunctivitis and swelling. In general, severity of infection is determined by the location of the larvae and how quickly and completely the patient can be rid of them.

Detection of larvae in the host's tissues constitutes diagnosis.

## Treatment

Surgical removal of the larva is the most dependable treatment. That several experimental drugs, such as praziquantel, have proven effective in the treatment of animals raises hope that chemotherapy may eventually be available for human use.

## Prevention

A major prevention is the proper cooking of freshwater fishes prior to eating. Also, application of animal flesh to human skin should be avoided, and questionable water, especially in endemic areas, should be boiled or filtered before humans drink it.

# HUMAN CYSTICERCOSIS

The fully developed cycticercus of *Taenia solium* is oval, about 0.5 cm or wider and usually enclosed by a capsule of host connective tissue (Fig. 13–2). In areas such as certain

**Figure 13–2**
**Cysticercus of *Taenia* spp.**

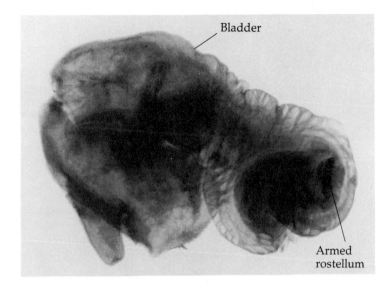

Bladder

Armed
rostellum

parts of the brain, the host capsule may be absent, and the
larva may attain a diameter of several centimeters. The ability of the cysticerci of *T. solium* to develop in practically any
organ in the body, and the severity of the resulting pathology, render it one of the most pathogenic species of tapeworms infecting humans (Fig. 13–3).

**Figure 13–3**
**Human cysticercosis.**
(a) Heart containing cysticerci
of *Taenia solium*. (b) *Taenia
solium* cysticercus close to bone.

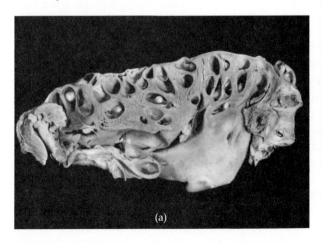

(a)

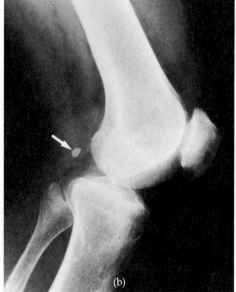

(b)

# Life Cycle

See Figure 12–5.

# Epidemiology

Prevalence of human cysticercosis predictably parallels the incidence of the adult worm. Relatively rare in the United States, it is quite common in Latin America (particularly in Mexico, where approximately 3 million people are infected), Africa, Indonesia, India, and China. Human infection with cysticerci occurs in several ways, perhaps the most common of which is direct ingestion of eggs. This may result from hand-to-mouth self-infection, from eating food contaminated with eggs by unsanitary food handling practices, or from consuming food or water contaminated with feces containing eggs. Internal autoinfection, whereby eggs are swept back into the stomach by reverse peristalsis, is another method of human infection, although of little epidemiological importance since only about 25% of patients with cysticercosis harbor the adult tapeworm. For some as yet unexplained reason, human males seem more prone to infection that human females. Eggs, whether ingested or swept back by reverse peristalsis, pass through the stomach and hatch in the small intestine. The escaping oncospheres penetrate the intestinal wall, enter the circulatory system, and are dispersed throughout the body.

# Symptomatology and Diagnosis

While the most common sites for infection by cysticerci are the skeletal muscles and the brain, they may be found in almost any tissue of the body, including the eyes, lungs, and subcutaneous tissue. Cysts are well tolerated in muscles and subcutaneous tissues, although heavy infections can produce muscle spasms, weakness, and general malaise. Developing cysts elicit a host inflammatory response resulting in fibrous encapsulation although, as noted earlier, such a capsule may not be formed when the cyst invades parts of the brain. Calcification of the cyst may occur after 1 year, after which time the disease may become asymptomatic. The most serious symptoms arise about 5 to 10 years after infection as a result of dead and dying cysticerci. The degenerating parasite tissues and associated fluid also elicit a host inflammatory reaction that can be very severe, even fatal.

In addition to precipitating host responses, cysts developing in the central nervous system, sense organs, or heart can exert mechanical pressure and cause severe neurological symptoms. Violent headaches, convulsions, local paralysis, vomiting, and optic disturbances are common and, again, are sometimes severe enough to be fatal.

Clinical diagnosis can be made by linking symptoms such as certain nervous disorders, for example, the late onset of epileptic convulsions, to a history of residency in an endemic area. Also, X-ray examination of infected muscles or central nervous system may be diagnostically useful if it reveals calcified cysts. Computer-assisted tomography (CAT) scans have been used to diagnose cysticerci in the brain.

## Treatment

Surgery is the recommended treatment for cysticerci in the fluid spaces of the body. However, in heavy infections of the central nervous system, while removal of some of the cysts has proven helpful, surgery is not generally beneficial. Praziquantel and some steroids (e.g., dexamethasone) are effective in reducing edema and alleviating some of the symptoms of cerebral cysticercosis. Preliminary results suggest that flubendazole, albendazole, and metrifonate may also be effective. Care must be taken during treatment for adult worms to avoid causing severe vomiting, which may induce reverse peristalsis.

## Prevention

The best preventive measures include strict attention to personal hygiene, sexual habits, and environmental sanitation. Removal of adult worms from the patient once infection has been ascertained is important in preventing autoinfection. Visitors to endemic areas should observe such preventive measures as the boiling of drinking water and avoiding salads and raw fruits and vegetables without rinds.

# HUMAN HYDATIDOSIS

As adults, member of the genus *Echinococcus* are among the smallest tapeworms, measuring 2 to 8 mm long with strobilae consisting of three or, rarely, four proglottids (Fig. 13–4). Usually one immature, one mature, and one gravid proglottid make up the strobila. The scolex bears a rostellum armed with a double row of 28–50 (usually 30–36) hooks,

**Figure 13–4**
**Morphology of adult**
*Echinococcus granulosus.*

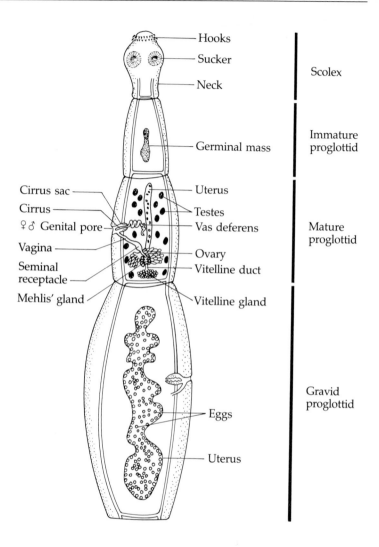

four prominent suckers, and a short neck region. Adult worms inhabit the small intestine of a wide variety of canines and, occasionally, cats. In heavy infections, it is not unusual to find hundreds of worms attached to a dog's small intestine.

## Life Cycle

The eggs, measuring 30 by 38 μm, reach the exterior by elimination of gravid proglottids with the host's feces (Fig. 13–5). Released when proglottids disintegrate, the eggs are

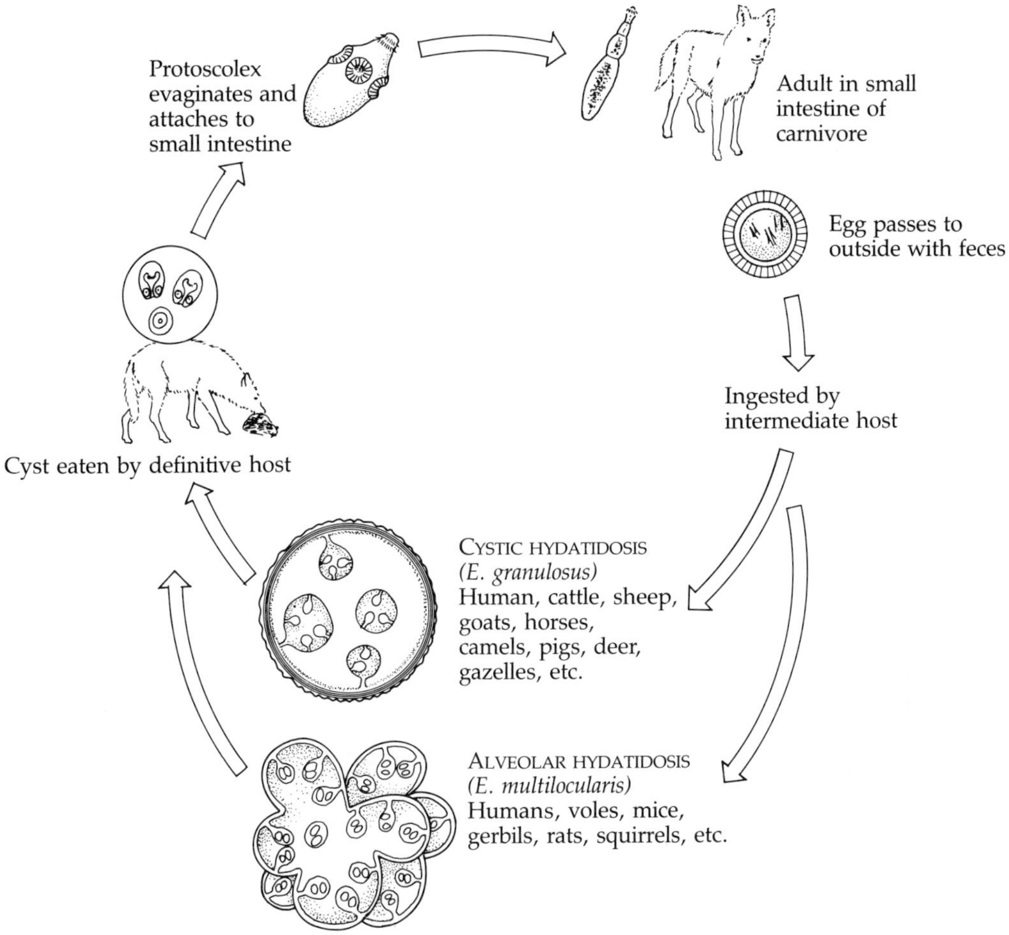
Protoscolex evaginates and attaches to small intestine
Adult in small intestine of carnivore
Egg passes to outside with feces
Ingested by intermediate host
Cyst eaten by definitive host
CYSTIC HYDATIDOSIS
(E. granulosus)
Human, cattle, sheep, goats, horses, camels, pigs, deer, gazelles, etc.
ALVEOLAR HYDATIDOSIS
(E. multilocularis)
Humans, voles, mice, gerbils, rats, squirrels, etc.

**Figure 13–5**
**Life cycle of *Echinococcus* spp.**

morphologically indistinguishable from other taeniid eggs, and each contains a fully developed oncosphere. These gain entry into the intermediate host by the intake of either water or forage contaminated with egg-containing feces. The usual intermediate host for *E. granulosus* is sheep, but cattle and other herbivores, as well as pigs, are sometimes utilized. Microtine rodents serve as intermediate hosts for *E. multilocularis*, while cats, foxes, and dogs that feed on rodents harbor the adults. Usually, human infection from eggs results from intimate contact with dogs, particularly when dogs are allowed to lick human faces after grooming themselves. Humans can also ingest eggs by putting contaminated fingers into the mouth or by eating raw plants contaminated with feces from infected foxes, cats, or dogs.

Once swallowed, eggs pass through the stomach and hatch in the small intestine. The freed oncospheres penetrate the intestinal wall, enter the mesenteric venules, and become lodged in capillary beds of various visceral organs. In humans, the developing hydatid cyst favors the liver, although other tissues—such as lungs, kidneys, spleen, heart, muscles, brain, and bone marrow—may be invaded. The hydatid cyst grows slowly, reaching a diameter of 10 mm in 5 months. However, it is not unusual for the cyst to reach the size of an orange or a small grapefruit and contain several liters of fluid. Within the fully formed cyst, minute larvae with inverted scolices develop. Since these immature, four-suckered scolices lack individual bladders, they are called **protoscolices** (singular, **protoscolex**)—not bladderworms or cysticerci, which contain a single scolex.

In humans and some domestic animals, the formation of hydatid cysts represents a dead end for the parasite. However, many wild animals, such as infected rabbits and squirrels, are potential intermediate hosts since the cysts are ingested when predators feed upon such animals. Upon reaching the small intestine of the definitive host (the predator), each protoscolex develops into an adult worm. The average life span of an adult worm is approximately 5 months, although some may survive as long as a year.

**Hydatid Cyst.** Hydatid cysts found in humans fall into three categories: (1) unilocular, (2) osseous, and (3) alveolar, the last representing a developmental stage of *E. multilocularis*. Of the three, the unilocular cyst is the most common and least pathogenic while the alveolar cyst is the most dangerous.

The diameter of the unilocular cyst may reach 20 cm or more in humans, although the usual diameter varies from 1 to 7 cm. At maturity, the cyst wall consists of two layers: a thick, laminated, noncellular outer tegument known as the **ectocyst** and an inner germinal epithelium that produces the protoscolices and is known as the **endocyst** (Fig. 13–6). Brood capsules attached to the germinal epithelium by a stalk, the **pedicel**, extend into the fluid-filled cavity of the cyst. In large cysts, these capsules may rupture, and the freed protoscolices, which sink to the bottom of the bladder, are commonly known as hydatid sand. Each brood capsule contains 10–30 protoscolices. Second-generation daughter cysts often form within the mother cyst. These are replicas

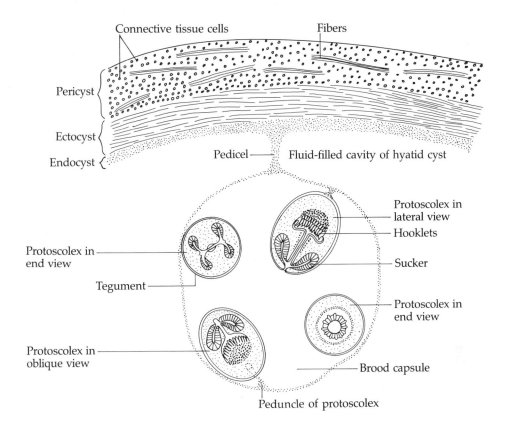

Figure 13–6
**Schematic representation of a section through part of a unilocular hydatid cyst.**

of the mother cyst and produce their own generation of protoscolices. Daughter cysts may, in turn, produce another generation of cysts. It is not surprising, then, that the average fertile primary cyst is estimated to contain more than 2 million protoscolices. If a cyst ruptures within a host, each liberated protoscolex can produce a daughter cyst. Whether the protoscolex develops into a cyst or whether small bits of germinal tissue cling to it and generate a new cyst is conjectural.

Osseous cysts are most commonly found in the ribs, vertebrae, and upper portions of long bones. These cysts usually develop in the marrow cavities. They are much smaller than unilocular cysts and contain little or no fluid and no protoscolices.

The outer membrane of alveolar cysts is very thin, laminated, and difficult to differentiate from surrounding tissues. Connective tissue septa divide the cyst into numerous irregular compartments, or alveoli, which are filled with a jellylike material. Alveolar cysts are found most commonly in the liver, where they tend to proliferate by evagination of the thin cyst wall. In humans, the cysts are usually sterile, lacking protoscolices.

## Epidemiology

Human hydatidosis is a zoonotic disease that results from intimate contact with dogs (Fig. 13–7). The percentage of infected dogs in countries throughout the world where dogs are used to herd domestic animals such as sheep may run as high as 50%, while the prevalence of hydatid cysts may be as high as 30% in sheep and cattle and 10% in hogs. Incidence among humans in Australia, Greece, Cyprus, Algeria, Yugoslavia, Argentina, Uruguay, and Chile is relatively high due to the close association with working dogs such as sheep dogs. Well-organized prevention programs have reduced the incidence in New Zealand and Tasmania. Scattered cases in the human population have been reported in the United States, especially in Mississippi, Utah, Arizona, and parts of California. Isolated areas of heavy incidence have also been recorded in the United Kingdom, especially in Wales and in some of the islands off the Scottish

**Figure 13–7**
**World distribution of hydatidosis.**

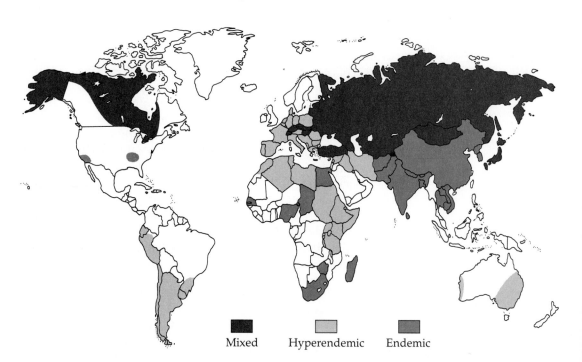

Mixed    Hyperendemic    Endemic

coast. Hydatid disease originating in the Middle East is spreading rapidly in Europe, especially in France and parts of Germany.

In nature, the carnivore–herbivore, predator–prey relationship—as in that between the wolf and moose, wolf and reindeer, or dingo and wallaby—enables *E. granulosus* to complete its life cycle. This is known as sylvatic echinococcosis. Humans are seldom involved in this type of cycle.

Certain unique, ethnic customs promote human infection. For example, members of certain primitive tribes in Kenya, where incidence of human hydatidosis is among the world's highest, utilize dogs not only to herd livestock but also to act as "nurse dogs." In this capacity, they protect babies and clean them after they defecate or vomit by licking their buttocks or faces.

The infection rate is also high among leather tanners in Lebanon, since dog feces is an ingredient of the tanning fluid used there. During the preparation process, the tanners' fingers become contaminated, and they accidentally ingest eggs by putting their unwashed fingers into their mouths.

Alveolar hydatidosis is common in such countries of the Northern Hemisphere as Japan, the USSR, western Alaska, and central Europe. Recently, human cases have also been documented in Iran, China, India, and the United States, countries previously free of the disease. In the midwestern United States, a cat-rodent life cycle has been reported for *E. multilocularis.*

## Symptomatology and Diagnosis

The presence of the unilocular cyst elicits a host inflammatory reaction that results in encapsulation of the cyst. The primary pathology of the unilocular cyst is impairment of organs from mechanical pressure (Fig. 13–8). Increased pressure resulting from cyst growth may cause surrounding tissues to atrophy. The symptoms, therefore, are not unlike those caused by a slow-growing tumor, varying according to the tissues affected. It may take many years for symptoms to appear. For instance, while the liver is the most commonly affected organ, symptoms such as jaundice may take as long as 20 years to emerge. Pulmonary infections characterized by a cough accompanied by allergic reactions also are common. The brain, kidneys, spleen, and vertebral column may also be invaded, producing symptoms ranging from seizures to kidney dysfunction over a protracted period.

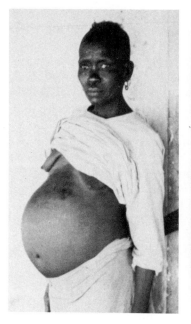

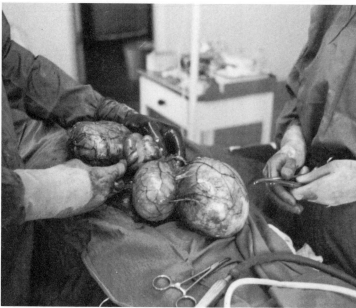

**Figure 13–8**
**Human hydatidosis.**
(a) Native Kenyan with disease.
(b) Removal of hydatid cysts by
surgical means.

Protoscolices, freed by the rupture of cysts, enter the circulatory system and are transported to tissues throughout the body where they produce secondary echinococcosis. This condition, which may not appear for 2–8 years, is far more serious than the primary infection. The rupture of cysts also releases hydatid fluid, which sometimes causes severe allergic reactions. If a significant amount of fluid enters the bloodstream, it can precipitate lethal anaphylactic shock.

The alveolar cyst usually is proliferative. While growth occurs at its periphery, its center may become calcified. Such cysts commonly occur in the liver and are often mistaken for hepatic carcinoma. They are difficult to extirpate, and the condition is usually fatal within 10 years.

The osseous cyst, because of its location, also is difficult to remove. Severe cases often display necrosis of diaphyses of long bones, spontaneous fracture, and distortion of cancellous tissue.

Diagnosis of hydatidosis is based upon a number of criteria, such as symptoms (hepatic hypertrophy, etc.), history of residence an endemic area, and close contact with dogs. X-ray examination is useful especially for revealing calcified cysts, and various ultrasound procedures may locate noncalcified cysts. Laboratory diagnosis, which might be more aptly termed "post-surgical confirmation" of hydatidosis, involves detection of protoscolices. Serologic tests are diagnostically useful, the indirect hemagglutination test being one of the most commonly used. The intracutaneous test (Casoni's intradermal test) is sufficiently sensitive to be helpful in screening for human hydatidosis. However, negative test results are more significant than positive test results since there is about an 18% incidence of false positives.

## Treatment

Surgery remains the preferred treatment for unilocular hydatidosis. Following drainage of the cyst fluid, replacement with 2% formalin (final concentration) for 5 minutes kills the protoscolices and the germinal epithelium. In any surgical procedure for cyst removal, care should be taken to avoid rupturing the cyst. Symptoms of allergic reaction respond best to treatment with antihistamines or epinephrine. Most recently, the benzimidazoles (albendazole and mebendazole) have been used successfully to reduce the size of both unilocular and alveolar cysts. It is anticipated that, at least in some cases, chemotherapy may eventually replace surgery. Several species of *Echinococcus*, notably *E. granulosus*, display a variety of developmental and physiological strains. Such variations must be considered when chemotherapy is prescribed since one regimen may be effective against one strain but not another.

## Prevention

Human hydatidosis can be prevented if contact is reduced between dogs and intermediate hosts such as sheep, hogs, and rodents, and if the public is informed of the danger of intimate contact with dogs, especially in endemic areas. As added measures, dogs should be treated regularly with anthelmintics and kept away from slaughterhouses, and refuse from slaughter houses should be disinfected.

## SELECTED READINGS

Gemmel, M. A. 1977. Experimental epidemiology of hydatidosis and cysticercosis. *Advances in Parasitology* 15, 311–369.

McManus, D. P., and Smyth, J. D. 1986. Hydatidosis: Changing concepts in epidemiology and speciation. *Parasitology Today* 2, 163–167.

# PART FOUR
## THE NEMATODA

# CHAPTER FOURTEEN

# GENERAL CHARACTERISTICS OF THE NEMATODA

After more than a century of debate, the place of nematodes, or roundworms, in the phylogenetic scheme remains unresolved. Considered by some to constitute an independent phylum, the Nematoda (or Nemata), they are regarded by others as members, together with such groups as the Rotifera and the Nematomorpha, of the phylum Aschelminthes. According to still another system of classification, the Nematoda and the Nematomorpha are designated as separate classes of the phylum Nemathelminthes. In the scheme followed herein, roundworms are assigned to a separate phylum Nematoda.

Parasitic nematodes are of great importance to biologists because they are abundant and widespread, frequently occur as endoparasites infecting a wide variety of invertebrate as well as vertebrate hosts, and often have a serious impact upon human health.

Nematodes that parasitize humans are assigned to either the Class Secernentea (= Class Phasmidia) or the Class Adenophorea (= Class Aphasmidia), distinguishable primarily by the presence or absence of minute sensory structures, known as **phasmids,** on the body surface. Most nematodes that infect humans belong to the class Secernentea.

While the origin of nematodes is obscure, there is marked similarity in structure and of elements of the life cycle among these organisms, whether free-living or parasitic. This consistency argues for "ancestral uniformity," a descendance from common ancestors. Since most nematodes are not host specific, they are probably largely independent of the evolution of their hosts, using them merely as vehicles for their own evolution. Life history studies have fostered the view that parasitic nematodes evolved at various times from free-living soil forms, with the free-living ancestor initially utilizing a host for transportation or protection only. Movements of such hosts isolated these nematode populations, preventing interbreeding with members of their free-living counterparts, thus providing the basis for speciation.

Significant preadaptation of the third-stage larva (see p. 287) to osmoregulation equips certain nematodes to utilize several environments during their life cycle. Such a third-stage larva is characteristic of all secernentean (phasmidian) parasites of animals and serves as a transfer stage from one environment to another. The third-stage larva of aphasmidians, on the other hand, is less diversified and plays no such role.

# STRUCTURE OF THE ADULT

Nematodes are generally elongate, cylindrical, and tapered at both ends. The basic body design is a tube within a tube, the outer tube being the body wall and underlying muscles and the inner tube the digestive tract (Fig. 14–1). Between

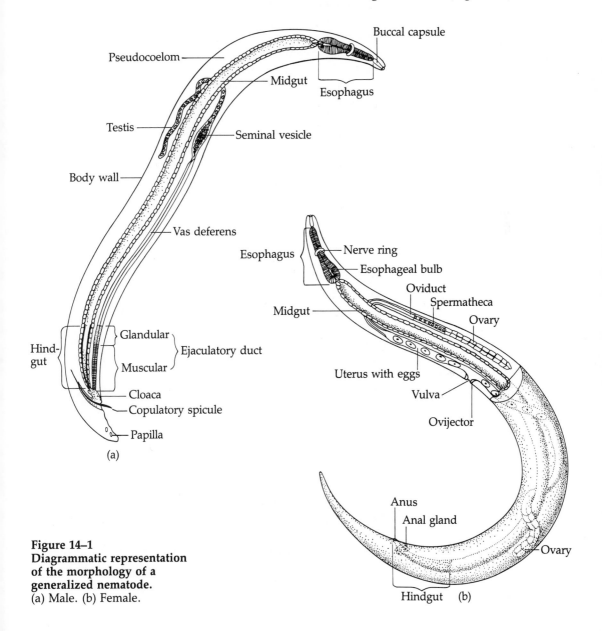

**Figure 14–1**
**Diagrammatic representation of the morphology of a generalized nematode.**
(a) Male. (b) Female.

the tubes is the fluid-filled pseudocoelom, in which the reproductive system and other structures are found. In certain species, the body is almost uniformly cylindrical and is extremely thin. Sexual dimorphism is evident: at the curved posterior end of the male there is a copulatory organ as well as other specialized organs such as alae and papillae, and males are usually smaller than females.

Parasitic nematodes vary widely in size according to species. While some are microscopic and others may reach more than a meter in length, most are between 1 mm and 15 cm long. Nematodes are colorless and vary from translucent (smaller nematodes) to opaque (larger nematodes) when examined alive. It is not uncommon for some to absorb colored matter from surrounding host tissues or fluids.

## Cuticle

An elastic **cuticle** covers the body surface of nematodes (Fig. 14–2). The presence of enzymes in the cuticle indicates that

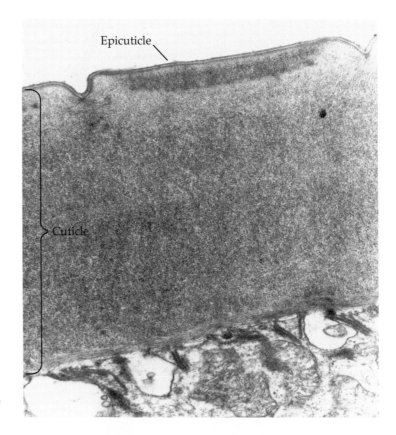

**Figure 14–2**
**Electron micrograph of cuticle of nematode.**

it is metabolically active, not an inert covering. Although the cuticle is generally smooth, various structures such as spines, bristles, warts, punctuations, papillae, striations, and ridges may be present on it. Some of these specialized structures are sensory and some aid in locomotion; their arrangement and position are of taxonomic importance.

The cuticle not only covers the entire external surface, but also lines the buccal cavity, esophagus (= pharynx), rectum, cloaca, vagina, and excretory pore. It consists of four basic layers: the **epicuticle**, the **exocuticle,** the **mesocuticle,** and the **endocuticle** (Fig. 14–3).

The epicuticle is a relatively thin layer and is a consistent component of all nematode cuticles. Typically, it is trilaminate, with a carbohydrate-containing glycocalyx. Its function is largely unknown, although it is believed to act, at least in part, as a protective barrier.

The exocuticle is usually composed of two distinct sublayers: the relatively homogeneous **external exocuticle,** with no visible substructure, and the radially striated **internal exocuticle.**

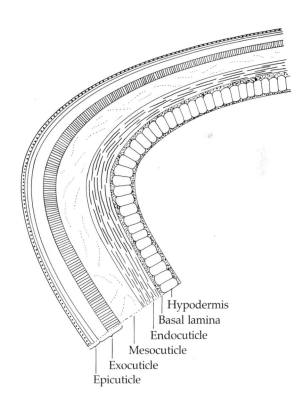

Hypodermis
Basal lamina
Endocuticle
Mesocuticle
Exocuticle
Epicuticle

**Figure 14–3**
**Diagram showing layers of nematode cuticle.**

The mesocuticle is the most diverse of the cuticular layers. It commonly consists of obliquely oriented, collagenous, fibrous sublayers that vary in number and in angular relationship to each other. The ability of the mesocuticular fiber sublayers to shift their angles of orientation provides flexibility to the cuticle. In some nematodes, the thickness of the mesocuticle is directly proportional to the age of the worm.

The endocuticle is the innermost layer of the cuticle. It is also fibrous, but the orientation of fibers is not as distinct as in the mesocuticle. Often, the pattern is disorganized, with a great deal of overlapping.

A basal lamina separates the cuticle from the underlying hypodermis.

## Hypodermis

Beneath the basal lamina lies the thin, cellular (in adenophoreans) or syncytial (in secernenteans) hypodermis. A major function of the hypodermis is formation of the cuticle. The hypodermis protrudes into the pseudocoelom along the

**Figure 14–4**
**Nematode morphology.**
(a) Portion of dorsal body wall showing relationship of dorsal cord to cuticle. (b) Cross-section through esophageal region. (c) Cross-section through midgut region.

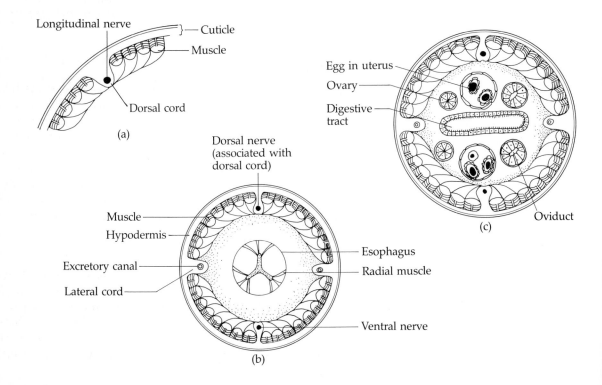

middorsal, midventral, and lateral lines to form the longitudinal **hypodermal cords.** These partially divide the pseudocoel into quadrants. Hypodermal organelles such as nuclei and mitochondria are confined to the cords. The lateral cords are the largest and contain the primary excretory canals when these are present, while the dorsal and ventral cords contain longitudinal nerve trunks (Fig. 14–4).

## Musculature

Within and closely associated with the hypodermis are one or more layers of longitudinally arranged muscle cells, the **somatic musculature.** Collectively, the cuticle, hypodermis, and somatic musculature make up the body wall. A convenient classification system to describe muscle cell arrangement has been devised based upon the number of rows of muscle cells per quadrant (Fig. 14–5). According to this system, an arrangement of multiple longitudinal rows of muscle cells in each quadrant is termed **polymyarian,** one with no more than two rows of cells is designated **holomyarian,** and one with two to five rows is called **meromyarian.** Each muscle cell comprises a contractile portion containing myofibrils and a noncontractile portion in which are found the various organelles, such as the nucleus, mitochondria, ribosomes, and endoplasmic reticulum, as well as stores of glycogen and lipid (Fig. 14–6). Sensory processes usually extend from the noncontractile portion of each cell to the longitudinal nerve trunks.

The somatic musculature connects to the cuticle by fibers that originate in the contractile portion of each cell, pass through the basal lamina, and attach to the endocuticle.

**Figure 14–5**
**Diagram showing arrangement of muscles in a nematode.**

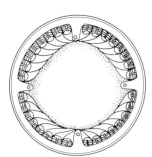

Polymyarian

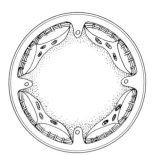

Holomyarian

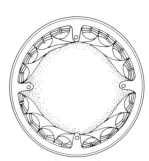

Meromyarian

**Figure 14–6**
**Schematic representation of one arm of a myocyton forming a junction with the nerve.**

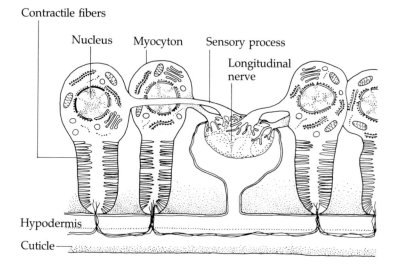

Contractile fibers

Nucleus    Myocyton    Sensory process

Longitudinal nerve

Hypodermis

Cuticle

## Digestive Tract

The digestive tract of nematodes is complete (Fig. 14–1). It consists of an anterior mouth, a gut that comprises three major regions, a cloaca, and a subterminal vent. The major regions of the gut are the foregut, midgut, and hindgut, each displaying a certain degree of specialization.

**Foregut.** The cuticle-lined foregut begins at the mouth, which, in many species, opens into a **buccal capsule** and continues as the esophagus. When present, the buccal capsule may contain ridges, rods, and plates for maintaining its shape as well as spears, stylets, or teeth for attachment to or penetration of the host or for acquiring food.

The buccal capsule, or the mouth if a capsule is absent, leads into the esophagus, an elongate structure of varying length and complexity. The lumen of the esophagus is characteristically triradiate in cross-section and is lined with cuticle. The structure of the esophagus varies within the phylum, but its similarity among members of each taxon makes it an important taxonomic feature (Fig. 14–7). It may be completely muscular or completely glandular, or the anterior half may be glandular and the posterior half muscular. Esophageal action is often enhanced by one or more muscular enlargements called **bulbs.** The glandular portion of the foregut ranges from a few unicellular glands to large, prominent glands lying along the esophagus. The glands secrete a number of digestive enzymes, including amylase, proteases, and cellulases. In a number of species, these enzymes initiate the digestive process, which is continued in the midgut until digestion is complete. Generally, nutrients are ingested and processed in the nematode foregut for eventual digestion and absorption in the midgut.

**Midgut.**    The esophagus empties into the midgut (or intestine) through a junction called the **esophago-intestinal valve.** The midgut is a straight tube lined with a single layer of cells bearing microvilli and a prominent glycocalyx. In smaller nematodes, it is interesting that the number of cells making up the midgut is fixed for each species. This phenomenon makes nematodes useful in certain developmental studies. The cellular layer rests on a basal lamina of connective tissue fibers and myofibers connected to the body wall by muscular extensions. The midgut is nonmuscular, the food being moved posteriorly by the muscular activity of the foregut and the overall body movements. The form of digestion varies among nematodes. In some, digestion is extracellular; in others, both intercellular and intracellular digestion occurs.

**Figure 14–7**
**Diagram showing variations in foregut of some nematodes.**
(a) *Rhabditis hominus.*
(b) *Strongyloides stercoralis.*
(c) *Ancylostoma duodenale.*
(d) *Enterobius vermicularis.*
(e) *Ascaris lumbricoides.*

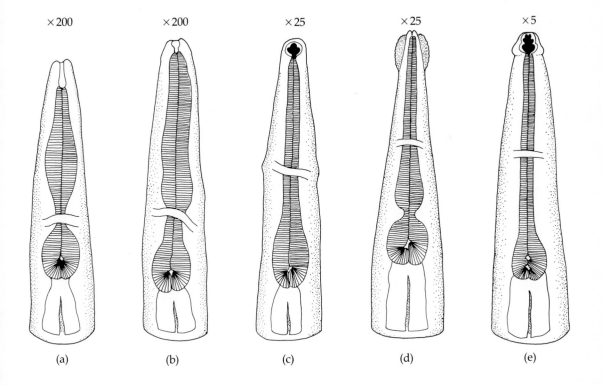

|   ×200   |   ×200   |   ×25   |   ×25   |   ×5   |
|   (a)   |   (b)   |   (c)   |   (d)   |   (e)   |

**Hindgut.** In females, the midgut empties into the cuticle-lined hindgut, or rectum—a short, flattened tube joining the midgut and the anus. In males, the posteriormost portion of the hindgut receives the products of the reproductive system via the vas deferens and is therefore called a **cloaca.**

## Nervous System

There are two major nerve centers in nematodes (Fig. 14–8). One, the **circumesophageal commissure,** or **nerve ring,** surrounds the esophagus. In at least one species, the commissure consists of four nerve cells and numerous supporting cells. Associated with the commissure are various ganglia from which longitudinal nerves emanate. The anterior longitudinal nerves innervate the anterior sense organs, such as oral papillae and amphids. The posterior longitudinal nerves, embedded in the dorsal and ventral hypodermal cords, innervate organs in the posterior regions of the body. The ventral longitudinal nerve is the largest nerve in the nematode body; it passes posteriorly as a chain of ganglia, the most posterior of which branches, continues dorsally from the hypodermal cord into the pseudocoelom, and encircles the rectum to form the second nerve center, the **rectal commissure.** Peripheral nerves branch from the main longitudi-

**Figure 14–8**
**Diagram of nematode nervous system.**
(a) Anterior end. (b) Posterior end.

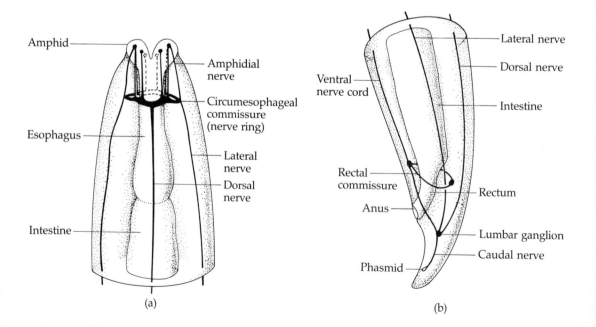

(a)                                    (b)

**Figure 14–9**
**Labial and cephalic papillae.**
*En face* view of nematode showing relationship of mouth, lips, amphids, and papillae.

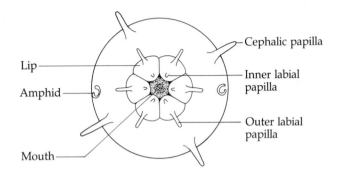

Lip

Amphid

Mouth

Cephalic papilla

Inner labial papilla

Outer labial papilla

nal trunks and supply sensory organs, such as the phasmids, in the cuticle.

Parasitic nematodes possess both mechano- and chemoreceptors. Located around the mouth are papillae of two main types: **labial papillae** on the lips surrounding the mouth and **cephalic papillae** behind the lips (Fig. 14–9). Papillae are mechanoreceptors and are innervated by **papillary nerves** derived from the circumesophageal commissure. Other papillae may be found at different levels of the nematode body. For example, **caudal papillae,** observed in many male nematodes, aid in copulation.

**Amphids** are chemoreceptors located in shallow, anterior depressions or pits at the same level of the body as the cephalic papillae. The sensory endings are modified cilia innervated by **amphidial nerves,** which are also associated with the circumesophageal commissure. **Phasmids** comprise another set of chemoreceptors that appear near the posterior end of many parasitic species as a pair of cuticle-lined organs. While morphologically resembling amphids, phasmids bear, in addition to the sensory nerve endings, a unicellular gland opening into the depression.

## Excretory System

The excretory system of nematodes, when present, is unique, the basic component(s) being one or two **renettes**—large unicellular glands that empty through an excretory pore (Fig. 14–10). The renettes and the excretory pore are usually located anteriorly at approximately the level of the circumesophageal commissure. Most frequently, renettes are associated with longitudinal excretory canals that course the length of the nematode body in the lateral hypodermis.

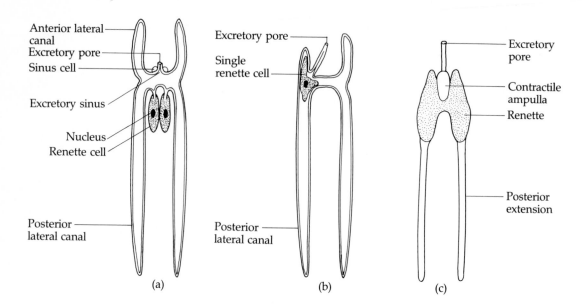

**Figure 14–10**
**Diagram of nematode excretory systems.**
(a) Rhabditoid. (b) Ascaroid. (c) Juvenile *Ancylostoma*.

In some genera, however, they empty independently to the exterior through an excretory pore, or two renettes join to form an H configuration, with a crossbar that connects with a common contractile ampulla, the pulsation of which causes expulsion of the excreta via a duct leading to the excretory pore. In yet another variation, two renettes join anteriorly, in which case excreta are emptied via a common duct through the excretory pore.

It has not been shown conclusively that this system serves as the primary excretory system. Indeed, there is strong evidence that the digestive tract is the principal excretory organ and that the system described above is chiefly osmoregulatory, with merely ancillary excretory and secretory functions.

## Reproductive Systems

Although some of the monoecious species are self-fertilizing hermaphrodites and others, such as *Strongyloides stercoralis* (see p. 307), are parthenogenetic, nematodes are usually dioecious.

**Male System.**    While there is usually a single testis, two are not uncommon (Figs. 14–1, 14–11). Tubular and usually convoluted and/or recurved, testes can be classified according to the location of their respective **germinal zones,** or regions of sperm formation. In the **telogonic** type, spermatogonial divisions occur at the blind end of the elongate testis, with the remaining portion of the testis making up the **growth zone;** in the **hologonic** type, the germinal zone extends the entire length of the testis. The **vas deferens** (sperm duct), a slender tube continuous at its proximal end with the testis, extends distally to the cloaca. Two specializations of the vas deferens are evident before it enters the cloaca. These are the **seminal vesicle,** in which sperm are stored, and the **ejaculatory duct.** In certain species, numerous unicellular **prostate glands** occur along the length of the ejaculatory duct.

Male nematodes are usually equipped with one or, more commonly, two **copulatory spicules** (Fig. 14–11).

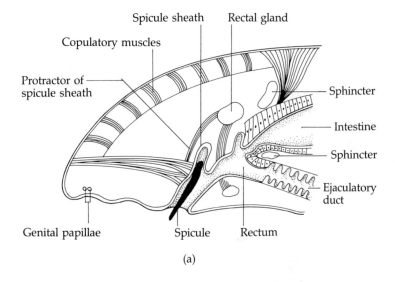

(a)

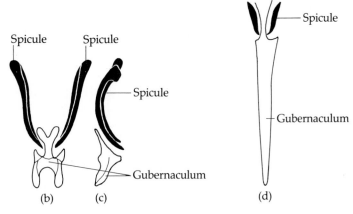

(b)     (c)     (d)

**Figure 14–11**
**Diagram of specializations of male nematode reproductive system.**
(a) Posterior portion of reproductive system of male nematode showing relationship of spicules to digestive tract.
(b)–(d) Various relationships of spicules to gubernaculum.

These cuticular structures, which usually resemble slightly curved, pointed blades, are encased within their respective spicule pouches located laterally in the cloacal wall. Each spicule contains a cytoplasmic core formed by cells lining the pouch. The spicules aid during copulation by keeping the female vulva open, thus facilitating the entry of sperm into the female reproductive tract.

In addition to spicules, other accessory structures may be present, such as a sclerotized **spicule guide,** or **gubernaculum.** This structure, located along the dorsal wall of the spicule pouch, typically has inwardly curved margins and serves to guide spicules when they are extended.

Nematode sperm have no flagella or acrosomes (Fig. 14–12). Sperm can be classified into several morphological types ranging from small, rounded cells that move by pseudopodia and display distinct anterior and posterior cytoplasmic areas to those with distinct heads and cytoplasmic extensions resembling nonmotile tails. Nematode sperm do not have nuclear envelopes. In some species, sperm are activated only after being introduced into the female reproductive tract.

**Female System.**    Female nematodes are usually **didelphic,** that is, equipped with two cylindrical ovaries and uteri (Figs. 14–1). **Monodelphic** species, with one ovary and one uterus, occur less frequently, and, rarely, there are **polydelphic** species, with multiple ovaries and uteri. The uteri in didelphic and polydelphic species unite to form a common **vagina** that opens through a gonopore, or **vulva,** usu-

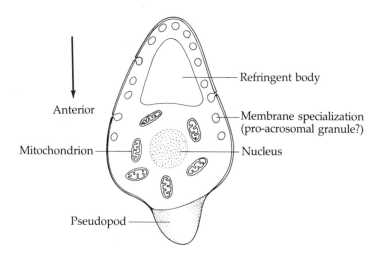

**Figure 14–12**
**Diagram of a generalized nematode sperm.**

Anterior

Mitochondrion

Refringent body

Membrane specialization (pro-acrosomal granule?)

Nucleus

Pseudopod

**Figure 14–13**
**Nematode eggs and larvae.**
(a) *Strongyloides stercoralis*
rhabditiform larva. (b) *Ascaris
lumbricoides* normal fertilized
egg with developing larva. (c)
*A. lumbricoides* unfertilized egg.
(d) Egg of hookworm. (e) Egg
of *Enterobius vermicularis*. (f)
Egg of *Trichuris trichiura*.

ally located near midbody. The ovary, a solid cord of cells attached to a central **rachis,** consitutes the first element in the linearly arranged female reproductive system. Oogonia are produced at the proximal end of the ovary, which is known as the **germinal zone.** As the oogonia develop into oocytes, they move distally along the rachis into the **growth zone.** Approaching the oviduct, the oocytes detach from the rachis and pass distally to a portion of the oviduct called the **spermatheca,** where sperm are stored. Initiation of meiosis and shell formation begin almost immediately after penetration by the sperm. The developing "egg" is moved down the tract by a combination of uterine peristalsis and hydrostatic pressure. The usually muscular, distal portion of the uterus, the **ovijector,** acts in conjunction with muscles of the vulva to expel ripe eggs.

Upon oviposition, the eggs of parasitic nematodes usually consist of three enveloping layers enclosing an embryo (Fig. 14–13) that may consist of a few blastomeres or a completely formed larva. Immediately following sperm penetration, the oocyte secretes a **fertilization membrane,** which

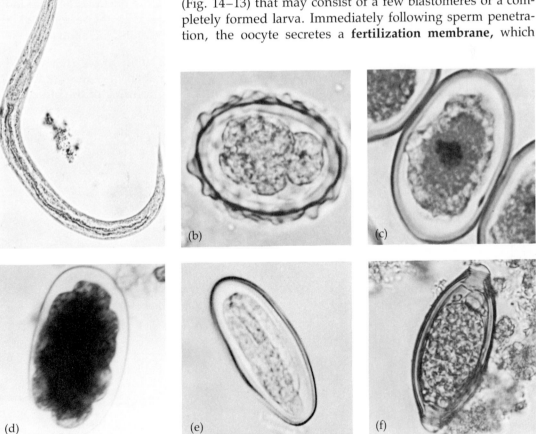

(a)

(b)

(c)

(d)

(e)

(f)

gradually thickens to form the chitinous **shell.** The inner membrane, the **lipid layer,** is also formed by the zygote. As eggs pass down the uterus, a **proteinaceous layer** is sometimes secreted by the uterine wall and deposited on the shell surface. This layer may be rough-textured (*Ascaris*) or smooth (*Trichuris*).

Eggs of parasitic nematodes may hatch either within the host or in the external environment. In the latter case, a first-stage larva usually emerges. Hatching of eggs in the external environment is controlled partially by such ambient factors as temperature, moisture, and oxygen tension and partially by the maturity of the larva. An egg will hatch only when external conditions are favorable, thus assuring that the emerging larva does not enter an unduly harsh environment.

The eggs of many nematodes hatch only after ingestion by a host, in which case hatching stimuli generated by the host may be carbon dioxide tension, salts, pH, and temperature. These conditions stimulate the enclosed larva to initiate its role in the hatching process with the secretion of enzymes to partially digest the enveloping membranes.

**Molting.**    Nematodes undergo four molts (Fig. 14–14), each of which involves (1) formation of a new cuticle, (2) loosening of the old cuticle, (3) rupturing of the old cuticle,

**Figure 14–14**
**Nematode growth pattern.**
H = hatch, M = molt, L = larvae.

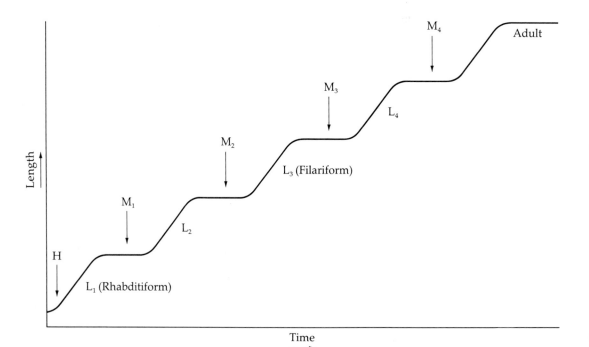

and (4) escape of the larva. This sequence of events is controlled by **exsheathing fluid** secreted by the larva. This fluid digests the cuticle at specific sites on the inner surface, causing it to loosen. Its ability to form new cuticle in the hypodermis before shedding the old one allows the nematode to develop continuously between molts; however, growth occurs most rapidly just after molting. This pattern of development strongly resembles that of the arthropods.

In some nematodes, there is a lag phase at some stage of development, during which a phase of the life cycle is temporarily arrested. Known as **hypobiosis,** this phenomenon is thought to be an adaptation that allows the larva to withstand adverse environmental conditions while awaiting access to a new host. Renewal of the life cycle following such interruption depends upon stimuli that accompany such events as penetration of host skin or being swallowed by the host. In some species, hypobiosis may occur in the definitive host.

## Larval Forms

Larval stages preceding each of the four molts in the life cycle of parasitic nematodes are generally referred to, respectively, as first-, second-, third-, and fourth-stage larvae (i.e., $L_1$, $L_2$, $L_3$, $L_4$), the first-stage larva being the stage prior to the first molt (Fig. 14–15). However, various other designations also are used for specific nematode larval forms as follows:

**Rhabditiform Larva** (Fig. 14–15a).   The first-stage larvae of such parasitic species as *Strongyloides* and hookworms are called **rhabditiform larvae.** The esophagus of this small larva is joined to a terminal esophageal bulb by a narrow isthmus.

**Filariform Larva** (Fig. 14–15b).   After molting twice, the rhabditiform larvae of *Strongyloides* and hookworms usually retain the remnants of their last cuticle and become ensheathed, third-stage or **filariform larvae,** in which the esophagus is typically elongate and cylindrical and has no terminal bulb. The filariform larva is usually the stage infective to the definitive host.

**Microfilaria** (Fig. 14–15c).   The prelarvae or advanced embryos of filarial nematodes such as *Wuchereria bancrofti* and *Loa loa* are known as **microfilariae.** The larval body surface is covered by a thin layer of flattened epidermal cells. The

**Figure 14–15**
**Diagrams of nematode larvae.**
(a) Rhabditiform. (b) Filariform.
(c) Sheathed larva of
*Wuchereria*. (d) Unsheathed
larva of *Onchocerca*.

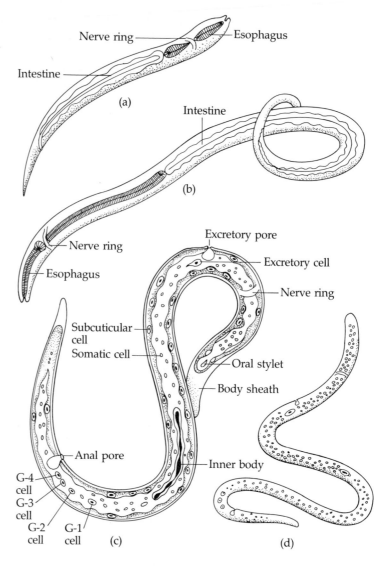

primordia of various adult structures are visible within the pseudocoelom in the form of a conspicuous cord of nucleated cytoplasm that extends the length of the body and represents the developing digestive tract. This larva, generally found in circulating blood and cutaneous tissues, is microscopic, usually measuring between 0.2 and 0.4 mm in length. Unlike tissue-dwelling microfilariae (see p. 335), microfilariae that live in host blood are usually surrounded by a thin, cuticular **sheath.**

# Physiology

Parasitic nematodes derive much of their energy from the metabolism of glycogen. This carbohydrate reserve is stored primarily in the hypodermis, the intestine, the noncontractile parts of the muscles, and parts of the reproductive system. It is difficult to establish with certainty whether adult intestinal nematodes are exclusively aerobic or anaerobic in their usage of carbohydrate or whether free-living larvae are invariably aerobic. Accumulated experimental data strongly suggest the advisability of determining not only whether each species uses oxygen but also what method of utilization each employs. For instance, intestinal nematodes belonging to the genus *Ascaris* can use oxygen if available; however, it serves only as a terminal electron acceptor in a system independent of an electron transport system or a functional Krebs' cycle. On the other hand, both larvae and adults of *Trichinella spiralis* use oxygen via the Krebs' cycle. Thus, the former organism generates ATP by means of substrate phosphorylation, while the latter organisms do so primarily through oxidative phosphorylation. The eggs and first- and second-stage larvae of *Ascaris* spp. exhibit aerobic metabolism with a functional Krebs' cycle. Indeed, optimal larval development in most species that have been studied is dependent upon relatively high concentrations of oxygen.

Some relatively large nematodes possess some sort of oxygen-binding system, including utilization of the respiratory pigments myoglobin and hemoglobin. Such pigments are usually found in the pseudocoelomic fluid and the hypodermis.

## SELECTED READINGS

Bird, A. F. 1971. *The Structure of Nematodes.* Academic Press, New York.

Gibbs, H. C. 1986. Hypobiosis in parasitic nematodes—An update. *Advances in Parasitology* 25, 129–174.

Lee, D. L., and Atkinson, H. J. 1977. *Physiology of Nematodes.* Columbia University Press, New York.

Rosenbluth, J. 1965. Ultrastructural organization of obliquely striated muscle fibers in *Ascaris lumbricoides. Journal of Cell Biology* 25, 495–515.

Rosenbluth, J. 1965. Ultrastructure of somatic cells in *Ascaris lumbricoides*. II. Intermuscular junctions, neuromuscular junctions, and glycogen stores. *Journal of Cell Biology* 26, 579–591.

Wright, K. A. 1987. The nematode's cuticle—Its surface and the epidermis: Function, homology, analogy—A current consensus. *The Journal of Parasitology* 73, 1077–1083.

# CLASSIFICATION OF THE NEMATODA*

## PHYLUM NEMATODA

Bilaterally symmetrical unsegmented pseudocoelomates; body generally elongate, cylindrical, covered by cuticle; mouth terminal, surrounded by lips; sexes separate; anterior body characteristically with 16 setiform or papilliform sensory organs and two amphids (chemoreceptors); digestive tract complete, with subterminal anus; excretory system, when present, empties through anterior, ventromedian pore; body musculature limited to longitudinally oriented muscles; no respiratory or circulatory systems; eggs with determinate cleavage, oviparous or ovoviviparous; stages in life cycle are egg, four larval stages, and adult.

### CLASS ADENOPHOREA

Amphids postlabial, variable in shape (porelike, pocketlike, circular, or spiral); cephalic sensory organs setiform to papilloid, postlabial and/or labial; setae and hypodermal glands commonly present; papillae usually present on body; hypodermal cells uninucleate; cuticle usually smooth, but transverse or longitudinal striations may be present; excretory organ, if present, single celled, ventral, and without collecting tubules; caudal glands (three) usually present (absent in most members of Dorylaimida, Mermithida, and Trichocephalida); usually two testes in males, with single ventral series of papilloid or tuboid preanal supplements; male tail rarely with caudal alae; parasitic species associated with invertebrates, vertebrates, and plants; many free living; most marine nematodes belong to this class.

#### Subclass Enoplia

When amphids occur as subcuticular pouches, external openings are transverse (cyathiform); when internal pouch is tubiform, external opening porelike, ellipsoid, or greatly elongated; cephalic sensory organs papilliform or setiform, with or without setae; caudal glands present (in most marine forms) or absent; subventral esophageal glands (five or more) commonly open into buccal cavity through teeth or at anterior esophagus; esophagus cylindrical, conical, or divided into narrow anterior portion and larger, glandular posterior portion; stichosome (a column of rectangular cells, called stichocytes, supporting and secreting into esophagus), esophagus (present in parasitic species); cuticle generally smooth, may bear transverse and/or longitudinal markings; with parasitic representatives.

*ORDER ENOPLIDA*

*ORDER ISOLAIMIDA*

*ORDER MONONCHIDA*

*ORDER DORYLAIMIDA*

---

*Only those taxa that include parasitic species are defined.

*ORDER TRICHOCEPHALIDA*
With protrusible axial spear in early larval stages; amphids adjacent to lip region; posterior esophageal glands in one or two rows along esophageal lumen, not enclosed by stichosome; stichosome and individual gland openings posterior to nerve ring; males and females with single gonad; germinal zones of male and female gonads extend entire length and form a serial germinal area on one side or around gonoduct; males with one or no spicule; eggs operculate; life cycle either direct (often requiring cannibalism), or indirect (involving arthropod or annelid intermediate host); adults parasitic in vertebrates.

*Superfamily Trichuroidea*
Stichosome of adults as single row on each side of esophagus (two rows in early larval development); body divided into elongate, narrow anterior end with esophagus with stichosome, and posterior half with reproductive system beginning at esophagointestinal junction; bacillary band (glandular and nonglandular cells of unknown function) occurs laterally; glandular tissue empty to exterior through cuticular pores; males and females with single gonad, reflexed; males with single spicule; eggs operculate—females oviparous, males small and degenerate in some species, in uterus of female; parasitic in humans and other mammals; life cycle direct or indirect. (Genus mentioned in text: Family Trichuridae[†]—*Trichuris*.)

*Superfamily Trichinelloidea*
Stichosome as single, short row of stichocytes; body not distinctly divided into two regions; no bacillary band present; female genital pore opening far anterior, in region of stichosome; ovary posterior to stichosome; males with single testis but no spicule; females viviparous. (Genus mentioned in text: Family Trichinellidae[†]—*Trichinella*.)

*ORDER MERMITHIDA*

*ORDER MUSPICEIDA*

**Subclass Chromadoria**

*CLASS SECERNENTEA*
Amphids usually open to exterior through pores located dorsolaterally on lateral lips or anterior extremity (in some species the amphidial apertures are oval, cleftlike, slitlike, or located postlabially); cephalic sensory organs are situated on lips and are porelike or papilliform, generally 16 in number arranged in two circles (a circumoral circle of 6 and an outer circle of 10), may be reduced in some species; caudal phasmids present; hypodermis uninucleate or multinucleate; cuticle from two to four layers, almost always transversely striated, laterally modified into a "wing" area marked by longitudinal striae or ridges, generally raised slightly above body contour; lateral alae may extend out a

---

[†]For diagnosis of families subordinate to the Nemata, see Maggenti, A. (1982). Nemata. In *Synopsis and Classification of Living Organisms* (S. P. Parker, ed.), pp. 879–929. McGraw-Hill, New York.

distance equal to body diameter; esophagus of most species have three esophageal glands, one dorsal (opening in anterior half of body) and two subventral (opening in posterior half of body); excretory system empties ventromedially through cuticularized duct on one or both sides of body; somatic setae or papillae absent on females; caudal papillae may occur on males; male preanal supplements paired and often elaborate; some males with medioventral preanal supplementary papillae; males commonly with caudal alae (known as copulatory bursa).

### Subclass Rhabditida

Esophagus of larvae divided into corpus, isthmus, and valved post-corporal bulb; lumen of esophageal bulb expanded into trilobed reservoir lined with cuticle; buccal cavity (stoma) without movable armature and composed of two parts (cheilostome and esophastome), each possibly subdivided into two or more sections; males generally with well developed bursae supported by cuticular rays or papillae.

#### ORDER RHABDITIA

Number of lips varies from six to none (6, 3, 2, 0); buccal cavity generally tubular but may be separated into five or more sections; esophagus divided into corpus, isthmus, and bulb; terminal excretory duct lined with cuticle and has paired, lateral collecting tubules running posteriorly; females with one or two ovaries; intestinal cells uni-, bi-, or tetranucleate; caudal alae (copulatory bursa), if present, contain papillae rather than supporting rays; parasites of invertebrates and vertebrates.

##### Suborder Rhabditina

Buccal cavity usually cylindrical, without distinct separation, generally two or more times as long as wide; lips usually distinct, with cephalic sensory papillae and porelike amphids; esophagus divided into corpus (procorpus and metacorpus) and postcorpus (isthmus and valved bulb); females with one or two ovaries; males generally with paired spicules and gubernaculum; caudal alae (copulatory bursa) common (absent in some families); parasites of invertebrates and vertebrates.

##### Superfamily Rhabditoidea

Well-developed cylindrical buccal cavity (stoma); lips vary from two to six; esophagus, at least in larvae, include muscular posterior bulb with rhabditoid valve; caudal alae of males supported by five to nine papilloid supplements; parasites of invertebrates and vertebrates. (Genus mentioned in text: Family Strongyloididae—*Strongyloides*.)

#### ORDER STRONGYLIDA

Labial region consists of three or six lips or may be replaced by corona radiata; stoma well developed or rudimentary (never collapsed and unobtrusive); esophagus of larvae typically rhabditiform (corpus, isthmus, bulb); esophageal bulb contains typical trilobed rhabdiform valve; esophagus of adults cylindrical to clavate; excretory system includes paired lateral canals and paired subventral glands; females with one or two ovaries and heavily muscular uterus; males with muscular copulatory bursa; with paired genital papillae; males with paired, equal spicules; adults parasitic in vertebrates.

*Superfamily Ancylostomatoidea*
Stoma thick-walled, globose, armed or unarmed anteriorly with teeth or cutting plates; without lips or corona radiata; copulatory bursae of males with greatly reduced branches; adults parasitic in intestine of mammals; $L_1$ and $L_2$ free living; commonly known as hookworms. (Genera mentioned in text: Family Ancylostomatidae[†]—*Ancylostoma*. Family Uncinariidae—*Necator*.)

*Superfamily Metastrongyloidea*
Oral opening may be surrounded by six well-developed or rudimentary lips; cuticle not adorned with longitudinal ridges; tail of females asymmetrical; copulatory bursa rays of males reduced and somewhat fused; adults parasitic in mammals. (Genus mentioned in text: Family Protostrongylidae[†]—*Parastrongylus*.

*ORDER ASCARIDIDA*
Oral opening usually surrounded by three lips (absent in some species); paired porelike amphids present; esophagus of some species with short swollen region in stomatal region, followed by cylindrical to club-shaped region, often ending in terminal bulb with three-lobed valve; in a few exceptions there are appendages (caeca) extending from posterior region of esophagus; excretory system with lateral collecting tubules, in some species extending posteriorly and anteriorly (H-shaped); males usually with two spicules (none or one in others); with or without gubernaculum; females usually with two ovaries (some have multiple ovaries); adults parasitic in vertebrates.

*Superfamily Ascaridoidea*
Bodies 1–40 cm long; cuticle thick in larger species, superficially annulated; terminal oral opening usually surrounded by three well-developed lips; porelike amphids on subventral lips; stoma poorly developed (collapsed); esophagus cylindrical to clavate; appendage (caecum) may extend from posterior portion of esophagus over anterior portion of intestine; second caecum may be present, extending forward past base of esophagus; females usually with paired ovaries; males with two spicules; small gubernaculum present in few species; adults parasitic in vertebrates; life cycle direct or indirect. (Genera mentioned in text: Family Ascarididae[†]—*Ascaris*. Family Toxocaridae—*Toxocara*. Family Anisakidae—*Anisakis*.)

*Superfamily Oxyuroidea*
Lips greatly reduced or absent; cephalic sensilla in whorl of eight or four; ventrolateral sensilla absent; stoma vestibular; esophagus variable but posterior bulb always valved; intestinal caeca absent; males may have precloacal suckers; copulatory

---

[†]For diagnosis of families subordinate to the Nemata, see Maggenti, A. (1982). Nemata. In *Synopsis and Classification of Living Organisms* (S. P. Parker, ed.), pp. 879–929. McGraw-Hill, New York.

spicules may be greatly reduced; adults usually parasites of amphibians, reptiles, and mammals. (Genus mentioned in text: Family Oxyuridae[+]—*Enterobius*.

## ORDER SPIRURIDA

Frequently with two lateral lips or pseudolabia (some species with four or more lips, rare species without lips); oral aperture variable in shape, encircled by teeth; amphids laterally situated on anterior extremity; stoma varies from cylindrical and elongate to rudimentary; esophagus generally divided into narrow anterior portion and expanded postcorpus enclosing multinucleate glands; hatched larvae generally provided with cephalic hook and porelike phasmids on tail; parasites of annelids, arthropods, molluscs, and terrestrial and aquatic vertebrates.

### Superfamily Filarioidea

Oral aperture circular or oval, usually surrounded by eight sensilla of external circle (internal circle absent or consisting of two or four papillae); stoma small and rudimentary esophagus with multincleate glands; corpus and postcorpus not distinct; vulva usually in anterior portion of body; copulatory spicules of males equal or unequal; caudal alae present or absent; no gubernaculum; parasites of amphibians, reptiles, birds, and mammals. (Genera mentioned in text: Family Filariidae[+]—*Wuchereria, Brugia, Onchocerca, Loa, Dirofilaria*.

### Superfamily Dracunculoidea

Stoma commonly reduced to small vestibule; full complement of sensilla surrounding oral opening, with internal circle comprised of six well-developed sensilla and external circle of eight 114 separate and well-developed sensilla; vulva in midbody region, atrophied in mature females; posterior intestine atrophied in females; males without well-developed caudal alae, small and postcloacal if present; adults are tissue parasites of fish, reptiles, and mammals. (Genus mentioned in text: Family Dracunculidae[+]—*Dracunculus*.)

---

[+]For diagnosis of families subordinate to the Nemata, see Maggenti, A. (1982). Nemata. In *Synopsis and Classification of Living Organisms* (S. P. Parker, ed.), pp. 879–929. McGraw-Hill, New York.

# CHAPTER FIFTEEN

## INTESTINAL NEMATODES

◇

# THE ADENOPHOREA

Parasitic nematodes belonging to the class Adenophorea possess neither phasmids nor an excretory system. Two parasites of the human intestinal tract, *Trichuris trichiura* and *Trichinella spiralis,* belong to this class.

## *Trichuris trichiura*

In adult *Trichuris trichiura* (Fig. 15–1), the anterior portion of the body is long and slender whereas the posterior portion widens abruptly and thickens, giving the worm the appearance of a bullwhip; hence its common name "whipworm." Males are slightly smaller than females, the latter measuring 30–50 mm in length. In both sexes, a capillarylike esophagus extends two-thirds of the body length and is encircled along much of its length by a series of unicellular glands, the **stichocytes.** The posterior extremity of males is characteristically coiled and equipped with a single spicule enclosed in a spinose, retractile cuticular sheath.

**Life Cycle** (Fig. 15–2).   Adult whipworms occur primarily in the human host's colon but also inhabit the appendix and rectum. The female deposits up to 10,000 eggs daily. These are typically barrel-shaped with two polar plugs. The eggs measure 50 by 22 μm and contain an uncleaved zygote at oviposition, after which the unembryonated eggs pass to the exterior in feces and develop slowly in warm, damp soil. An unhatched, infective, third-stage larva develops in three to six weeks.

New human hosts become infected when these embryonated eggs are ingested with contaminated food or water or from fingers. The larvae hatch in the upper portions of the small intestine and quickly burrow into the cells of the intestinal villi near the crypts of Lieberkühn, where they mature and molt in about 3–10 days. They subsequently migrate to the caecal region, molting en route, and develop to sexual maturity in 30–90 days from the time eggs are ingested. As adults, they embed the long, slender anterior part of their bodies deeply into the colon submucosa. While these worms normally have a life span of approximately 5 years in the human host, there have been reports of infections lasting 8 years or longer.

**Figure 15–1**
*Trichuris trichiura* **adult worms.**
(a) Male. (b) Female.

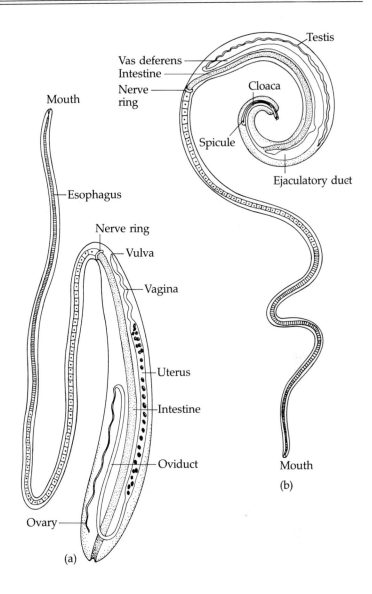

**Epidemiology.** Whipworm infection occurs worldwide, most frequently in tropical countries, and while the prevalence is very high (estimated numbers of infections are several hundred million, making it the third most common nematode infecting humans), worm burdens, fortunately, are low in the majority of cases. In the United States, it is the second most common nematode infecting humans (after *Enterobius)* and is found predominantly in the Southeast, paralleling human *Ascaris* infections. Generally, the worm is

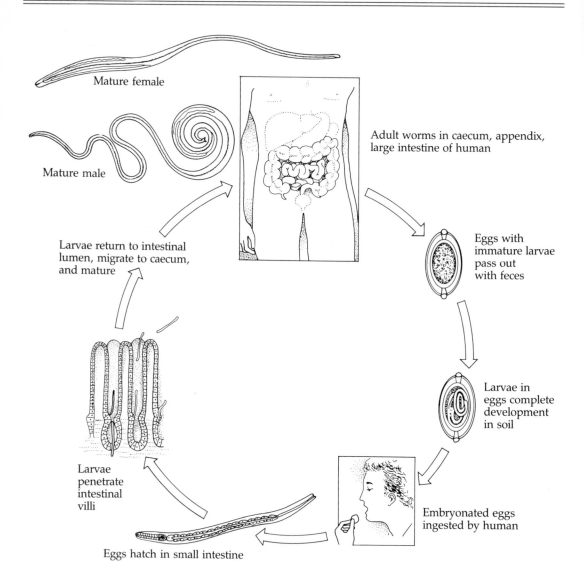

Mature female

Mature male

Adult worms in caecum, appendix, large intestine of human

Eggs with immature larvae pass out with feces

Larvae in eggs complete development in soil

Embryonated eggs ingested by human

Larvae return to intestinal lumen, migrate to caecum, and mature

Larvae penetrate intestinal villi

Eggs hatch in small intestine

**Figure 15–2**
**Life cycle of** *Trichuris trichiura.*

found in areas of warm climate, heavy rainfall, dense shade, and sanitary conditions conducive to soil pollution.

Children are more likely to be infected than adults because they are more apt to come into close physical contact with contaminated soil.

**Symptomatology and Diagnosis.**   Most infections are light with no clinical symptoms. Chronic infections, however, produce such characteristic symptoms as bloody stools, pain in the lower abdomen, weight loss, rectal prolapse, nausea, and anemia. In the case of rectal prolapse, adult worms can be observed externally, embedded in the rectal mucosa. Anemia results primarily from hemorrhage when the worms penetrate the intestinal wall, although some blood loss may be attributed to the worms ingesting host blood. In heavy infections, secondary bacterial infections are common, a result of the worms' penetration of the mucosal lining providing entry for pathogenic bacteria. Mixed infections of whipworm and *E. histolytica,* hookworm, or *Ascaris lumbricoides* are fairly common.

Identification of eggs from fecal material constitutes diagnosis.

**Treatment.**    Mebendazole, the drug of choice, is most effective when administered orally for three consecutive days. Mebendazole is one of the benzimidazolecarbamate class of compounds that generally causes degenerative changes in the nematode intestine. It is believed to have a depolymerizing effect on cytoskeletal elements, such as microtubules.

## *Trichinella spiralis*

Small and slender, adult trichina worms are rarely observed (Fig. 15–3). The male, measuring 1.5 by 0.04 mm, has a curved posterior end with two lobed appendages called **alae.** The male reproductive system, with its single testis, is located in the posterior third of the body. The female, measuring 3.5 by 0.06 mm, has a bluntly rounded posterior end and is monodelphic, with the vulva in the anterior fifth of the body.

**Life Cycle** (Fig. 15–4).    *Trichinella spiralis* requires only one host in its life cycle, with larvae and adults occurring in different organs. Infection results from the consumption of meat, most commonly poorly cooked pork, containing encapsulated first-stage larvae. Once ingested, these larvae are released in the duodenum by the action of the host's digestive enzymes. Shortly thereafter, the freed larvae penetrate the absorptive and goblet cells of the mucosa. There, within 24–30 hours, they reach sexual maturity.

Soon after copulation, the male passes out of the host, while the female burrows deeper into the mucosa and submucosa, sometimes entering the lymphatic ducts to be carried to the mesenteric lymph nodes. About 5 days after initial ingestion of infected larvae by the host, the adult

**Figure 15–3**
*Trichinella spiralis* **adult worms.**
(a) Male. (b) Female.

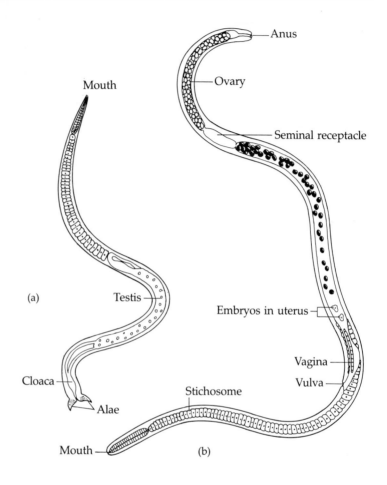

ovoviviparous female begins depositing first-stage larvae. It is estimated that one female, in a period of 9–16 weeks, produces about 1,500 larvae. Eventually, the female dies, while the first-stage larvae, about 0.1 mm long, are carried by the lymphatic and blood vessels to the right side of the heart in venous blood.

From the heart, the larvae enter the peripheral circulation and are carried to various tissues of the body. It is only in striated muscles—especially those of the diaphragm, jaws, tongue, larynx, and eyes—that larvae develop into the infective stage. Penetration of muscle cells and establishment as intracellular parasites within myofibers occurs about 6 days after initial infection. Usually a single larva occupies each muscle fiber (Fig. 15–5). On or about the seventeenth day, the larva begins to coil. It absorbs nutrients from the host muscle sarcoplasm and becomes surrounded by a nu-

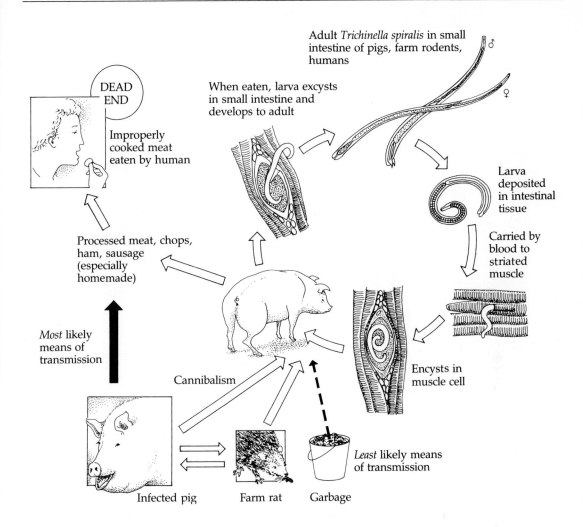

Adult *Trichinella spiralis* in small intestine of pigs, farm rodents, humans

When eaten, larva excysts in small intestine and develops to adult

DEAD END

Improperly cooked meat eaten by human

Larva deposited in intestinal tissue

Carried by blood to striated muscle

Processed meat, chops, ham, sausage (especially homemade)

*Most* likely means of transmission

Cannibalism

Encysts in muscle cell

*Least* likely means of transmission

Infected pig     Farm rat     Garbage

**Figure 15–4**
**Life cycle of *Trichinella spiralis*.**

cleated mass known as a **nurse cell.** Growth is rapid, the larva reaching a length of about 1 mm in approximately 8 weeks, at which time it becomes infective. Encapsulation begins about the twenty-first day as the larva is gradually enveloped by a double, ellipsoidal capsule of host origin 0.25–0.5 mm long. The outer capsule membrane is derived from the sarcolemma, while the inner membrane is a combination of degenerative myofibers and other cells such as fibroblasts. Capsule formation is completed in about 3 months.

Eventually, the capsule becomes calcified, a process that may begin as early as 6 months after initial infection and that requires about 18 months for completion. If calcification is delayed, a *T. spiralis* larva can remain viable for several

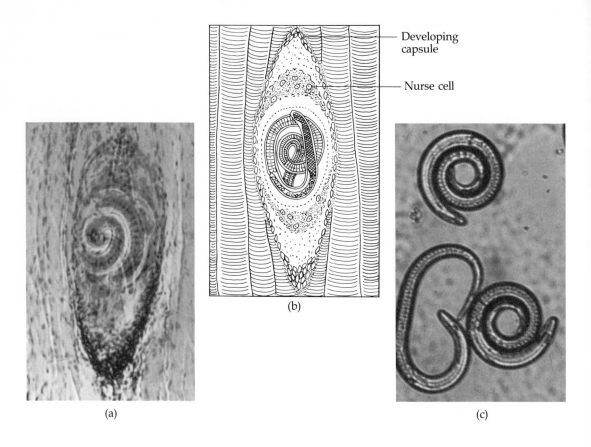

(a)

(b)

(c)

Developing capsule

Nurse cell

**Figure 15–5**
***Trichinella spiralis* encysted larva in skeletal muscle fiber.**
(a) Larva–nurse cell complex. (b) Schematic representation of larva–nurse cell complex. (c) *T. spiralis* larvae freed from nurse cells by pepsin–HC1 digestion; unstained, living.

years. During capsule formation, the enclosed larva enters developmental arrest, a state in which it can survive indefinitely. When muscle harboring the encapsulated larva is eaten by a carnivorous mammal, the larva excysts and reinitiates the life cycle.

**Epidemiology.**    The term **sylvatic trichinellosis** denotes the cycling of the disease between wild carnivores and their prey or carrion. **Urban trichinellosis,** on the other hand, is the term used to designate the cycling of the disease among humans, rats, and pigs. Rats and pigs feeding on garbage that includes infected pork waste, become infected in turn. Dead or dying infected rats are themselves eaten by the pigs. Raw or poorly cooked pork, usually sausage, harboring infective larvae then becomes the vehicle for human infections. In nature, the cycle is also maintained by cannibalistic rats.

In Alaska, where polar and black bears are common sources of human infection, there is overlapping of sylvatic and urban trichinellosis. The disastrous 1897 André hydrogen balloon expedition to the Arctic provides dramatic evidence of trichinellosis in polar bears. A book and a movie, both titled *The Flight of the Eagle*, recount the story of these ill-fated Swedish explorers who, having lost most of their supplies, perished after they resorted to eating the meat of a polar bear they had killed. Lacking any means of kindling fires, they were forced to eat the meat raw. Unfortunately, the meat was infected, and the explorers died, not from exposure but from trichinellosis. Evidence of the cause of the tragedy was discovered 33 years later in the frozen, stored carcass of the bear.

Trichinellosis is a cosmopolitan disease that occurs most commonly in Europe and the United States, where there are estimated to be about 150,000 to 300,000 cases a year, but the number of cases reported clinically is less than 150. The disease is rare in parts of the tropics and subtropics for the opposite reason that it is found in the United States: a low consumption of pork, and of meat in general, by protein-deprived peoples whose diet consists primarily of fish. However, there are parts of the tropics where the people are not protein-deprived yet the disease is rare. Religious bans keep still other peoples—such as Jews, Hindus, and Moslems—free of the disease; and, obviously, vegetarians are not exposed to infection.

**Symptomatology and Diagnosis.** The primary symptoms of trichinellosis are the result of larval invasion of muscle and other tissues and the hyperimmune reaction of the host to the metabolic by-products and secretions of the larvae. While relatively few victims have infections heavy enough to produce clinical symptoms, those infections that do occur appear during three clinical phases: (1) mild, during penetration of adult females into the mucosa; (2) severe, during migration of larvae; and (3) moderate, after penetration and encapsulation of larvae in muscle cells. Symptoms usually abate after 30 days.

Symptoms resulting from the first phase appear 12 hours to 2 days following ingestion of infective larvae. The microscopic lesions formed as a result of penetration become inflamed from host reactions against concomitant bacterial invasion and the worms' excreta. Nausea, fever, perfuse perspiration, and diarrhea commonly occur. Some facial edema may be present, accompanied by a slight rash. These symptoms subside within 5–7 days following onset.

The second phase may last for 3 weeks and is characterized by symptoms resembling such diseases as rheumatism, pneumonia, encephalitis, pleurisy, meningitis, myocarditis, and peritonitis.

During the third phase, there may be intense muscular pain, difficulty in breathing, swelling of facial muscles, weakening of blood pressure and pulse, heart damage, and nervous disorders, including hallucinations. Death may result from heart failure, respiratory complications, peritonitis, or cerebral involvement.

Most cases of human trichinellosis are asymptomatic and go undetected. In suspected cases, several diagnostic laboratory procedures are available. Positive skin and serological tests are significant. Negative tests, especially in the early stages of the disease, are inconclusive. Intradermal tests using a suspension prepared from larvae are sensitive enough to give positive results within an hour provided the suspected infection is at least 2–3 weeks old. The appearance of a wheal of about 5 mm in diameter indicates exposure to the worm. Several other serological procedures, such as flocculation and agglutination tests, are available and are similar in levels of sensitivity.

The definitive diagnostic procedure is the demonstration of live larvae in a piece of biopsied muscle. In such a demonstration, usually performed about the third or fourth week of infection, a muscle section is placed either between two slides or in a muscle press and examined microscopically, or the muscle section can be first digested with pepsin and then examined microscopically for larvae.

**Treatment.**   There is no satisfactory chemotherapeutic regimen for trichinellosis. The therapeutic value of thiabendazole and mebendazole are still under debate. Bed rest and supportive treatment, such as administration of analgesics to relieve symptoms, are beneficial. In selected cases involving the heart or the central nervous system, steroid therapy has been used successfully to relieve inflammatory symptoms.

**Prevention.**   Education of the public is the most effective way to control the disease in the human population. Additionally, laws governing pork production should be strengthened. For instance, there should be widespread legislation, as in California, requiring that garbage containing raw scraps intended for use as hog feed first be sterilized. Also, although costly, microscopic examination of pork should be reinstituted and updated. Finally, the public should be informed of the need to cook pork products thoroughly (at temperatures higher than 58.3°C), to the point at which none of the meat shows pink, in order to kill the infective larvae. Microwave cooking of pork, especially roasts, should be avoided until more precise specifications of temperature settings, time, etc., are established.

# THE SECERNENTEA

The second group of nematodes infective to humans belongs to the class Secernentea. Although species belonging to this class exhibit morphological and life cycle differences, all possess **phasmids**—minute, usually paired, chemoreceptors located posterior to the anus. The adult forms of five nematodes that infect the human intestine are discussed: the thread worm *Strongyloides stercoralis,* the two hookworms *Ancylostoma duodenale* and *Necator americanus,* the large intestinal roundworm *Ascaris lumbricoides,* and the pinworm *Enterobius vermicularis.*

## *Strongyloides stercoralis*

*Strongyloides stercoralis* and other members of this genus are unique in that they may exhibit either a **direct,** or **homogonic,** exclusively parasitic life cycle or an **indirect,** or **heterogonic,** life cycle in which free-living generations may be interrupted by parasitic generations, depending upon environmental conditions. Both the homogonic life cycle and the parasitic phase of the heterogonic life cycle involve only parthenogenetic females, while the free-living life cycle involves both males and females.

Parthenogenetic, parasitic females are 2.0–2.5 mm long (Fig. 15–6a). The esophagus, lacking a posterior bulb, extends one-third the body length, and there is a shallow buccal capsule. The vulva lies in the posterior third of the body, and the didelphic uteri contain few eggs at any one time. Males (Fig. 15–6b) are about 1.0 mm long; free-living females (Fig. 15–6c), about 2.0 mm. The uteri of a free-living

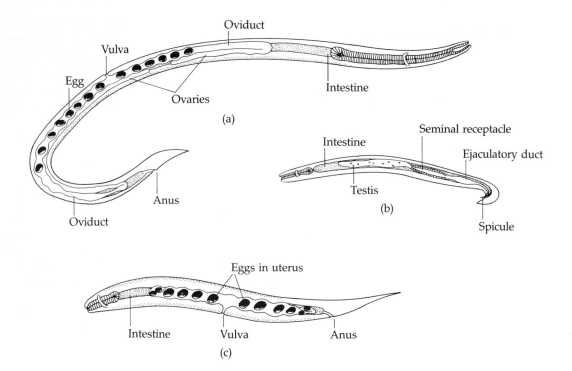

**Figure 15–6**
**Morphology of *Strongyloides stercoralis*.**
(a) Parasitic female. (b) Free-living male. (c) Free-living female.

female contain many more eggs than do those of its parasitic counterpart. The free-living female is also somewhat larger, with the vulva situated in the midsection of the body.

**Life Cycle** (Fig. 15–7). The life cycle of *S. stercoralis* can be divided into three phases: free-living, parasitic, and auto-infectious.

*Free-living Phase.* Free-living *S. stercoralis* dwell in moist soil in warm climates. Copulation occurs in the soil. When the sperm penetrates an oocyte, its nucleus disintegrates. Sperm penetration merely activates the oocyte to develop parthenogenetically with no contribution to the genetic material of the developing embryo. Following oviposition, the first-stage, rhabditiform larvae are well developed and require only a few hours for complete development. The eggs hatch in the soil, where the liberated larvae feed actively on organic debris, pass through four molts, and develop into sexually mature adults.

This free-living, or heterogonic, cycle may continue without interruption. However, if the environment becomes inhospitable, the rhabditiform larva molts twice to become a nonfeeding, filariform larva, the form infective to humans.

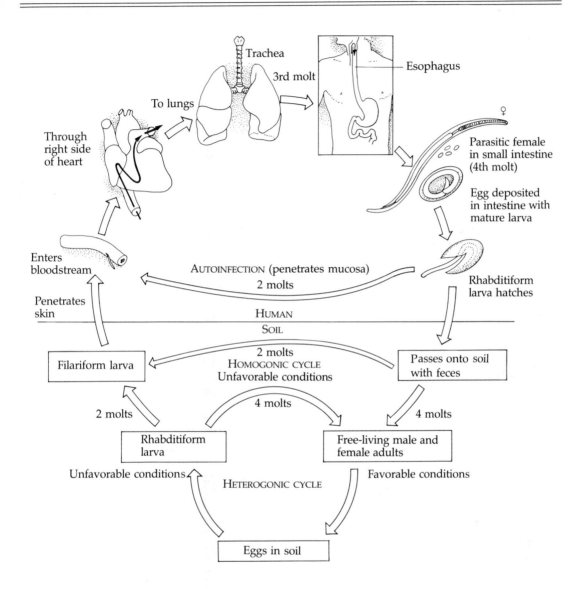

Trachea

3rd molt

To lungs

Esophagus

Through
right side
of heart

♀

Parasitic female
in small intestine
(4th molt)

Egg deposited
in intestine with
mature larva

Enters
bloodstream

AUTOINFECTION (penetrates mucosa)
2 molts

Rhabditiform
larva hatches

Penetrates
skin

HUMAN

SOIL

Filariform larva

2 molts
HOMOGONIC CYCLE
Unfavorable conditions

Passes onto soil
with feces

2 molts

4 molts

4 molts

Rhabditiform
larva

Free-living male and
female adults

Unfavorable conditions

HETEROGONIC CYCLE

Favorable conditions

Eggs in soil

**Figure 15–7**
**Life cycle of** *Strongyloides*
*stercoralis.*

*Parasitic Phase.*    When filariform larvae encounter a human or other suitable host, they readily penetrate the skin and are carried by the lymphatics or the small cutaneous veins to the postcaval vein, whence they enter the right side of the heart and are carried to the lungs via the pulmonary artery. In the lungs, following a third molt, the larvae rupture from the pulmonary capillaries and enter the alveoli.

From the alveoli, the larvae move up the respiratory tree to the epiglottis. Abetted by coughing and subsequent swallowing by the host, they migrate over the epiglottis to the esophagus and down to the small intestine, where they undergo a final molt and become sexually mature females. Parasitic males have been observed only rarely. Only females burrow into the mucosa of the small intestine and produce embryonated eggs parthenogenetically. The eggs average 54 by 32 μm and possess a thin, transparent shell. These hatch in the mucosa into first-stage rhabditiform larvae, which feed during passage through the lumen of the intestine and exit the host body with feces. Eggs are seldom found in feces. Under conditions favorable for development, the larvae become established in the soil, undergo four molts, and become free-living adults. However, under adverse conditions, the rhabditiform larvae metamorphose into infective filariform larvae after two molts.

*Autoinfection.*    During passage through the host digestive tract, rhabditiform larvae may rapidly undergo two molts into filariform larvae and, by penetrating the intestinal mucosa or perianal skin, enter the circulatory system and continue their parasitic lives without ever leaving the host. Such a cycle is not uncommon and accounts for some World War II veterans having harbored infections for more than 40 years, as well as for the development of increasingly heavy, even lethal, infections.

**Epidemiology.**    Humans usually contract infection through contact with infective larvae in the soil, less frequently from larvae in contaminated water. It has been estimated that human cases of strongyloidiasis currently number 34.9 million worldwide. There are an estimated 21 million cases in Asia, 900,000 in the USSR, 8.6 million in Africa, 4 million in tropical America, 400,000 in North America, and 100,000 in the Pacific islands. The free-living forms thrive best in warm, moist climates where sanitation is lacking. Among residents of mental institutions, the prevalence in feces of infective larvae or larvae capable of rapidly becoming infective, combined with poor sanitation and/or unsanitary personal habits, results in a high incidence of infection. A study of 1,437 mental patients in New York City institutions revealed an 18% rate of infection.

Since dogs and cats also serve as sources of human infection, the disease can be considered zoonotic.

**Symptomatology and Diagnosis.**    Symptoms of human strongyloidiasis appear in three phases: cutaneous, pulmonary, and intestinal.

The cutaneous phase is characterized by slight hemorrhaging, swelling, and intense itching ("ground itch") at sites that have been invaded by infective filariform larvae. Occasionally, the invasion sites are secondarily invaded by infectious, microbial agents, resulting in severe inflammation.

Larval migration through the lungs produces the pulmonary phase. Lung damage due to massive, cellular reactions to the migrating larvae may delay or prevent further migration. When this happens, the larvae may develop in the lungs and commence reproducing as they would in the intestine, in which case the patient develops burning sensations in the chest, a cough, and other symptoms of bronchial pneumonia.

Intestinal symptoms appear when female worms become embedded in the mucosa and, rarely, beyond the muscularis. Moderate to heavy infections produce pain and intense burning in the abdominal region, accompanied by nausea, vomiting, and intermittent diarrhea. Long-standing infections result in chronic dysentery and weight loss. Very heavy infections may be fatal, attributable, in most instances, to massive invasion of tissues by filariform larvae, to secondary bacterial infections from ulceration of intestinal mucosa, or to immunosuppression (as in AIDS patients).

The surest means of diagnosis is microscopical identification of rhabditiform, and sometimes filariform, larvae in feces. Accurate diagnosis requires that larvae of *S. stercoralis* be distinguished from those of hookworms, which they resemble (Fig. 15–8). Occasionally, eggs are passed in the feces, in which case these also must be distinguished from hookworm eggs (Fig. 14–13). The same is true when duodenal fluid is aspirated for examination. Sputum should also be examined for larvae.

Serological tests have proven useful. Enzyme-linked immunosorbent assays (ELISA), which produce few cross-reactions, have been used successfully.

**Treatment.**    Oral administration of thiabendazole over a period of 2–7 days, depending upon resistance of the worms, is the therapy of choice. Relapses of the intestinal phase have been reported, especially in patients who are immunologically compromised (irradiated cancer patients, tissue transplant patients, etc.).

**Prevention.**    Prevention requires the sanitary disposal of human excrement, protection of skin from contact with contaminated soil, and appropriate treatment in cases of autoinfection.

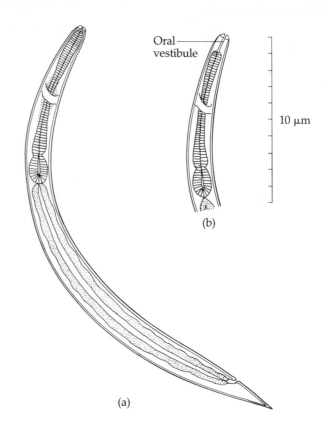

Oral
vestibule

10 μm

(b)

(a)

**Figure 15–8**
**Rhabditiform larvae.**
(a) *Strongyloides stercoralis.*
(b) Anterior portion of
rhabditiform larva of
hookworm. Note the elongated
oral vestibule.

# HUMAN HOOKWORM

Hookworm disease has been, and remains, among the most prevalent and important of human parasitic diseases. Unlike malaria, amoebiasis, or schistosomiasis, hookworm disease may not be clinically spectacular; yet it can profoundly affect entire populations by gradually sapping the victims' strength, vitality, and overall well-being. As commonly seen in certain parts of the Near and Far East, and until recently in the southeastern United States, victims become lethargic and nonproductive, resulting in economic losses beyond calculation. While great progress has been made in combating this scourge, hookworm disease has by no means been controlled or eradicated but remains a major public health problem in many parts of the world, especially in developing countries.

Adults of two species of hookworms, *Ancylostoma duodenale* and *Necator americanus*, cause infection among hu-

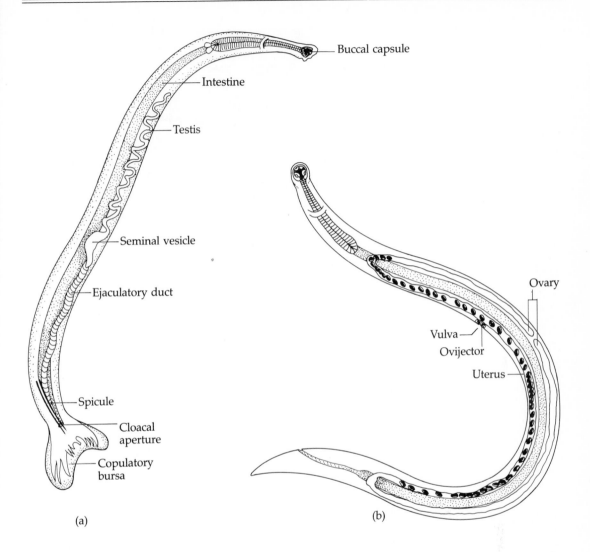

**Figure 15–9**
**Morphology of adult hookworms.**
(a) Male. (b) Female.

mans. Since these worms are similar in morphology and life cycle, they will be described together with notations on dissimilarities (Fig. 15–9).

## Ancylostoma duodenale

Adults are somewhat larger than those of *N. americanus*. Female adults measure about 9–13 mm long, while males are 5–11 mm long. The female reproductive system is didelphic; males have a single testis. The posterior end of the male has an umbrella-shaped bursa with riblike rays that expands over and envelops the vulva of the female to anchor the

**Figure 15–10**
**Copulatory bursa of male**
**hookworm.**

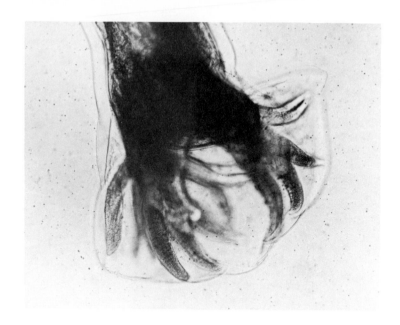

male during copulation (Fig. 15–10). The vulva is located in the anterior half of the body in female *N. americanus* and in the posterior half in *A. duodenale*. There are chitinous specializations in the buccal capsules of both species (Fig. 15–11). *N. americanus* has a conspicuous pair of semilunar cutting plates on the dorsal wall, a concave tooth on the dorsal medial wall, and a pair of triangular lancets deeper on the ventral wall of the buccal capsule; *A duodenale*, on the other

**Figure 15–11**
**Comparison of hookworm**
**buccal capsules.**
(a) *Ancylostoma.* (b) *Necator.*

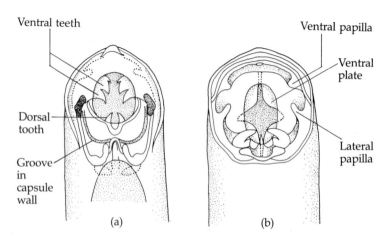

hand, has two pairs of teeth on the ventral wall of its buccal capsule.

Eggs of the two species are indistinguishable other than that those of *N. americanus* are slightly larger, measuring 64–76 μm long and 36–40 μm wide. Eggs from both species have thin, transparent shells and bluntly rounded ends and upon oviposition, enclose uncleaved embryos.

**Life Cycle** (Fig. 15–12).   Humans, almost exclusively, are hosts for *A. duodenale,* while dogs are also common hosts for *N. americanus.* Eggs are passed out in feces; under optimal conditions (temperature of 23–33°C, shade, and a sandy soil rich in organic materials), a rhabditiform larva matures

**Figure 15–12**
**Life cycle of hookworm.**

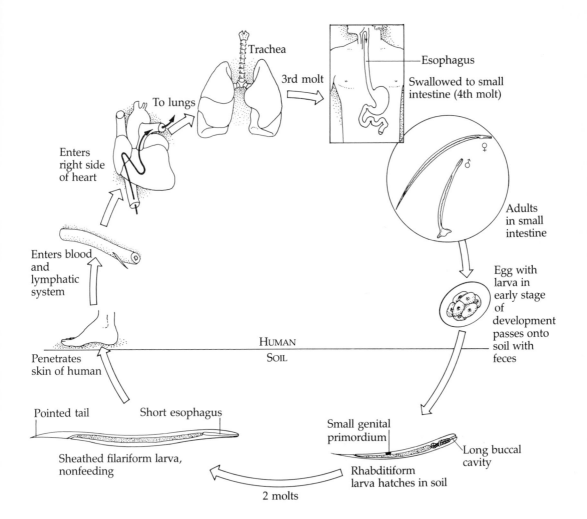

in 1–2 days and hatches from the shell. The newly hatched larva, about 275 μm long, feeds on bacteria and organic materials in the soil and doubles its size in 5 days. After two molts, the rhabditiform larva becomes a nonfeeding, infective, filariform larva. The cuticle of the last molt is retained and encloses the larva as a sheath.

These active filariform larvae inhabit the upper 10 cm of soil, usually remaining within 50 cm of the initial site of oviposition, where they can live up to 6 weeks. Human infection occurs when ensheathed filariform larvae penetrate the skin, usually that of the feet and legs. Entry is most often through hair follicles, pores, and skin abrasions. Upon penetration, the larvae enter the host's lymphatic system, migrate to the right side of the heart, and then enter the lungs via the pulmonary artery. Rupturing from lung capillaries, they enter the alveoli and migrate up the respiratory tree, molting en route, and then are coughed up and swallowed. This migratory period lasts about one week. At the third molt, each larva develops a temporary buccal capsule, enabling it to develop into a feeding, adolescent worm. Once the larvae reach the small intestine, they actively burrow into the intervillar spaces where, at about the thirteenth day, they undergo their fourth molt. They become sexually mature adults 5–6 weeks post-penetration.

**Epidemiology.**    An estimated 72.5 million humans harbor *A. duodenale*, the majority (59 million) in Asia. Some 384.3 million humans are infected with *N. americanus* worldwide, of which one million live in the United States.

*A. duodenale*, commonly known as the Old World hookworm, occurs in southern Europe, North Africa, India, China, Japan, and southeast Asia. It also has been reported in the New World among Paraguayan Indians, in isolated areas of the United States, and in the islands of the Caribbean. Infection confirmed among coal miners in Belgium and Great Britain produces a classic form of anemia. Similarly, tunnel construction workers in Switzerland, Germany, and Italy are commonly infected.

## Necator americanus

The New World, or American, hookworm, is found in the southern United States, Central and South America, and the Caribbean islands. This species is also indigenous to Africa, India, southeast Asia, China, and the southwestern Pacific islands. It is believed to have been introduced into the Americas during the slave trade era or even earlier.

Four essential factors in the spread of hookworm are (1) shaded sandy or loamy soil; (2) sufficient moisture to assure development of eggs and larvae, that is, rainfall of 75–125 cm during the warm months of the year; (3) contamination of the soil by feces containing eggs, introduced as a result of poor sanitation and/or the use of human excrement for fertilizer; and (4) a population that, by choice or necessity, comes in contact with contaminated soil.

**Symptomatology and Diagnosis.**    The course of human hookworm disease can be divided into three phases: invasion, migration, and establishment in the intestine.

Invasion commences when infective larvae penetrate human skin. Although little damage is inflicted upon the superficial skin layers, cellular reaction that is stimulated during blood vessel penetration may isolate and kill the larvae. Local irritation from invading larvae, combined with inflammatory reaction to accompanying bacteria, stimulates the appearance of an urticarial condition commonly known as **ground itch.**

The migration phase is the period during which larvae escape from capillary beds in the lung, enter the alveoli, and progress up the bronchi to the throat. This migration can produce severe hemorrhaging when large numbers of worms are involved; otherwise, a dry cough and sore throat may be the only symptoms.

The most serious stage of hookworm infection occurs when the parasites become established in the host's intestine. Upon reaching the small intestine, young worms use their buccal capsules and "teeth" to burrow through the mucosa, where they begin vigorously feeding on blood (Fig. 15–13). Salivary secretions of the worms contain anticoagulants to facilitate blood-feeding. When more than 25 *N. americanus* or 10 *A. duodenale* are present, even if 40% of the iron removed by the worms is reabsorbed by the host, an iron-deficiency anemia develops, accompanied by intermittent abdominal pain, loss of appetite, and a craving to eat soil (geophagy). Heavy infections often produce severe anemia, protein deficiency, dry skin and hair, edema, distended abdomen (especially in children), stunted growth, delayed puberty, mental dullness, cardiac failure, and even death.

Diagnosis based on clinical symptoms can be misleading because the same symptoms may result from nutritional deficiencies or from a combination of infection and such

**Figure 15–13**
**Photomicrograph of hookworm**
**buccal capsule.**

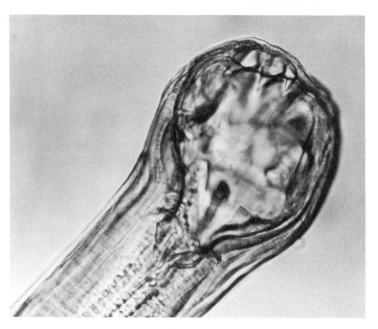

deficiencies. Positive diagnosis requires identification of eggs in feces. For light infections, concentration-type diagnostic techniques, such as zinc sulfate flotation or several modifications of the formalin–ether method, are employed.

Meticulous care in identification of larvae is essential, especially from stools that are several days old, since the rhabditiform larvae of hookworms strongly resembles that of *Strongyloides* (Fig. 15–8) and even of ruminant parasites such as *Trichostrongylus* spp., which occasionally infect humans.

**Treatment.**   Several drugs provide effective treatment for both human hookworm species. One, mebendazole, given orally for three consecutive days, results in a very high cure rate. When severe anemia has developed due to hookworm infection, the anemia should be treated first. While oral administration of iron prior to treatment for hookworm quickly restores hemoglobin levels, reversing the course of treatment delays hemoglobin restoration to normal levels for months.

**Prevention.**   Obvious precautions are required to prevent the spread of hookworm infection: improved sanitation, including proper disposal of human excrement; treatment of infected individuals; protective measures to prevent contact with infective larvae; and correction of nutritional deficiencies to reduce susceptibility. Proper disposal of dog feces is important in programs to control *N. americanus*. Finally, education of the people is always an important aspect of control programs.

## Cutaneous Larval Migrans

Similar to the manner in which animal schistosome larvae attack humans, infective filariform hookworm larvae of animals, for which humans are incompatible hosts, often penetrate human skin. Such larvae normally fail to pass beyond the stratum germinativum, instead persisting and migrating for some time at that level, causing a skin condition not unlike schistosome dermatitis known as **cutaneous larval migrans,** or **creeping eruption** (Fig. 15–14). The most common

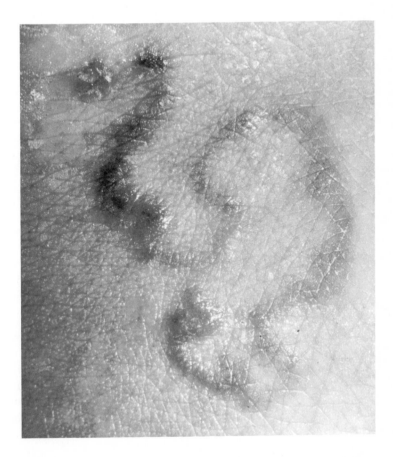

**Figure 15–14**
**Cutaneous larval migrans.**

agents are the cat and dog hookworms *Ancylostoma braziliense* and *A. caninum.*

**Epidemiology.**    Creeping eruption is prevalent in many parts of the world, particularly in tropical and subtropical regions. In the United States, incidence is high along the Gulf Coast and in the southern Atlantic states. Humans become infected with animal hookworms by contact with soil upon which infected dogs and cats have defecated. A frequent source is children's sandboxes, which, during summer days, afford optimum conditions of shade, sandy soil, and warmth. Infective larvae also thrive in the soil under houses. It is not surprising, therefore, that infection rates are highest among children, plumbers, electricians, etc.

**Symptomatology and Diagnosis.**    The feet, arms, and face are the most common sites of infection; however, any part of the body that comes in contact with contaminated soil is susceptible. Red, itchy papules develop at the invasion site, and the migratory paths of the larvae appear as slightly elevated ridges. These ridges represent an inflammatory response to the cutaneous tunnels made by the burrowing larvae. This tunneling phenomenon, probably due to larvae seeking a point of entry into the circulatory system, produces intense itching along the migratory pathways. The larval infection may persist for weeks or even months, and secondary bacterial infection is common.

**Treatment.**    Treatment is generally directed toward alleviating symptoms, such as the intense itching, rather than destroying the larvae. A topical ointment consisting of a 10% suspension of thiabendazole has proven effective, and light infections often respond to chilling of the active portion of the lesion with ethyl chloride. The latter treatment must be administered with extreme caution since prolonged exposure to ethyl chloride can produce second degree burns. Any accompanying microbial infection should be treated with antibiotics and/or fungicides.

**Prevention.**    Obviously, prevention of cutaneous larval migrans caused by hookworms depends upon avoiding contact with soil contaminated with feces from infected dogs and cats. Toward that end, animals should be denied access to underhouse crawl spaces, sandboxes should be kept covered when not in use, and pets should be treated with appropriate anthelmintics.

## *Ascaris lumbricoides*

Among *Ascaris lumbricoides*, known as the large intestinal roundworm of humans, females may attain lengths of 40 cm, while male worms may reach 30 cm (Fig. 15–15). In both sexes, the mouth is surrounded by one dorsal and two ventrolateral lips. The posterior end of the female is straight, while that of the male curves ventrally. The didelphic female reproductive system is located in the posterior two-thirds of the body, with the vulva situated about one-third of the body length from the anterior end. The female is prodigious in egg production, depositing about 200,000 daily. The uterus may contain up to 27 million eggs at a time. The fertilized egg measures 45–75 μm long and 35–50 μm wide.

**Life Cycle** (Fig. 15–16).   Adult worms live in the lumen of the small intestine and draw nourishment from the semidigested food of the host. Copulation occurs at this site, and eggs are passed with feces. The outer, albuminous coat of the egg is golden brown due to bile pigment absorbed from feces (see Fig. 14–13c). Among the oval, fertilized eggs are found numerous unfertilized eggs, identifiable by their elongated shape and the absence of an albuminous coat. When fertilized eggs are deposited, the zygote is uncleaved, and it remains in this state until the eggs reach soil. Eggs deposited in soil are resistant to desiccation and low temperature but are vulnerable to temperatures slightly above that of the host's body. The zygote within the eggshell develops when the environmental (soil) temperature (about 25°C) is lower than the body temperature of the host (i.e., 37°C). However, development ceases at temperatures below 15.5°C, and eggs are killed at temperatures above 38°C.

After 2–4 weeks in moist soil with proper temperature and oxygen levels, the embryo molts at least once in the shell and develops to an infective larva. Eggs containing infective larvae may remain viable in the soil for two years or longer.

After being ingested by a human, infective eggs hatch in the duodenum. The larvae actively burrow into the mucosal lining, enter the circulatory system, and are carried via the venous system to the liver, through the right side of the heart, and on to the lungs by way of the pulmonary arterial flow. This migration requires approximately one week. The larvae remain in the lungs for several days, molting twice during this sojourn, eventually rupturing from the pulmo-

**Figure 15–15**
*Ascaris lumbricoides.*
(a) Male and female adults, external view. (b) Female reproductive system teased out of body. (c) Cut-away view of adult male.

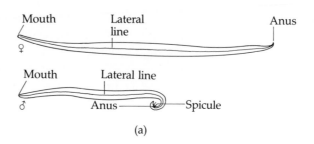

(a)

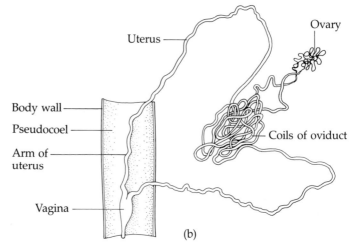

(b)

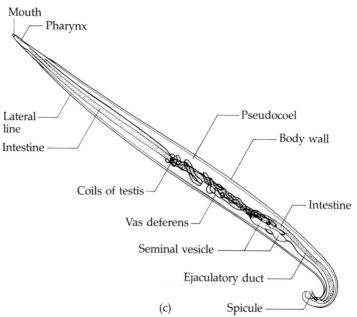

(c)

nary capillaries, and entering the alveoli. From there, they move up the respiratory tree and trachea to the epiglottis to be coughed up, swallowed, and passed down again to the small intestine. During this complex migratory process, individual worms increase from 200–300 μm to approximately ten times that length. A fourth molt occurs in the small intestine, and only worms that undergo this final molt survive in the intestine and develop to sexual maturity. The interval

**Figure 15–16**
**Life cycle of *Ascaris lumbricoides.***

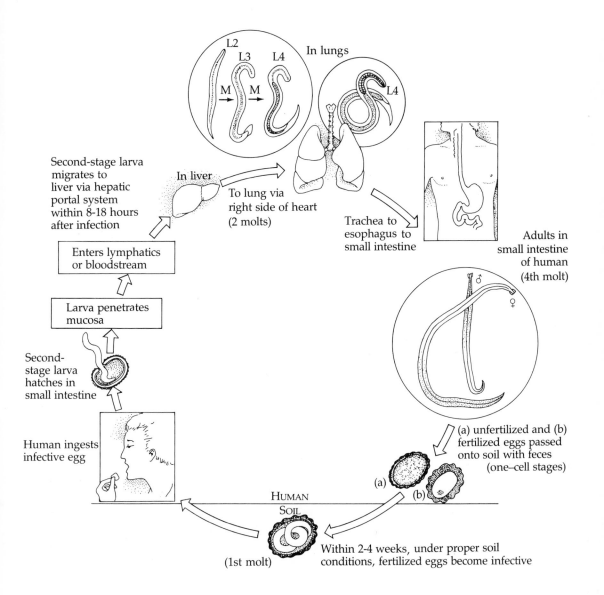

from ingestion of infective eggs to the appearance of sexually mature worms in the small intestine is about 3 months.

**Epidemiology.**    Distribution of *A. lumbricoides* is worldwide, but it is more prevalent in warmer climates. Dependent upon poor sanitation for its spread, human ascariasis has been described as a household and backyard infection. As estimated 1,008 million people are infected, making it the most common nematode parasitizing humans. It is most prevalent in children, particularly between the ages of 5 and 9 years, the group most frequently exposed to contaminated soil and least likely to observe basic sanitary practices such as washing hands before eating and keeping hands out of the mouth. Hand-to-mouth transmission is most common; however, in countries where human excrement is used as fertilizer, contaminated vegetables are also a common source of infection. Water is rarely implicated in transmitting *A. lumbricoides.*

Since ascariasis is more prevalent in humid climates than in arid ones, its occurrence is often patchy within individual countries. For instance, prevalence in Nigeria ranges from 0.9 to 98.2%; in India, from 8.0 to 90.6%; and, in Ghanaian villages, from 0 to 76%. Generally, prevalence is highest in Africa and Asia, with 40% of the population infected. Latin America follows closely, with 32%.

**Symptomatology and Diagnosis.**    About 85% of ascariasis cases are symptomless; however, the most frequent symptom is upper abdominal discomfort of varying intensity. Symptoms such as asthma, insomnia, eye pain, and rashes represent allergic responses of the host to metabolic excretions and secretions of adult worms, as well as to dead and dying worms. Little damage results from larval penetration of the host's intestinal mucosa. However, aberrant larvae migrating in such organs as the spleen, liver, lymph nodes, and brain usually elicit an inflammatory response. Also, larvae escaping from capillaries in the lungs and entering the respiratory system cause small, hemorrhagic foci accompanied by coughing, fever, and difficulty in breathing. When larvae occur in large numbers, numerous small blood clots may develop, leading to potentially fatal pneumonitis if large areas of the lungs are affected.

Large numbers of worms sometimes cause mechanical blockage of the intestinal tract, and worms may penetrate the intestinal wall or appendix, causing local hemorrhage, peritonitis, and/or appendicitis. Adult female worms may even wander up the bile duct to the liver, causing abcesses, or down the pancreatic duct, causing fatal, hemorrhagic pancreatitis. Loss of appetite and insufficient absorption of digested food also occur as a result of heavy infections. Migration of worms can also be promoted by high fever, chemotherapy, administration of anesthesia, etc.

Diagnosis is made by identification of eggs in feces (Fig. 14–13). Since egg production is fairly constant (about 200,000 eggs per female daily), egg counts can provide a fairly accurate estimate of the number of adult worms present provided standard-sized samples are used.

**Treatment.**    For treatment of individual patients not requiring hospital care, piperazine citrate is highly effective, about 85% of infections responding to a single dose. The drug paralyzes the worm, nullifying its normal ability to counter intestinal peristalsis and causing it to be passed out of the host. For general control, however, mass treatments of the populace with broad spectrum anthelmintics—such as mebendazole, thiabendazole, pyrantel embonate, or albendazole—two or three times a year are most effective.

**Prevention.**    The most reliable preventive measure consists of a multipronged attack emphasizing scrupulous personal hygiene, public sanitation, health education, and environmental sanitation, especially the processing of night soil. For optimal effectiveness, such a program should be combined with mass treatment of the population.

## Visceral Larval Migrans

**Visceral larval migrans** usually results from migration of second-stage larvae of ascaroids, the adults of which normally are found in dogs and cats, within the internal organs of accidental hosts, primarily young children. Most commonly, human visceral larval migrans develops following ingestion of infective eggs of *Toxocara canis*, although several other nematode species, such as *Bayliascaris procyonis and T. cati*, can also cause the condition. In humans, second-stage larvae hatching from the eggs penetrate the intestinal wall and quickly invade the liver. Although the majority of these larvae remain in the liver, some pass on to the lungs and, sometimes, the central nervous system and eyes. Although most of the larvae eventually gravitate to a single location and become encapsulated by host tissues, for a period of at least several weeks they actively migrate through tissues, leaving long trails of inflammatory and granulomatous reaction cells.

It should be emphasized that, while hookworms of nonhuman hosts are the usual suspects in cases of cutaneous larval migrans, and *T. canis* is most often implicated in visceral larval migrans in humans, location of lesions and even presence of characteristic symptoms are not completely reliable criteria for specific identification of the etiologic agent.

**Epidemiology.**    Since symptoms of visceral larval migrans are imprecise and inconsistent and since dog parasites were long considered noninjurious to humans, confirmed cases of this disease have been rare. However, available reports indicate that the disease occurs worldwide and probably involves several nematode species. In the United States, a high percentage of puppies and kittens are infected with *Toxocara*, perhaps as many as 98% according to some reports. The life cycle of *T. canis* appears to occur only in puppies. In adult dogs, the second-stage larva encysts in various tissues. In pregnant bitches, these larvae can become activated and migrate, crossing the placenta, infecting the fetal pup, and there completing the life cycle. The close association of young children with their pets has been cited frequently as a factor in the transmission of parasitic disease; hence, it is not surprising that this segment of the population is the most vulnerable to this disease. The ubiquitous sandbox provides an ideal setting for survival of eggs, as do park areas and beaches where owners walk their dogs.

**Symptomatology and Diagnosis.**    The degree of pathology is related to the number of eggs ingested and the site where the larvae settle. Most infections are light, and symptoms include fever, pulmonary congestion, and eosinophilia.

Characteristic lesions most often occur in the liver and are accompanied by concentrations of various leukocytes, especially eosinophils. The lesion is a protective response of the host, but it also protects the larva since it isolates the parasite from further contact with host defense mechanisms.

In heavy infections, some children develop anemia from the excessive leukocyte buildup. Ocular disease may develop when larvae become trapped in the eye. The severest consequences of the infection are usually allergic reactions, especially if the patient is hypersensitive to metabolites produced by the larval nematodes, although in rare instances death due to toxicariasis has been reported.

Diagnosis is complicated because of the lack of a specific body of symptoms. Eosinophilia and hepatomegaly occurring in conjunction with a history of proximity to pets are clinically significant. While the only definitive diagnosis is identification of the larvae, this is exceedingly difficult to obtain since they are usually too few in number to be retrieved by needle biopsy. An effective ELISA test is currently being used to detect antibodies directed against the excretory–secretory antigens of *Toxocara* larvae.

**Treatment.**    Most infections are self-limiting, and only severe cases are treated. Thiabendazole, sometimes with corticosteroids when allergic symptoms also occur, is the drug of choice.

**Prevention.**    Generally, children should be protected from exposure by routine treatment of pets for worms. Puppies and kittens should be treated every 6 months and adult pets every 2 months. Sandboxes should be covered when not in use.

## *Anisakis* spp.

Anisakid nematodes include a number of ascaroid species that normally infect the stomach and intestines of a variety of marine animals—fishes, birds, and such fish-eating mammals as dolphins, whales, seals, and porpoises. Third-stage larvae, usually measuring about 2–3 cm long and 0.5–1.0 mm wide, are found in the body cavities, liver, or musculature of a number of marine fishes that serve as intermediate or paratenic hosts in the life cycle of the worms.

*Anisakis* and certain other anisakid nematodes, especially *Pseudoterranova* and *Phocanema*, represent a public health concern in many parts of the United States for humans who eat raw or inadequately cooked fish harboring infective larvae in their flesh. It is a major parasitologic problem in Japan and parts of Scandinavia, and was once so in the Netherlands. Human anisakiasis has essentially disappeared from the Netherlands due to new laws regulating fish processing that prohibit holding fish on boats without immediate refrigeration. When left at ambient temperature, anisakid larvae migrate from the intestinal tracts of fishes into the flesh, where they are more likely to be accidentally eaten by humans.

**Figure 15–17**
**Photomicrograph of a section through the esophagus of an *Anisakis* larva in the human intestinal tract.**

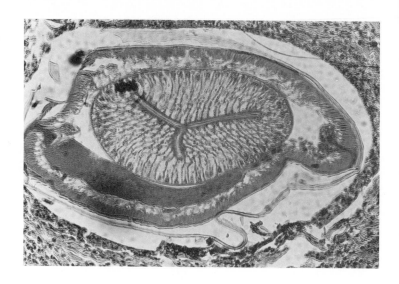

When ingested by a human, larvae burrow into the stomach or intestinal walls and cause inflammatory responses varying from localized granulomata to massive, eosinophilic, hemorrhagic, tumorlike growths (neoplasms with larvae at the center of the lesion) (Fig. 15–17). Consequent swelling of the intestinal wall may cause intestinal obstruction, peritonitis, and the development of abcesses. Most cases have been reported from countries where fish, such as herring in Scandinavia and sashimi in Japan, are eaten raw. The spreading popularity of sushi restaurants in the United States (especially California and Hawaii) has caused an increase in anasakiasis. A number of human deaths have been attributed to anisakiasis.

## *Enterobius vermicularis*

This nematode, commonly known as the pinworm or seatworm, is parasitic only to humans (Fig. 15–18). It is familiar to parents of young children worldwide. Female *Enterobius vermicularis*, measuring 8–13 mm long by 0.4 mm wide, are characterized by the presence of winglike expansions (**alae**) of the body wall at the anterior end, distension of the body due to the large numbers of eggs in the uteri, and a pointed tail. Males, smaller in size, are 2–5 mm long and possess a curved tail.

**Figure 15–18
Morphology of adult
*Enterobius vermicularis.*
(a) Male. (b) Female.**

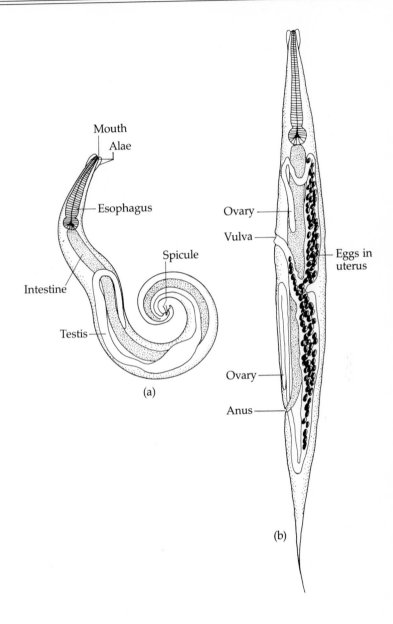

(a)

(b)

**Life Cycle** (Fig. 15–19).    Sexually mature worms usually inhabit the ileocaecal area of the human intestinal tract, but they can spread to adjacent regions of the small and large intestines. Adhering to the mucosa, the worms feed on bacteria and epithelial cells. Males die following copulation, while egg-bearing females with up to 15,000 eggs in their uteri migrate to the perianal and perineal regions. There,

**Figure 15–19**
**Life cycle of *Enterobius vermicularis*.**

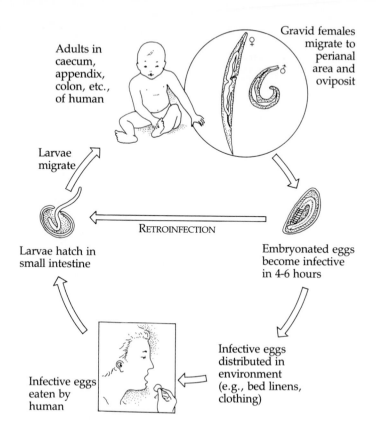

Adults in caecum, appendix, colon, etc., of human

Gravid females migrate to perianal area and oviposit

Larvae migrate

RETROINFECTION

Larvae hatch in small intestine

Embryonated eggs become infective in 4-6 hours

Infective eggs eaten by human

Infective eggs distributed in environment (e.g., bed linens, clothing)

stimulated by the lower temperature and the aerobic environment, they deposit their eggs and then also die. More eggs are released when the female's body ruptures. The elongate eggs, each measuring approximately 50–60 by 20–30 μm, are characteristically flattened on one side and contain, upon deposition, an immature larva. The infective, third-stage larva develops within the egg several hours after leaving the body of the female worm. Infection and reinfection occur when eggs containing the infective larvae are ingested by the host. Such eggs are usually picked up from bedclothes or fingernails contaminated when the host scratches the perianal zone to relieve the itching caused by nocturnal migration of the female worms. However, the lightweight eggs are sometimes airborne and so can also be inhaled. Retroinfections occur when third-stage larvae hatch from perianally located eggs and migrate back up the host's intestinal tract.

Ingested eggs usually hatch shortly after reaching the duodenum. The escaping larvae undergo molts and development as they migrate posteriorly, becoming sexually mature when they arrive at the colon. The life cycle of *E. vermicularis* is generally completed in about 2 months. While vulnerable to even moderately high temperatures, eggs are highly resistant to drying and remain viable for a week or more under cool, humid conditions. There are claims that eggs can remain viable for years under suitable conditions.

**Epidemiology.**    Children, especially of early school-age, are most frequently infected with *E. vermicularis*. Geographic distribution of the worm is global. It is especially prevalent in temperate zones, where an estimated 500 million persons are infected. Prevalence, however, varies with each locale. For instance, Alaskan Eskimos display a 51% prevalence; elementary students in and around Tallahassee, Florida, 27%; preschool pupils in San Francisco, 58%; Sicilian children, 77%; children overall in the United States, 33%. It is the most common nematode parasitizing humans in the United States.

Infections occur in one of four ways: (1) retroinfection when hatched larvae migrate back into the large intestine; (2) self-infection when the infected person is reinfected by hand-to-mouth transmission; (3) cross-infection when infective eggs are ingested, either with contaminated food or from fingers that have been in contact with a contaminated surface; or (4) inhalation of airborne eggs. In households with heavily infected individuals, infective eggs have been found in samples of dust taken from chairs, tabletops, dresser tops, floors, baseboards, etc. In a survey to determine the distribution of airborne pollen in public places such as theaters, pollen and pinworm eggs were found on sample plates not only from arm rests and baseboards but also from chandeliers high above the seats; most of these eggs, however, were no longer viable. Experiments show that at room temperature or above, fewer than 10% of such eggs survive more than 2 days, probably accounting for the less than universal infection in such environments.

**Symptomatology and Diagnosis.**    Pinworms are not usually very pathogenic. Clinical symptoms such as itching and irritation are caused by the migration of gravid females around the perianal, perineal, and vaginal areas. Heavy infections in children may also produce such symptoms as sleeplessness, loss of weight, hyperactivity, grinding of teeth, abdominal pain, and vomiting. Gravid females may also migrate up the female reproductive tract, become trapped in the tissues, and produce granulomata in the uterus and fallopian tubes. They may also migrate to the appendix, the peritoneal cavity, or even the urinary bladder.

Diagnosis is verified when adult worms and/or eggs are detected. The female worms emerge at night and are usually visible in the perianal and perineal regions. Adult worms are often observed on the feces as well; however, eggs are found in the feces in only about 5% of cases. The most reliable procedure for finding eggs is to press a strip of scotch tape on the perianal skin, remove it, and place it on a clean microscope slide for examination. Negative results from this method for seven consecutive days constitute confirmation that the patient is free of infection.

**Treatment.**    Following positive diagnosis in any individual member, treatment should be administered to all members of a household. Several relatively inexpensive and essentially nontoxic drugs are available. One frequently used is mebendazole in tablet form; it is usually administered twice at two-week intervals. It is contraindicated for pregnant women, however, since it is teratogenic in experimental animals.

A currently favored drug is pyrvinium pamoate. Available in both tablet and liquid form, it also is usually administered twice at two-week intervals. While free of serious, adverse side effects, it may cause nausea in some cases.

**Prevention.**    Complete eradication of pinworm infection from a population is virtually impossible. Careful personal hygiene is the most effective means of control. Fingernails should be cut short, and hands should be washed thoroughly after the toilet is used and before food is prepared or eaten. Since it is most prevalent in urban areas where relatively large populations intermingle, education of parents has proven most effective. Parents should be informed that it is a self-limiting, nonfatal infection widespread among children and that no social stigma should be attached to it. There is no evidence that dogs can transmit the infection. Infected children as well as other members of the household should be treated promptly. Bedclothes and towels from infected homes should be carefully laundered in hot water and aired in sunlight.

# SELECTED READINGS

Cheng, T. C. 1982. Anisakiasis. In *Handbook Series in Zoonoses*. Vol. II, Sect. C. "Parasitic Zoonoses" (J. H. Steele and M. G. Schultz, eds.), pp. 37–54. CRC Press, Boca Raton, Florida.

Crompton, D. W. T. 1988. The prevalence of ascariasis. *Parasitology Today* 4, 162–169.

Meyers, W. M., Connor, D. H., and Neafie, R. C. 1976. Strongyloidiasis. Inne *Pathology of Tropical and Extraordinary Diseases* (Binford, C. H., and Connor, D. H., eds.). Armed Forces Institute of Pathology, Washington, D.C.

Miller, T. A. 1979. Hookworm infection in man. *Advances in Parasitology* 17, 315–384.

Oshima, T. 1987. Anisakiasis—Is the sushi bar guilty? *Parasitology Today* 3, 44–48.

Smith, J. H., and Wootten, R. 1978. *Anisakis* and anisakiasis. *Advances in Parasitology* 16, 93–163.

Zimmerman, W. J. 1971. The trichinosis problem: Facts, fallacies, and future. *Iowa State University Veterinarian* 33, 93–97.

# CHAPTER SIXTEEN

# BLOOD AND
# TISSUE NEMATODES

Seven nematodes belonging to the superfamily Filaroidea are parasitic to humans. Generally referred to as filarial worms, these are *Wuchereria bancrofti, Brugia malayi, Onchocerca volvulus, Loa loa, Mansonella perstans, M. ozzardi,* and *M. streptocerca.* The life cycles of these parasites are essentially similar, so only significant variations will be noted in the discussion of each species.

A nematode parasitic in the cutaneous tissues of humans, *Dracunculus medinensis,* belongs to the superfamily Dracunculoidea. Its life cycle is significantly different from that of the filarial worms and is discussed separately (see p. 348). Two other nematodes, human tissue parasites belonging to the genus *Parastrongylus,* are also discussed.

## LIFE CYCLE

The long, threadlike, adult filarial worms are found in the lymphatic glands, tissues, and body cavities of the host (Fig. 16–1). Females are ovoviviparous, the larvae hatching in the uterus. At the time of larviposition, the larvae, known as **microfilariae,** are less well developed than typical first-stage larvae and are considered prelarvae or advanced embryos (Fig. 14–15). Once deposited by the female, microfilariae migrate into the blood vessels via the thoracic lymph duct or by penetrating the walls of the lymph vessels to invade neighboring small blood vessels. Larvae can survive in blood up to several years until ingested by the insect vector.

Blood-inhabiting microfilariae are usually **sheathed,** retaining the flexible eggshell as a covering membrane. However, in tissue-inhabiting species, the sheath is usually sloughed and the larva is said to be **unsheathed.**

After being ingested in a blood meal of a suitable insect vector, microfilariae develop in the digestive tract of the insect into first-stage, rhabditiform larvae. These larvae penetrate the midgut into the hemocoel and migrate to the thoracic muscles, where they undergo two molts and metamorphose within 3 weeks into the infective, third-stage, filariform larvae. Filariform larvae migrate to the proboscis sheath and gain access to the human bloodstream through the puncture made by the feeding insect. In the human, larvae undergo two molts, metamorphosing into adult worms during migration to the definitive site of infection. Approximately 6 months later, microfilariae appear in the bloodstream.

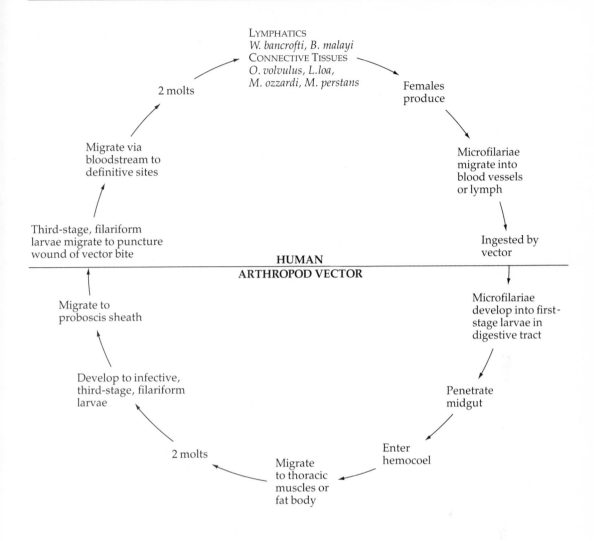

**Figure 16–1
Generalized life cycle of
filarial worms.**

# PERIODICITY

In 1879, Patrick Manson, while studying *W. bancrofti* infections among inhabitants of southern China, noted a nocturnal surge in the microfilarial population in the peripheral circulation. Later observed in a number of species of filarial worms, this periodicity varies with species (or strain) and even with endemic area. For instance, while microfilariae of *W. bancrofti* in the Caribbean islands, parts of South and North America, Africa, and Asia are nocturnal, those of the strain endemic to the South Pacific islands are **diurnally** subperiodic; that is, while they are present in the peripheral circulation throughout an entire 24-hour period, their numbers increase during the daytime. In the Philippines, on the other hand, this same species shows a modified nocturnal periodicity in that twice as many larvae are present at night as during the day. When microfilariae vacate the peripheral circulation, they accumulate in the small vessels of the lungs and liver.

Evolution of the phenomenon of microfilarial periodicity is of obvious survival value since it enhances opportunity for the microfilariae to be ingested by the insect vectors at certain times. It is not surprising that the surge of microfilariae coincides with the active feeding periods of the various insect vectors. For instance, in the examples presented above, the nocturnal *W. bancrofti* strain is associated with the nocturnal mosquito *Culex fatigans,* while the subperiodic strain is associated with a diurnal feeder, *Aedes polynesiensis.*

Although numerous studies have been undertaken to determine the mechanism(s) responsible for microfilarial periodicity, the explanation for this aspect of helminth physiology remains elusive. It is known that periodicity is not dependent on light and dark conditions, but rather on the 24-hour activity pattern, or circadian rhythm, of the definitive host. For example, if the routine is altered so that the host sleeps by day and is active at night, the periodicity of microfilariae is reversed. The sleeping period of the host is characterized by decreases in body temperature and oxygen tension, increases in carbon dioxide tension and body acidity, lower excretion of water and chlorides by the kidneys, less adrenal activity, etc. Some or all of these physiologic changes may trigger the rhythmic behavior of microfilariae, but it should be re-emphasized that different species and strains of microfilariae respond differently to similar stimuli.

# FILARIAL WORMS

## *Wuchereria bancrofti*

This filarial worm, parasitic only to humans, causes Bancroft's filariasis, characterized by extensive enlargement of extremities (Fig. 16–2). Ancients likened the thickened skin to that of elephants; hence the misnomer **elephantiasis** (which literally means "caused by elephants" rather than

**Figure 16–2**
**Human from South Pacific**
**severely affected by**
**elephantiasis.**

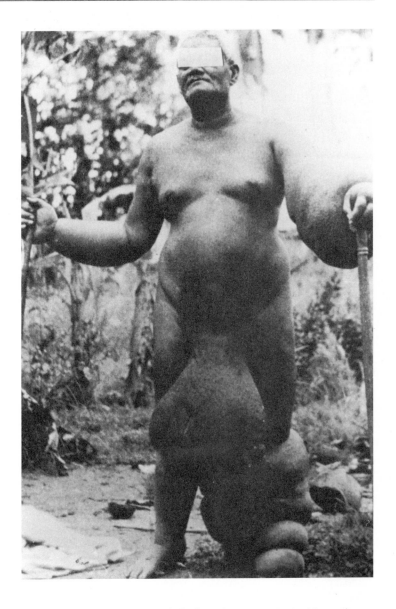

"like" elephants). The adult female worm is 8–10 cm long, with the vulva situated anteriorly near the middle of the esophagus. Male worms are smaller, attaining a length of only 40 mm, and are distinguishable further by their curved posterior ends and genital spicule apparatus.

**Life Cycle** (Fig. 16–1). Adults live coiled together in the major lymphatic ducts. Sheathed microfilariae, following deposition, utilize mosquitoes of several genera as vectors, including *Culex, Aedes, Mansonia, Anopheles,* and *Psorophora.* Development in the mosquito requires 1–3 weeks. Once introduced into the definitive host, larvae molt twice and migrate to the varices of lymphatics of the groin glands and epididymis of males and labial and mammary glands of females, where they mature in 6 or more months.

**Epidemiology.**   This widely distributed, common parasite occurs throughout a broad belt encircling the globe and including the Nile delta, central Africa, Turkey, India, southeast Asia, the Philippines, Pacific islands, Indonesia, Australia, Caribbean islands, and parts of South and Central America (Fig. 16–3). It was probably introduced into the New World during the slave trade. It is certain that infection was introduced into the United States via slaves brought to Charleston, South Carolina, and that it persisted in the Southeastern United States until the 1920's. The Pacific strain occurs throughout the Pacific islands except Hawaii.

Human infection is closely related to the ecology of the mosquito vectors as well as to human habits. For instance, the occurrence of periodic filariasis, found in areas of dense population and poor sanitation, parallels the distribution of its principal vector, *Culex fatigans,* which breeds in sewage-contaminated water. On the other hand, subperiodic filariasis in the Pacific islands often occurs in rural areas, and

**Figure 16–3**
**Distribution of *Wuchereria bancrofti.***
( + = islands; black areas = concurrent *Brugia malayi.*)

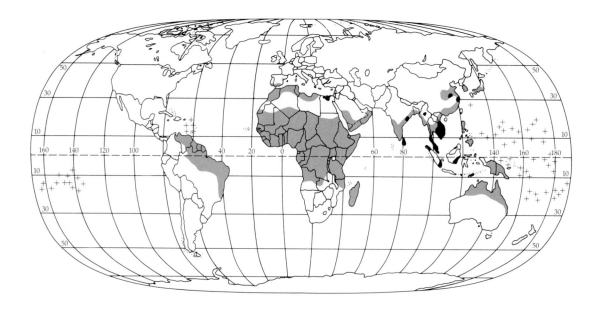

this correlates ecologically with its principal vector, *Aedes polynesiensis*, a mosquito that breeds in the brush.

**Symptomatology and Diagnosis.**    Pathology in *W. bancrofti* infection is due largely to living, dead, and degenerating adult worms. As lymph vessels and glands become blocked by such worms, edema develops; in time, the accumulation of connective tissue cells and fibers contributes to the enlargement of limbs, scrotum, and other extremities.

Clinically, the disease is divided into **incubation, acute** (inflammatory), and **obstructive** phases. The incubation phase is largely asymptomatic and may last for a year or more. Symptoms that appear are usually mild and may include low-grade fever caused by lymphatic inflammation. In time, the adult worms die, microfilariae disappear, and the patient is often unaware of having been infected. In endemic areas, children frequently harbor microfilariae in their blood while exhibiting few symptoms. During World War II, United States armed forces in the south Pacific were constantly exposed to infection, but surprisingly few showed any microfilariae in the peripheral circulation.

The acute phase commences when the female parasites reach maturity and begin releasing microfilariae. This phase is actually an allergic response to the products of dying and degenerating adult worms and is characterized by intense inflammation of the epididymis, testes, and lymph areas of the lower body. Chills, fever, and toxemia, accompanied by localized swellings in the arms and legs, may persist for days and/or recur at frequent intervals.

The obstructive phase is characterized by a blockage of lymph flow resulting from acute granulomatous response in the lymphatic system surrounding dead and degenerating adult worms. This phase may eventually lead to elephantiasis; however, only about 10% of the infected population manifests this chronic condition, and, even then, it develops only after many years of continual filarial reinfection. Elephantiasis is rarely seen in people less than 25 years old and is most prevalent in humans older than 40 years.

Diagnosis requires demonstration and accurate identification of microfilariae in the blood. The time of day (or night) at which blood should be collected and examined for motile microfilariae depends upon the strain involved. Stained thick and thin blood smears are used for species identification. Such criteria as presence or absence of sheath and distribution of internal nuclei and organ primordia are discernible after staining. In early infections, before microfilariae are present in the blood, intradermal tests using antigen prepared from *Dirofilaria immitis* (the dog heartworm) are almost 100% accurate. Diagnostic procedures should be supplemented with a complete history of patient exposure in endemic areas.

**Treatment.** Daily oral administration of diethylcarbamazine for 14–30 days is usually lethal to microfilariae. Administered with care, it also can kill adult worms. Metranidazole is useful as a backup when diethylcarbamazine proves to be ineffective.

Edema may be alleviated by pressure bandaging of the affected region to force excessive lymph from the area. Granulomatous tissue can sometimes be removed surgically, but such treatment is rarely attempted in advanced cases of elephantiasis.

**Prevention.** Control of and protection from mosquitoes in endemic areas should accompany mass chemotherapy of the indigenous population. The use of screens, insect repellents, and insecticides coupled with mass treatment with Hetrazan has proven effective in controlling Bancroft's filariasis in the U.S. Virgin Islands, Puerto Rico, and Tahiti.

## *Brugia malayi*

Until 1960, several species of filarial worms with similar microfilariae were assigned to the genus *Wuchereria*. In that year, based on the study of adult worms, the genus *Brugia* was established to designate the "malayi" group—including *B. malayi*, which is a parasite of primates, including humans, as well as cats.

The adult worms closely resemble *W. bancrofti*, although they are only about half as large. Females are about 55 mm long; males, about 23 mm. The sheathed microfilariae usually appear nocturnally in the peripheral circulation, but there is also a subperiodic strain. The nocturnal strain is host-specific, infecting humans exclusively, while the subperiodic strain infects not only humans but also cats, macaque monkeys, and leaf monkeys.

**Life Cycle.** The life cycle of *B. malayi* closely parallels that of *W. bancrofti*. The principal mosquito vectors are members of the genus *Mansonia*. However, members of the genera *Aedes*, *Culex*, and, occasionally, *Anopheles* also serve in this capacity.

**Epidemiology.**   The Pacific geographic range of *B. malayi* overlaps that of *W. bancrofti*, extending from India to China, Japan, Formosa, Malaysia, and Indonesia (Fig. 16–3). It is found most often in low-lying regions, which provide optimal breeding conditions for the vectors.

**Symptomatology and Diagnosis.**   While *B. malayi* rarely affects the genitalia, the adult worms live in the lymphatics and, otherwise, cause the same symptoms as *W. bancrofti*, culminating in elephantiasis. Diagnosis is identical to that for *W. bancrofti*.

**Treatment and Prevention.**   Treatment and prevention are also the same as for *W. bancrofti*.

## Onchocerca volvulus

Female worms can attain a length of 50 cm, while the males are only about 42 cm long. The male has a transversely striated cuticle reinforced externally with spiral thickenings.

**Life Cycle.**   Adult worms are found in fibrous tumors called **onchocercomas** in the subcutaneous connective tissues and viscera of humans (Fig. 16–4), who are the only known hosts for this species. Usually, there are a male and

**Figure 16–4**
*Onchocerca volvulus.*
(a) Section through a nodule showing adult worms with microfilariae.
(b) Onchocercomas on native in Zaire. Arrows point to those on elbow, hips, and knees.

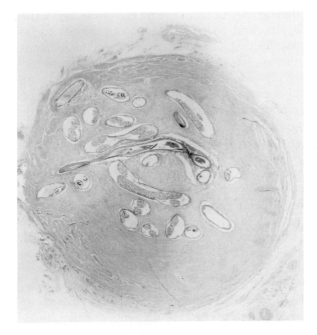
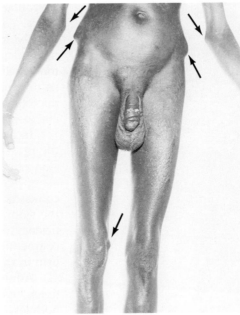

a female coiled in each nodule but, occasionally, several worms are observed coiled within a single onchocercoma. Immediately upon deposition, eggshells rupture, and the unsheathed microfilariae migrate to the lymphatics or, more often, to the connective tissues of the skin and eyes. Since they do not live in the blood, they are not periodic, but are positively phototactic. Blackflies, *Simulium* spp., serve as vectors, and the average developmental time for the infective larvae is 2 weeks.

**Epidemiology.**   Worldwide, there are an estimated 17 million cases of onchocerciasis, with 80 million people being at risk for the disease. Most of these cases are in tropical Africa, although there are significant numbers in the highlands of western Guatemala, Colombia, and northeastern Venezuela. The disease also occurs in Mexico and the Near East. In endemic areas in Central America, infected flies abound and breed in the high mountain streams, usually at 1,000–4,000 feet above sea level. Infection is common among workers in the highland coffee plantations. Recent estimates show that, although it is being controlled to some extent in Central and South America, prevalence is increasing in Africa as a result of the development of irrigation and hydroelectric dams.

**Symptomatology and Diagnosis.**   In victims of the disease, which is commonly known as "river blindness," *O. volvulus* microfilariae invade the cornea, causing inflammation of the sclera, cornea, iris, and retina. Formation of fibrous tissue usually follows, leading to impaired vision or total blindness. Ocular disease has been attributed to a number of factors, including physical activity of the microfilariae as well as microfilarial secretions and, perhaps, toxicity from dead microfilariae and/or adult worms. In any event, ophthalmic changes are gradual and require 7–9 years to develop fully.

In addition to the dramatic condition described above, the presence of microfilariae in the connective tissues of the skin often produces severe dermatitis resulting from either allergic responses or toxicity. Affected areas of the skin become thickened, depigmented, wrinkled, and cracked. Since the symptoms resemble those accompanying vitamin A deficiency, it has been suggested that they reflect the parasite's competition for vitamin A or interference with its metabolism in the host.

Adult worms may also cause minor pathological alterations. Specifically, adult worms often cause subcutaneous nodules, especially over bony prominences (Fig. 16–4).

Onchocercomas caused by the Venezuelan and African strains of *O. volvulus* usually appear in the pelvic area but also occur less frequently on the chest, spine, and knees. On the other hand, infection with the Central American strain more commonly produces nodules above the waist, especially on the head and neck. Although subcutaneous onchocercomas are readily excised, adult worms in deep-seated nodules continue to produce microfilariae that can migrate to the surface for transmission and can continue to damage the eyes.

Superficial nodules, cutaneous reactions, eosinophilia, or ocular symptoms in patients from endemic areas are strong indicators of onchocerciasis. Microscopic demonstration of microfilariae from dermal lymph or skin biopsy is proof positive, as is the identification of adults in skin nodules.

**Treatment.** Administration of diethylcarbamazine rapidly destroys microfilariae but does not affect adult worms. Since rapid destruction of microfilariae can produce such profound allergic responses as dermatitis, edema, and conjunctivitis, simultaneous treatment with corticosteroids and antihistamines is advocated. This regimen is usually followed by suramin treatment to eliminate adult worms. While the nature of suramin action is not wholly understood, it has been suggested that its effectiveness in treating adult *O. volvulus* derives from its ability to block active sites of several enzymes essential to the worms' metabolism. Suramin may produce such adverse side effects as loss of consciousness and severe nausea and is contraindicated in patients with ocular involvement. In brief, the suggested chemotherapeutic protocol for treatment of onchocerciasis is administration of diethylcarbamazine to destroy microfilariae, followed by suramin treatment if recurrence of microfilariae indicates the continuing presence of live adult worms. Currently, a less toxic agent, ivermectin, is being tested on 65,000 patients in 12 countries in West Africa. A single tablet destroys all larvae in the body within 2–3 days, and one dose annually is sufficient. This drug paralyzes the microfilariae, allowing macrophages to remove them before they can degenerate and release toxic materials into the blood. Chemotherapy is usually preceded by surgical removal of all accessible onchocercomas, since ivermectin has little effect on adult worms.

**Prevention.** Preventive measures are threefold: surgical and chemical treatment of infected patients to prevent further spread of the disease, control of the insect intermediate host population, and protection of susceptible persons. Patient treatment has already been discussed. Control of *Simulium* requires judicious use of insecticides on aquatic larvae, especially during the dry seasons, and on vegetation along the banks of swift-moving streams and rivers. Protective netting and screening and use of insect repellents effectively shield individuals from the bite of infected flies.

## Loa loa

Adult female *Loa loa* are 50–70 mm long, with the vulva located at the extreme anterior end; adult males measure 30–35 mm in length. The adults live in the subcutaneous tissues of the body, where they migrate freely. Because their movement is often visible beneath the conjunctiva, these parasites are known as African eye worms.

**Life Cycle.**    Humans and baboons are the only definitive hosts of *Loa loa*. The sheathed microfilariae are diurnal, retreating to the capillaries of the lungs at night. Various members of the mango fly genus *Chrysops* serve as intermediate hosts in which the developmental period is approximately 10–12 days. Within 1 hour after introduction into the definitive host, third-stage larvae penetrate to the subcutaneous and muscle tissues where, over the next 12 months, they molt twice and metamorphose into adult worms. The life span of adult worms is estimated to be 4–17 years.

**Epidemiology.**    An estimated 13 million patients suffer from loaiasis. Although the parasite was introduced into the Caribbean islands during the slave trade era, it did not persist, and the disease is now limited to the African equatorial rain forest and southern Sudan. The intermediate host breeds in muddy ponds and swamps; not surprisingly, infection rates are highest in those regions.

**Symptomatology and Diagnosis.**    *Loa loa* is only mildly pathogenic. Adult worms wander throughout the body, moving through the tissues at a maximum rate of about 1.5 cm/minute. The most troublesome infection sites are the conjunctiva (Fig. 16–5) and the bridge of the nose, where impaired vision, irritation, and pain may result. Most symptoms are general inflammatory reactions to adult worms and microfilariae and are often transient, appearing and disappearing at irregular intervals. A typical manifestation takes the form of transient, painful, subcutaneous swellings, com-

**Figure 16–5**
**Adult female *Loa loa* under conjunctiva.**

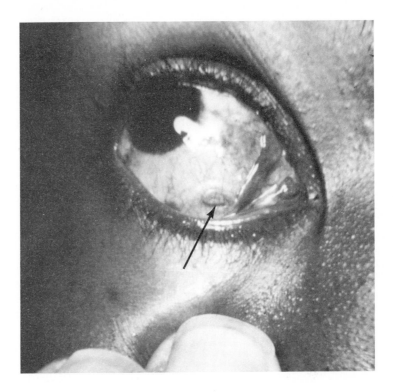

monly termed **fugitive** or **Calabar swellings,** which are most often seen on the hands or forearms or near the eyes and may grow to the size of a hen egg.

Sheathed microfilariae in the spleen can cause eosinophilia and fibrosis. Victims of the infection commonly exhibit a wide range of symptoms attributable to the wandering worms, such as low-grade fever, dermatitis, pain in the limbs, edema, and eosinophilia.

Diagnosis is usually based on sightings of the wandering worm in the conjunctiva, the presence of Calabar swellings, eosinophilia, and/or diurnal demonstration of microfilariae in blood. Antigens prepared from *Dirofilaria immitis* are useful diagnostic tools when other methods fail.

**Treatment.**    Surgical removal of wandering adult worms from the conjunctiva is advisable. Treatment with diethylcarbamazine as described for other filarial infections is also recommended.

**Prevention.**    The protocol recommended for control and prevention of infection with *O. volvulus* and other filarial worms applies for *L. loa* infection as well.

## Mansonella ozzardi, M. perstans, and M. streptocerca

In the genus *Mansonella,* the precise number of species infective to humans has not been firmly established. There are striking similarities among all these species, and the validity of assigning them to separate species may warrant challenge. In all instances, members of the fly genus *Culicoides* serve as vectors, and adult worms reside in the body cavities of the definitive hosts. *M. ozzardi* favors visceral adipose tissues, while *M. perstans* prefers the peritoneal cavity and, occasionally, the pericardial cavity. The unsheathed microfilariae of the three species display no periodicity and are readily visible in blood and other tissues of the host. *M. ozzardi* is endemic in northern Argentina, the northern coast of South America, and Central America. *M. perstans* is seen primarily in tropical Africa but also, to a lesser degree, in South America and the Caribbean region. *M. streptocerca* is common in East Africa, including Uganda, Kenya, and southern Sudan.

Other than local tissue reaction in the form of hydrocoels, no dramatic symptoms are associated with infection by these parasites.

## THE GUINEA WORM

### Dracunculus medinensis

Awareness of *Dracunculus medinensis* dates back to antiquity. The "fiery serpent" of the biblical Israelites, it is today commonly called the guinea worm or Medina worm. Long and thin, the adult female measures 500–1200 mm by 0.9–1.7 mm and the adult male 12–29 mm by 0.4 mm.

**Life Cycle.**    Adult worms inhabit the body cavity, its surrounding membranes, and the connective tissues of the human host. Male worms are rarely observed. The vulva, positioned equatorially in young females, is atrophied and nonfunctional in adults. The branched, gravid uterus, filled with thousands of larvae, compresses the intestine of the female and renders it nonfunctional. Gravid females migrate to the subcutaneous tissues of infected humans.

In the subcutaneous tissues, gravid worms direct their heads toward the skin and secrete an irritant that causes papules to form in the host's dermis, most frequently on the ankles or wrists (Fig. 16–6). As the papule grows, it assumes the external appearance of a blister, eventually rupturing and leaving a cup-shaped ulcer in the skin. When the open ulcer comes in contact with water, a loop of the worm's uterus prolapses, either through the broken anterior end of the body or through the mouth, and ruptures, releasing numerous first-stage, rhabditiform, larvae into the water. The larvae can survive in the aquatic environment for several days. Cold water stimulates contractions of the female body wall, causing larvae to be ejected in spurts. As the larvae are ejected, the body wall continually eases out of the ulcer and atrophies, and the remaining worm shortens proportionately. Larvae ingested by a suitable species of the copepod genus *Cyclops* burrow through the midgut and enter the hemocoel. The presence of more than five or six larvae is fatal to the arthropod.

Within the *Cyclops* hemocoel, the larvae undergo two molts, metamorphosing into infective, sheathed, third-stage larvae in approximately 20 days. When drinking water contaminated with infected *Cyclops* is swallowed, the larvae,

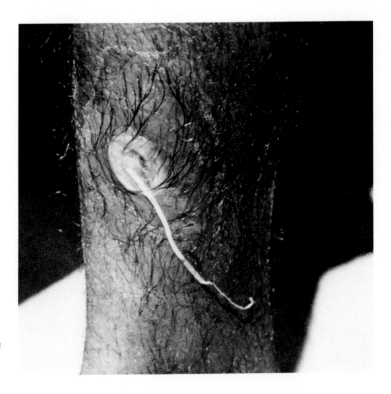

Figure 16–6
Female *Dracunculus medinensis* partially protruding from blister on leg.

freed from the arthropod during digestion, exsheath in the duodenum of the human host. The larvae then burrow through the mucosa, undergo two more molts, and lodge in the liver, body cavity, or subcutaneous tissues, where they mature in 8–12 months. The adult female is fertilized about 3 months post-infection; males usually die and degenerate 3–7 months after infection. A period of 10–14 months elapses between time of initial infection of a human host and the appearance of the skin blister.

**Epidemiology.**   Human infection occurs throughout most of Africa, except for the southern regions, as well as in southwestern Asia (including southern India), northeastern South America, and the West Indies. Two conditions are requisite for completion of the life cycle: (1) ingestion of infected copepods and (2) contact of the infected human host with water. In drought-stricken areas of Africa, pools of stagnant water abundant with copepods provide sources of infection for natives in search of drinking water. In southern India, the step-well is a prime source of infection. The practice of standing ankle or knee deep in the well to fill water containers allows gravid female worms in open ulcers of infected persons to release their larvae. Copepods, previously infected by larvae released the same way, are simultaneously withdrawn with the drinking water, providing a source of new infections.

**Symptomatology and Diagnosis.**   *Dracunculus medinensis* infections cause a broad spectrum of nonspecific symptoms such as eosinophilia, nausea, diarrhea, asthma, and fainting, which are believed to result from absorption of metabolic wastes produced by female worms during papule formation. In addition, cutaneous ulcers caused by female worms are common sites for secondary bacterial and fungal infections.

Female worms failing to reach host skin sometimes cause reactions in deeper tissues of the body. Commonly, they degenerate or become calcified; during these processes, the worms may release strongly antigenic molecules that can cause fluid-filled abscesses, or worms that calcify near a joint may produce a type of chronic arthritic condition.

Appearance of localized blisters or ulcers or microscopical identification of the female worm or larvae constitute diagnosis. X-ray examination may reveal calcified worms.

**Figure 16–7**
*Dracunculus medinensis* **female worm slowly withdrawn from ulcer on foot with twig.**

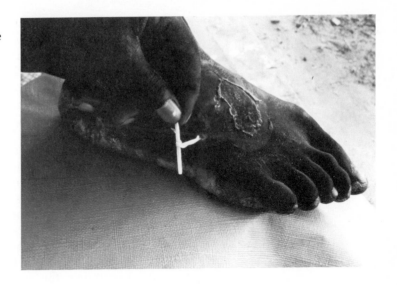

**Treatment.**    Both chemotherapeutic and mechanical techniques, including surgical, are employed for removal of adult worms. The drug of choice is metronidazole administered over a 7-day period. Metronidazole not only acts on the worm itself, but also acts as an anti-inflammatory agent. Mechanical withdrawal of the gravid female from the ulcerated area requires painstaking care, and the worm must be extracted slowly. If the worm breaks during the extraction process, larvae escape into the subcutaneous tissues, causing severe and painful inflammation. The ancient method, dating back to biblical days, of rolling the worm on a stick is still used in parts of Africa and Asia (Fig. 16–7). During the procedure, the worm is coiled around a stick, which is slowly turned, withdrawing the worm a few centimeters a day. Applying cold water to the area hastens the process by causing expulsion of more larvae to the exterior and allowing exposure of an additional 5 cm or so of the worm. The caduceus, the official emblem of the medical profession, includes a pair of serpents wrapped around a staff. It is not inconceivable that it may have been derived from this ancient method of *D. medinensis* removal.

**Prevention.**    As with other parasitic diseases, prevention and control require interruption of the life cycle. It is essential that the practice of bathing and washing in sources of drinking water be discontinued. Water suspected of being contaminated should be boiled before use, and, whenever possible, drinking water should be obtained from swift-running waterways that are usually free of copepods. Chemical treatment of water with chlorine or copper sulfate to destroy *Cyclops* is an alternative.

## *Parastrongylus* spp.

Normally a parasite in the pulmonary arteries and heart of rodents, *Parastrongylus cantonensis* is now known to cause a type of eosinophilic meningoencephalitis in humans. This delicate nematode, the males of which are 16–19 mm long and the females 20–25 mm long, uses aquatic and terrestrial gastropods as the intermediate host. Humans become infected when molluscs and a variety of paratenic hosts or their body fluids containing third-stage larvae are ingested raw. After entering the human, the parasite eventually reaches the meninges and brain, where it causes inflammation. Parastrongylosis in humans results in severe headache, fever, partial paralysis, stiff neck, coma, and even death.

Parastrongylosis occurs in southeast Asia; Taiwan; the Pacific islands, including Hawaii; and Madagascar; and the parasite has been reported from Australia and Puerto Rico.

A related species, *Parastrongylus costaricensis,* has been reported from humans in Costa Rica. This nematode matures in the mesenteric arteries and causes thickening and necrosis of the intestinal wall. Abdominal pain and high fever are the common symptoms. Humans become infected by ingesting third-stage larvae in molluscan intermediate hosts. This parasite occurs in cotton rats in Texas.

## SELECTED READINGS

Bhaibulaya, M. 1982. "Angiostrongylosis" [old designation for Parastrongylosis]. In *Handbook Series in Zoonoses* (J. H. Steele, ed.), pp. 25–36. CRC Press, Boca Raton, Florida.

Denham, D. A., and McGreevy, P. A. 1977. Brugian filariasis: Epidemiological and experimental studies. *Advances in Parasitology* 15, 244–309.

Duke, B. O. L. 1984. Filtering out the guinea worm. *World Health* 3, 29.

Trent, S. 1963. Reevaluation of World War II veterans with filariasis acquired in the South Pacific. *American Journal of Tropical Medicine and Hygiene* 12, 877–887.

# PART FIVE

# THE ARTHROPODA

# CHAPTER SEVENTEEN

# ARTHROPODS AS VECTORS

Members of the phylum Arthropoda probably constitute the largest number of individuals and species of any phylum in the animal kingdom. There are at least 760,000 known species of arthropods. According to current classification systems, the phylum is divided into four subphyla: Trilobitomorpha, Chelicerata, Crustacea, and Uniramia. This chapter deals with the role of Chelicerata (ticks and mites) and Uniramia (insects) as vectors of human disease-producing organisms (Fig. 17–1).

Although most arthropods generally are of little or no medical importance, they are of considerable biological interest, particularly to parasitologists. In addition, parasitic arthropods, such as ticks, mites, and certain insects, are of considerable medical and veterinary importance not only because they inflict direct injury upon their hosts but also because many serve as vectors for various pathogenic microorganisms and viruses.

# SIGNIFICANCE OF ARTHROPODS AS VECTORS

Disease-producing organisms transmitted to humans by arthropods have significantly influenced the history and demography of the human race. The plague, or Black Death, that so tragically decimated the population of Europe in the fourteenth century is vivid documentation of the toll such a disease can exact. Trench fever, the scourge of World War I, also attests the gravity of vector-borne diseases. Other such diseases that have had dramatic impact upon other historic events and eras are trachoma during Napoleon's invasion of Egypt, malaria and yellow fever during the construction of the Suez and Panama Canals in the nineteenth century, and African trypanosomiasis and malaria during the European explorations of Africa in the nineteenth century.

The disease agents transmitted by various arthropods vary widely in size and degree of pathogenicity. The smallest are submicroscopic viruses no larger than a large protein molecule and are obligate parasites of cells. Rickettsiae, currently considered a highly specialized form of bacteria, are somewhat larger than most viruses, although their size range overlaps the larger viruses and smaller bacteria. Like viruses, rickettsiae are obligate parasites, and they are at

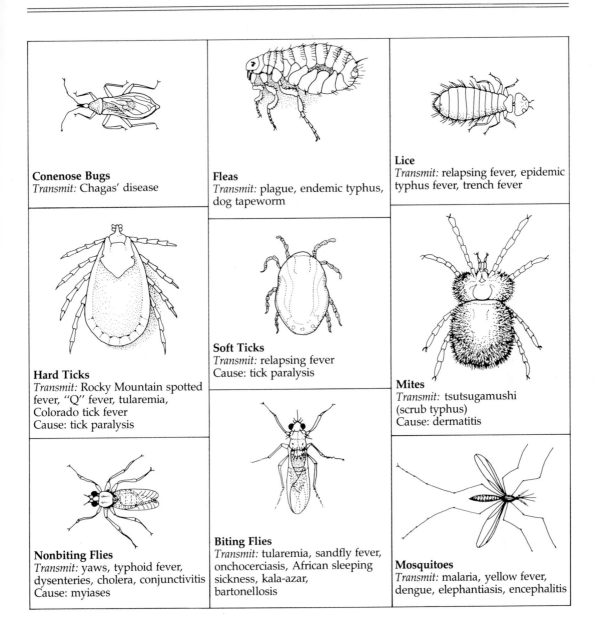

**Conenose Bugs**
*Transmit:* Chagas' disease

**Fleas**
*Transmit:* plague, endemic typhus, dog tapeworm

**Lice**
*Transmit:* relapsing fever, epidemic typhus fever, trench fever

**Hard Ticks**
*Transmit:* Rocky Mountain spotted fever, "Q" fever, tularemia, Colorado tick fever
Cause: tick paralysis

**Soft Ticks**
*Transmit:* relapsing fever
Cause: tick paralysis

**Mites**
*Transmit:* tsutsugamushi (scrub typhus)
Cause: dermatitis

**Nonbiting Flies**
*Transmit:* yaws, typhoid fever, dysenteries, cholera, conjunctivitis
Cause: myiases

**Biting Flies**
*Transmit:* tularemia, sandfly fever, onchocerciasis, African sleeping sickness, kala-azar, bartonellosis

**Mosquitoes**
*Transmit:* malaria, yellow fever, dengue, elephantiasis, encephalitis

**Figure 17–1**
**Some arthropods that transmit pathogens of human diseases.**

some time dependent upon arthropods for transmission. Unlike viruses, but similar to many bacteria, rickettsiae are susceptible to antibiotics. Next in order of size, bacteria inhabit a wide range of environments and display a wide variety of metabolic patterns and host relationships. While many bacteria are free-living, many form symbiotic relationships of commensalistic, mutualistic, or parasitic nature. The role of insects in the transmission of protozoans such as *Plasmodium, Leishmania,* and *Trypanosoma* and nematodes such as *Wuchereria, Onchocerca,* and *Brugia* has already been discussed. Likewise, a number of tapeworm infections are arthropod-transmitted. For instance, *Dipylidium caninum* is transmitted by fleas, *Diphyllobothrium latum* by copepod crustaceans, and *Hymenolepis diminuta* by beetles. The lung fluke *Paragonimus westermani* uses a crustacean as the second intermediate host in its life cycle.

The manner in which the various organisms parasitic to humans are transmitted dictates the types of associations arthropods establish with the parasites. The simplest relationship is one in which the arthropod is a **mechanical vector,** functioning merely as a passive carrier of the etiologic agent. For instance, typhoid organisms and *Entamoeba histolytica* cysts from contaminated excreta adhere to body parts of the common housefly and roach or pass through their digestive tracts and are subsequently transferred to food and drink touched by the insects. As a **biological vector,** the arthropod is used by the disease-producing organism not only as a means of transmission but also as a vehicle for development and/or reproduction before it becomes infective.

Biological transmission is of four types. In **propagative biological transmission,** the disease-producing organism reproduces in the arthropod, but undergoes no further developmental changes; examples are the plague bacillus in the flea and the yellow fever virus in the mosquito. In **cyclo-propagative biological transmission,** the disease-producing organism undergoes cyclical changes and reproduces in the arthropod. Plasmodia transmitted by mosquito vectors and trypanosomes by tsetse flies are examples of this type. In **cyclodevelopmental biological transmission,** the disease-producing organism must undergo cyclical changes in the arthropod vector but does not multiply there. For example, filarial worms must spend a portion of their life cycle in their mosquito vectors but reproduce elsewhere. Finally, in **trans-ovarial transmission,** certain disease-producing organisms, such as rickettsiae that cause Rocky Mountain spotted fever and scrub typhus, are transmitted from the infected parent arthropods (i.e., ticks and mites) to their offspring.

Once the etiologic agent is infective to humans, there are several means by which it gets from arthropod to human host. In some blood-sucking flies, infective forms leave the insect's mouthparts during the blood meal and enter the human skin through the puncture. The malarial parasite uses a more efficient mechanism to reach its human victim: the infective form is carried to the salivary gland of the mosquito and enters the human blood stream via saliva secreted by the insect into the human skin while feeding. Other insect-transmitted infections—such as viral encephalitis, yellow fever, dengue, and sleeping sickness—are transmitted in similar fashion. In some non–blood-feeding arthropods, the feeding larva (e.g., maggot) ingests the agent, retaining it in the digestive tract during metamorphosis; later, the resulting adult arthropod transmits it to the human via vomit or excreta on food and drink.

## GENERAL STRUCTURAL FEATURES

In the early stages of evolution, primitive arthropods were conspicuously multisegmented, each segment equipped with a pair of appendages; in present forms, some segments are fused, the number of appendages is reduced, and some have even evolved wings, all of which markedly enhance their mobility. In insects, the most successful of terrestrial animals, the body is divided into three regions (Fig. 17–2): the **head,** with a variety of mouthparts and sense organs; the more or less rigid **thorax,** bearing wings and three pairs of walking appendages; and the segmented **abdomen,** lacking appendages. Acarines—the ticks and mites—represent the second most successful terrestrial arthropod group. They also have three body regions, but they are wingless and possess four pairs of walking appendages (Fig. 17–3). Segmentation in ticks and mites is so indistinct that they appear to be unsegmented.

Arthropods have a chitinous exoskeleton, the **cuticle,** that extends to all external openings. The rigid cuticle limits growth so that periodic molting is required. The **open circulatory system** consists of a dorsal tubular heart that slowly pumps hemolymph through large sinuses that make up the major body cavity or **hemocoel.** Hemolymph is not always involved in oxygen transport; in many terrestrial forms, gaseous exchange between cells and environment is accomplished through a system of branched tubules, or **tracheae.**

The nervous system consists of a pair of ventral nerve cords with segmentally arranged ganglia; the typical "brain"

**Figure 17–2**
**Anatomy of typical insect.**
(a) External. (b) Internal.

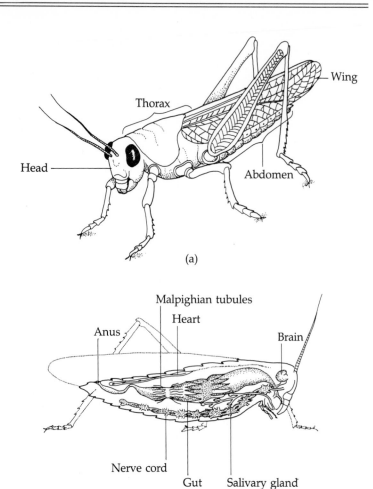

(a)

(b)

is a major ganglion located dorsally in the head region and connecting with the nerve cords by circumesophageal connectives from the anteriormost ventral ganglion. Nitrogenous wastes are excreted by terrestrial insects and most acarines in the form of uric acid, which is produced in **Malpighian tubules** that empty into the hindgut.

Arthropods acquire disease-producing organisms primarily during feeding. Because they obtain food from a wide variety of sources, the mouthparts of arthropods likewise vary widely. The mouthparts of primitive insects were adapted for chewing, and many extant species retain that adaptation. Grasshoppers, bees, ants, wasps, cockroaches,

**Figure 17–3**
**Anatomy of typical acarine.**
(a) External. (b) Internal.

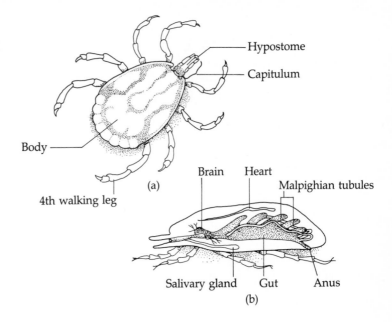

and termites retain the basic mouthparts of chewing insects. Although chewing insects are ineffective as biological transmitters of organisms that produce human disease, knowledge of their basic mouthparts is essential to an understanding of the evolutionary modifications that have produced the more specialized feeding apparatuses.

Lying directly behind the "upper lip," or **labrum,** are the first of the true mouthparts, the paired **mandibles,** which are heavily sclerotinized and bear jagged teeth along their medial margins. Behind them are the paired, jointed **maxillae.** The **hypopharynx** is not a true mouthpart but an unsegmented, tubular outgrowth of the body wall arising from the ventral, membranous floor of the head. The "lower lip" of insects is the heavily sclerotinized, segmented **labium.** The mandibles masticate the food, and the maxillae and labium push the pulverized food into the mouth.

In more advanced insects, the major evolutionary modification of the feeding apparatus is from the chewing type to one of several cutting and/or piercing types (Fig. 17–4).

The **cutting-sponging type,** characteristic of horseflies, features sharp-bladed mandibles and long, stylelike maxillae. The mandibles cut and tear the skin of the host, and the spongelike labium collects the blood and conveys it to the esophagus via a tube formed partially by the hypopharynx.

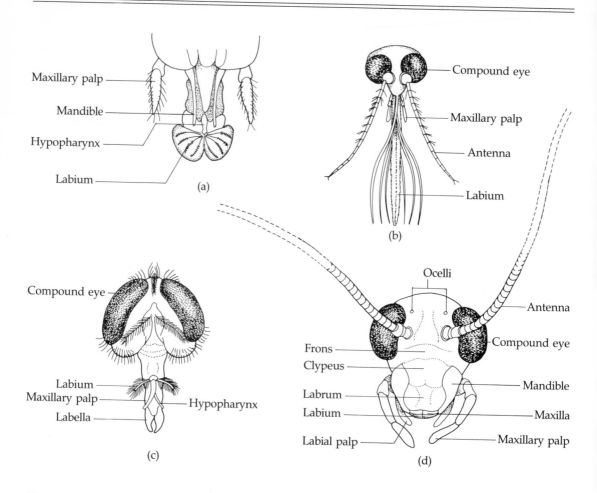

**Figure 17–4**
**Types of some insect mouthparts.**
(a) Cutting–sponging.
(b) Piercing–sucking.
(c) Sponging. (d) Chewing.

The mouthparts of most nonbiting dipterans, such as the common housefly, are of the **sponging type,** similar to the cutting-sponging type except that the mandibles and maxillae are nonfunctional. The remaining parts form a proboscis with a spongelike apex called the **labella.** Liquid food is conducted to the mouth via minute capillary channels on the labella. Solid food is ingested only after being dissolved or suspended in deposited saliva.

The **piercing-sucking type,** characteristic of mosquitoes, flies, lice, and bedbugs, features mandibles, maxillae, and hypopharynx modified into a long, thin, tubular, sharp-tipped stylet for piercing skin. This narrow tube is enclosed by the labrum to form a **stylet bundle** that is held in a groove on the labium. Together, the stylet bundle and the labium make up the **proboscis.** While not itself penetrating the skin, the labium guides the bundle into the wound site.

During insect feeding, the stylet bundle pierces the skin of the host like a hypodermic needle, and blood is withdrawn through it. The hypopharynx usually contains the salivary gland duct.

Among acarines, mites are more versatile in their feeding habits than ticks. While mites may feed on decaying animal matter, feces, plants, animal secretions, and blood, ticks feed only on the blood of reptiles, birds, and mammals. Since the mouthparts of ticks and mites are similar, those of the former will serve to illustrate both groups (Fig. 17–5).

The **capitulum** is a small anterior projection bearing the three structures that make up the mouthparts: that is, the elongate **hypostome,** a pair of segmented **chelicerae,** and a pair of segmented **pedipalps.** The hypostome, usually toothed, is medially located, ventral to the mouth with its free end projecting anteriorly. Bilateral chelicerae are located in the dorso-lateral surfaces of the hypostome, flanking the mouth. The free end of each chelicera is forked—one branch forming a fixed, dorsal, toothed digit, the **digitus externus,** the other a lateral, movable **digitus internus.** With these appendages, the host's skin is pierced and/or torn, and either the entire capitulum or, at least, the toothed hypostome is inserted into the opening. The appendages also serve as anchors when the parasite is attached. Paired pedipalps arise from the base of the capitulum at its antero-lateral margin. During feeding, the pedipalps either bend outward ("soft

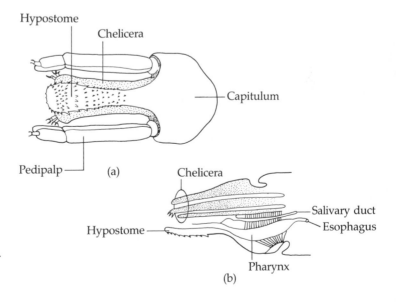

**Figure 17–5**
**Mouthparts of ticks.**
(a) Ventral aspect of capitulum.
(b) Longitudinal section
through tick head.

ticks") as the chelicerae and hypostome penetrate the flesh or remain rigidly and intimately associated with the hypostome ("hard ticks") during skin penetration. In either instance, the pedipalps serve as counteranchors while the tick is attached to the host.

# THE DIPTERANS

While the previous sections dealt with structural modifications in arthropod vectors and some of the means by which the vectors transmit pathogens, the following sections emphasize specific arthropods and some of the human pathogens they transmit. Numerous arthropod-transmitted pathogens have been discussed in preceding chapters devoted to protozoans and helminths, and appropriate references are made to those earlier chapters.

Because of their overwhelming numerical preponderance and the medical importance of the pathogens they transmit, dipterans are treated separately from other insects. Alone they may transmit about as many disease organisms as all other insects combined.

## BITING DIPTERANS

### Mosquitoes

A number of species of the mosquito family Culicidae are active transmitters of organisms responsible for human disease. Two groups in this family, the anophelines and the culicines, are quite distinct biologically. For instance, the cigar-shaped anopheline eggs are equipped with side floats and are usually deposited diffusely over water. Culicine eggs, on the other hand, possess no side floats and may be deposited in raftlike arrays on the surface of water (*Culex*), in cushionlike arrangements under water plants (*Mansonia*), or on damp surfaces to await heavy rains (*Aedes*) (Fig. 17–6).

While anopheline larvae appear immediately under and parallel to the surface of the water, culicine larvae hang from breathing tubes anchored either to the water surface (*Culex* and *Aedes*) (Fig. 17–7) or to the stems of aquatic vegetation (*Mansonia*). Adults are distinguishable by the configuration and angle of their body parts (Fig. 17–8). Anopheline body

**Figure 17–6
Mosquito eggs.**

| Eggs of *Anopheles* | Eggs of *Aedes aegypti* | Eggs of *Culex* |
|---|---|---|
| | | |
| With floats | No floats | No floats |
| Eggs laid singly on water | Eggs laid singly on dry surface | Eggs laid in rafts on water |

parts are aligned in a straight line, inclined at an angle to the surface upon which they alight, while those of culicine adults are bent into a hump-backed posture.

Pathogenic organisms transmitted to humans by mosquitoes can be divided into three groups, one of which includes the causative agents of malaria, *Plasmodium* spp. The role of the anopheline mosquito in the transmission of human malaria has already been discussed (see p. 115). Although there are approximately 350 known species of *Anopheles* throughout the world, only about two dozen are major

**Figure 17–7
Mosquito larvae.**
(a) *Culex* adhering to water by its breathing tube. (b) *Aedes.*
(c) *Anopheles.*

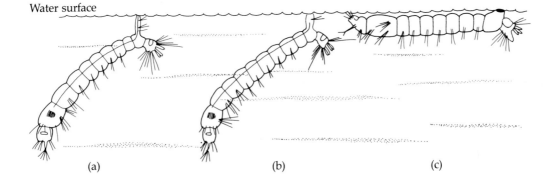

Water surface

(a)                    (b)                    (c)

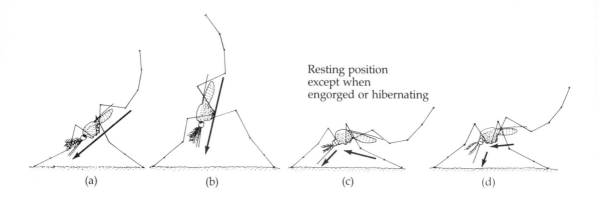

Resting position
except when
engorged or hibernating

(a)                    (b)                    (c)                    (d)

**Figure 17–8**
**Resting positions of common mosquitoes.**
(a), (b) *Anopheles.* (c) *Aedes.*
(d) *Culex.*

transmitters of human malaria. Many species are genetically or ecologically incompatible with the malarial organism. For example, differences in susceptibility of mosquito populations to *Plasmodium* sometimes reflects variations in gene frequency in different geographic areas. Also, ecological hazards, such as storms and droughts, influence the mosquitoes' feeding habits and oviposition and, therefore, affect the life span of the vector and its ability to harbor the parasite effectively.

Filarial worms, the causative agents of human filariasis, constitute a second group of these mosquito-borne pathogens. Numerous anopheline and culicine species serve as vectors for these organisms. It has been previously noted (see p. 338) that the ecology of the mosquito, especially its feeding cycle, is inextricably linked to the periodicity of microfilarial surge in the human host. For instance, the principal vector of the nocturnally surging *Wuchereria bancrofti* is the nocturnally feeding mosquito *Culex fatigans,* while the subperiodic variety employs the diurnal feeder *Aedes polynesiensis.*

The third group of pathogens are the arboviruses, arthropod-borne viruses transmitted from one person to another by insects or acarines. More than 200 diseases are transmitted in this manner, approximately three-quarters of them by mosquitoes, a few by biting flies, and the rest by ticks. The most serious of the arboviral diseases are the hemorrhagic fevers and the encephalitides. In hemorrhagic fever, increased permeability of capillary walls caused by the viruses precipitates bleeding from kidneys, lungs, gums, nose, etc. In viral encephalitis, viral attacks upon the central nervous system cause symptoms ranging from minor back pain to temporary paralysis, with sometimes lingering spastic effects.

**Yellow fever** is probably the most prevalent of the hemorrhagic diseases. During building of the Panama Canal, yellow fever caused such widespread illness among the workers that the project came to a halt. It was then that the Yellow Fever Commission, under the leadership of Dr. Walter Reed and his associates Drs. James Carroll, Jesse W. Lazear, and A. Agramonte, won acclaim by proving Dr. Carlos Finlay's hypothesis that the pathogen is transmitted by *Aedes aegypti.*

Female mosquitoes acquire the virus while feeding on the blood of the yellow fever victims. A single female ingests thousands of viruses at one feeding and usually remains infective for the rest of her normal life—200 to 240 days. Under field conditions, the normal incubation period in the mosquito is 12 days; however, this is subject to alterations influenced by fluctuations in temperature. For instance, in mosquitoes exposed to temperatures of 36.8°C, the incubation period is reduced to 4 days; at 21°C, the period is lengthened to 18 days. In addition to *Aedes aegypti,* other mosquito species serve as natural vectors for yellow fever; among these are *Aedes vittatus* in Egypt and *Aedes simpsoni* and *Aedes africanus* in eastern Africa. Jungle animals, especially monkeys, serve as natural reservoirs for the yellow fever virus.

Currently, world incidence of the disease, as reported by the World Health Organization, fluctuates from one hundred to several thousand cases annually. Vector control and mass inoculation have virtually eliminated endemicity in the Americas and have greatly reduced the incidence in Africa.

Two hemorrhagic fevers, **hemorrhagic dengue** and **breakbone fever,** are transmitted by several species of *Aedes.* The former is endemic in southeast Asia, where native children are the prinicpal victims. It has a mortality rate of about 7%. Breakbone fever is nonlethal and is characterized by a rash, high fever, and pain in the joints. It has been reported in Japan, New Guinea, northern Australia, the Philippines, and Hawaii.

In the United States and parts of Latin America, viral encephalitides, such as **Western** and **Eastern equine encephalitis, St. Louis encephalitis,** and **Venezuelan equine encephalitis,** are usually nonlethal. Culicine mosquitoes are the principal vectors, and transmission is from birds to horses or humans, both of which are dead ends in the transmission sequence. A similar but more serious disease, **Japanese B. encephalitis,** occurs in Japan.

**Figure 17–9**
Blackfly, *Simulium damnosum,*
biting human.

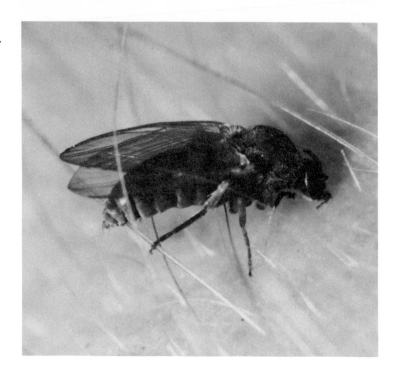

## Blackflies

*Onchocerca volvulus* (Fig. 17–9), the causative agent of **human onchocerciasis** (see p. 343), is transmitted by the blackflies *Simulium damnosum* and *S. neavei* in Africa and *S. ochraceum, S. callidum,* and *S. metallicum* in Mexico, Central America, and South America. Females of *Simulium* spp. lay eggs in fast-flowing water ranging from streams to large rivers—in the latter, most abundantly where rapids occur and in areas below dams. The hatched larvae and resulting pupae remain in the aquatic habitat. Adult female flies feed on the blood of a variety of mammals, including humans. In addition to transmitting onchocerciasis to humans, the bites of the blackflies can themselves be troublesome, frequently producing severe reactions.

## Sandflies

Phlebotomine sandflies (Fig. 17–10) transmit three different types of organisms pathogenic to humans. The viral disease **sandfly fever** occurs in the Mediterranean region, central Asia, south China, parts of India, Sri Lanka, and parts of

**Figure 17–10**
**Stages in life cycle of**
*Phlebotomus.*

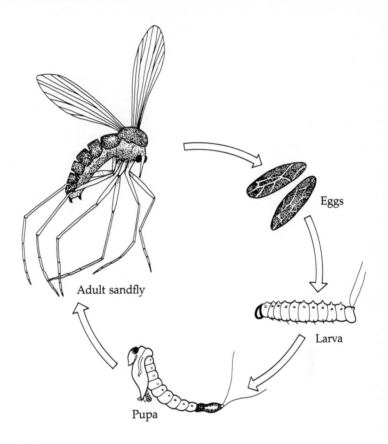

Eggs

Adult sandfly

Larva

Pupa

South America. Of short duration, it is not considered seri-ous. In the northwestern regions of South America, sand-flies transmit the bacterium *Bartonella bacilliformis*, the caus-ative agent of **Corrion's disease** (= **bartonellosis**), a severe, often fatal illness. The third group of pathogens transmitted by sandflies are those that cause the various types of **leish-maniasis** (see pp. 88–97).

The phlebotomine sandflies that are vectors for these pathogens generally belong to two genera: *Phlebotomus* in the Eastern Hemisphere and *Lutzomyia* in the Western Hemisphere. A small insect, measuring 1.25–2.5 mm long, the sandfly has long, slender legs and has short setae cov-ering most of its body parts and wings. The females use piercing-sucking mouthparts to extract juices from plants and blood from various vertebrates. Sandflies are not strong fliers, usually remaining close to their breeding sites in damp areas rich in organic debris, for example, under logs and dead leaves, inside hollow trees, and in animal burrows.

**Figure 17–11**
**Tsetse fly, *Glossina*.**
(a) *G. palpalis*. (b) Pupa.
(c) *G. morsitans*.

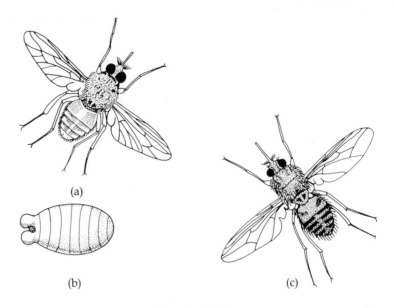

(a)

(b)                    (c)

## Tsetse Flies

Members of the genus *Glossina* (Fig. 17–11) are a menace not only because they are vectors for **African trypanosomiasis** (see p. 98–105) but also because both male and female flies feed on blood, their bites inflicting large welts on their hosts (Fig. 17–12). Although *Glossina* was once widely distributed, it is now limited to continental Africa south of the Tropic of Cancer. During the life cycle of this important vector, the female harbors in her body a supply of fertilized eggs that hatch at intervals into larvae that feed from specialized "milk glands." The developing fourth-stage larva is deposited in a shady spot, usually at the base of a tree or shrub, and immediately burrows into the soil and pupates. A single female tsetse fly deposits 8 to 10 larvae, one at a time, at intervals of about 10 to 12 days each. The adult fly emerges in 3–4 weeks.

While several species will feed on human blood, they appear to prefer that of wild game. The various species of *Glossina* are ecologically adapted to different localities according to feeding preferences and site choices for larviposition. For instance, the two species that serve as transmitters of trypanosomiasis breed either under trees near rivers and lakes, taking their blood meals from people at drifts or watering places (West African sleeping sickness), or in open woodland, feeding mainly on large game (East African sleeping sickness).

**Figure 17–12**
**Tsetse fly welts on human skin.**

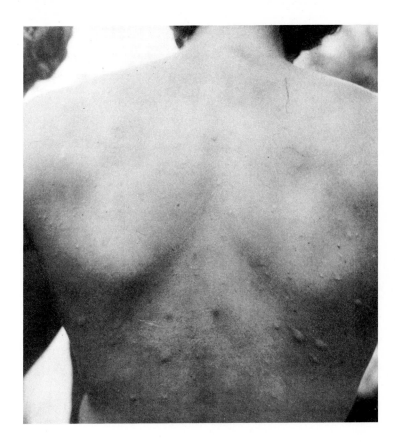

## Tabanid Flies

Tabanid flies (Fig. 17–13) are large, stoutly built, and often beautifully colored. Strong fliers, they viciously attack a variety of mammals, including humans. Since only the adult females are blood feeders, only they have mouthparts adapted for cutting and piercing. Members of two genera, *Chrysops* and *Tabanus*—commonly known, respectively, as deerflies and horseflies—serve as major transmitters of human pathogens.

Tabanid flies are prominent among the arthropod vectors of such bacterial diseases of humans and/or animals as **tularemia** and **anthrax.** Tularemia, a disease of humans in the United States, Canada, northern Europe, the USSR, Turkey, and Japan, is caused by *Pasteurella tularensis,* for which wild rabbits often serve as reservoir hosts. One of the vectors for *P. tularensis* is *Chrysops discalis.* Anthrax, a much dreaded disease of cattle caused by *Bacillus anthracis,* is also

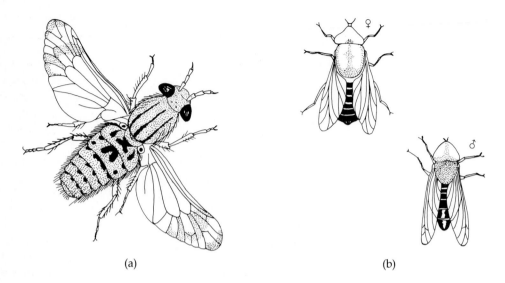

**Figure 17–13
Tabanid flies.**
(a) *Chrysops.* (b) *Tabanus* (male and female).

a serious disease among humans. *Tabanus striatus* and other tabanid flies are common vectors. **Loaiasis,** caused by the African eye worm *Loa loa* (see pp. 346–47) is transmitted to humans by several diurnally feeding species of *Chrysops,* including *C. dimidiata* and *C. silacea.*

## NONBITING DIPTERANS

The common housefly (*Musca*), the bluebottle fly, and a number of blowflies (*Calliphora*) are examples of nonbiting dipterans. While adults are nonparasitic and are primarily considered household and farm pests, they are, nonetheless, capable of the mechanical transmission, via contaminated appendages, of a variety of human pathogens, including the bacteria that cause **typhoid fever** (etiologic agent, *Salmonella typhi*) and **bacillary dysentery** (etiologic agents, *Shigella dysenteriae* and certain strains of *Escherichia coli*). In addition, the causative agents of two eye diseases, **trachoma** and **conjunctivitis,** are transmitted by this group of dipterans. The etiology of these diseases has not been established conclusively. Trachoma is probably caused by a virus of the psittacosis-lymphogranuloma group, while conjunctivitis can be attributed to several different bacteria. These flies are also suspected of transmitting other agents of human diseases, such as *Vibrio comma,* the bacterium responsible for **cholera,** and *Treponema pertenue,* the spirochete that causes **yaws.**

A number of other organisms that produce disease in humans are also commonly associated with these flies, although there is no direct evidence that they act as major transmitters. In fact, one body of opinion holds that only two types of diseases, certain intestinal and ocular disorders, are transmitted by flies and that, like the bedbug, these flies are much maligned as transmitters of other pathogens.

## OTHER INSECTS

A significant factor in the epidemiology of diseases transmitted by nondipteran insects is the vastly limited mobility of the three groups in this category (reduviid bugs, fleas, and lice) compared to dipterans. Although reduviid bugs possess functional wings, they are poor fliers. Fleas and lice are wingless.

### Reduviid Bugs

There are about 2,500 known species of reduviid, or assassin, bugs (Fig. 17–14). A short, three-jointed proboscis is attached to the tip of the head, and the insects feed primarily on body fluids of other insects, although some attack humans and other animals. They are comparatively large insects, measuring 1.5–2 cm long, and some are brightly

**Figure 17–14**
**Some blooksucking reduviids.**
(a) *Triatoma.* (b) *Rhodnius.*
(c) *Panstrongylus.*

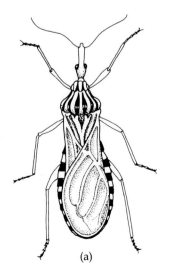

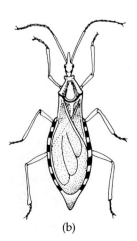

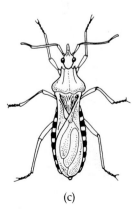

(a)                    (b)                    (c)

**Figure 17–15**
**Distribution of reduviids and**
**Chagas' disease.**

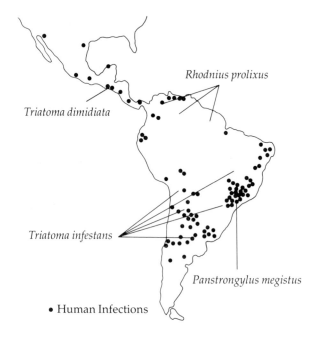

*Rhodnius prolixus*

*Triatoma dimidiata*

*Triatoma infestans*

*Panstrongylus megistus*

• Human Infections

colored. Members of three genera—*Triatoma, Panstrongylus,* and *Rhodnius*—are the major vectors for **Chagas' disease** (see pp. 105–109). While several dozen species belonging to these genera occur in various countries of North and South America (Fig. 17–15), they are like the *Plasmodium*-transmitting mosquitoes in that relatively few actually serve as significant vectors for Chagas' disease. Most species are arboreal and feed on wild animals, and their importance lies in maintaining the infection in sylvatic reservoirs. Species that commonly inhabit or occasionally intrude into human dwellings are the major transmitters to humans. Such insects, unlike transient mosquitoes, actually invade a home and establish stable colonies in cracks and crevices of walls and in thatched roofs. The adults emerge at night for a blood meal once or twice a week. Their bites are painful, often resulting in itchy swellings from toxins injected during feedings. The female lays her eggs in wall crevices, furniture, and roofs, and wingless nymphs hatch in about 8–30 days. Development to adulthood generally progresses through five nymphal instars to sexual maturity. The cycle is temperature-dependent and may require from 6 months to 2 years for completion.

# Fleas

While the parasitologist's interest in fleas (Fig. 17–16) usually centers on their blood-sucking habits and their role as intermediate hosts for helminth parasites, the primary concern here is with their role as vectors for pathogenic organisms.

Fleas constitute a small, highly specialized order of insects of obscure origin and evolution. Eggs are deposited by females a few at a time, usually 3 to 20, either on or off the host. When deposited on the host, they soon fall off since they are not adhesive; therefore, they are commonly found in the host's abode. A cephalic spine expedites the hatching of a whitish, vermiform larva with distinct head and no legs

**Figure 17–16**
**Fleas.**
(a) Male of the cat flea *Ctenocephalides felis*. (b) Female *C. felis*. (c) Male of the Oriental rat flea *Xenopsylla cheopis*. (d) Female *X. cheopis*.

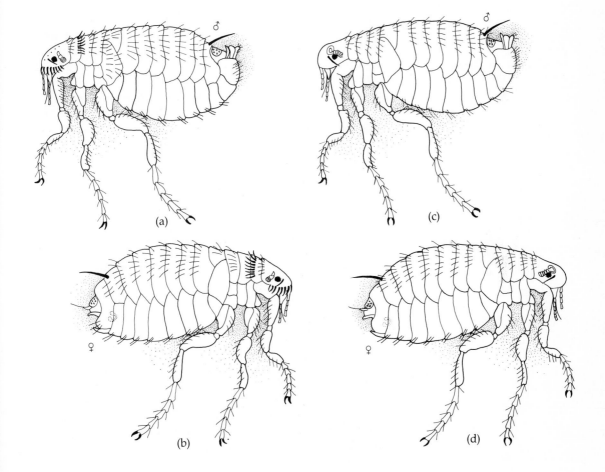

that, at this stage, resembles larvae of certain dipterans. The mouthparts of the larva are of the chewing type, and nourishment is derived from decaying vegetable and animal matter. The larval growth period varies from 9 to 200 days, depending on such environmental conditions as humidity, temperature, and oxygen tension. Flea larvae usually undergo two molts, which alternate with growth periods prior to pupation. Duration of the pupation period also depends upon environmental conditions, varying from 7 days to a year.

The adult flea is flattened laterally, is wingless, and has muscular hind legs for jumping. The body is covered with spurs and bristles, directed backward, that facilitate its movement through the fur or feathers of the host. While many fleas are host-specific in their blood-feeding habits, others display little specificity.

A notorious organism transmitted by fleas is the bacillus *Yersinia pestis,* which causes **bubonic plague.** During the fourteenth century A.D., the **Black Death,** as bubonic plague was commonly called, killed a quarter of the the population of Europe. Epidemics in the sixth century A.D. and the **Great Plague** of London in 1665 likewise took heavy tolls in human lives. These epidemics probably originated in central

**Figure 17–17**
**Distribution of plague throughout the world as of 1969.**

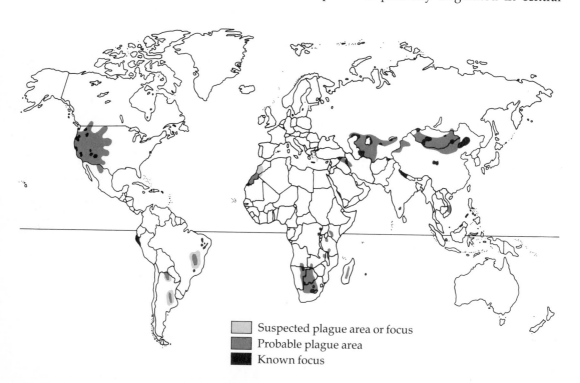

Suspected plague area or focus
Probable plague area
Known focus

Asia and spread via caravans and, later, international shipping. Epidemics recurred as late as the nineteenth century. According to WHO statistics, there are now about 1,000 to 6,000 cases of plague annually, and the use of modern antibiotics and other medications has reduced the annual mortality rate to 100–200. Presently, in the sparsely populated regions of the western and southwestern United States, large numbers of sylvatic reservoirs harbor the disease-producing bacterium, representing a continual danger of infection to humans who encroach on these environs (Fig. 17–17).

In the usual course of the infection, there is an interchange of fleas between wild, infected rodents and domestic rats. The disease spreads rapidly among the domestic rat population, killing a high percentage. Transfer of the infection from rats to humans requires that the flea feed upon both. The common human flea *Pulex irritans*, while capable of parasitizing both humans and domestic animals, rarely feeds on rats and, therefore, is not an important vector of the plague bacillus in nature. However, several species of the genus *Xenopsylla* do feed on both humans and other animal hosts, including rats. *Xenopsylla cheopis*, the Asiatic rat flea, is the most commonly encountered species in this genus and is the major vector for plague bacilli. Presumed to have originated in the Nile valley, it has spread throughout the world on rat hosts. Male and female fleas acquire the bacilli during feeding on infected rats. The ingested bacilli proliferate in the flea's digestive tract and form a semisolid plug, blocking the gut and rendering the flea unable to swallow food (Fig. 17–18). In spite of increasing hunger, the flea's repeated attempts at obtaining blood are futile, and during each attempt, ingested blood is regurgitated into the

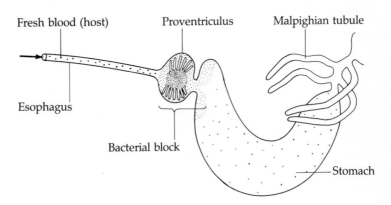

**Figure 17–18**
**Diagram of foregut of flea showing bacterial block. Esophagus is distended due to accumulation of host blood.**

**Figure 17–19**
**Plague buboes on human patient.**

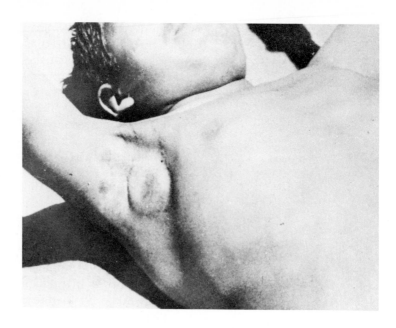

host bloodstream along with portions of the bacterial plug, resulting in the introduction of large numbers of bacilli into the host.

In humans, plague bacilli proliferate in the blood, causing highly lethal **septicaemic plague.** Bacilli usually localize in swellings, called **buboes** (Fig. 17–19), in the groin and armpits, and the bacterial count in the blood is low, rendering bubonic patients virtually noninfectious to fleas or other humans. This is not the case, however, with the highly contagious and lethal **pneumonic plague,** the form of the disease that occurs when lungs become infected. Interhuman transmission of the bacilli occurs through air-borne, contaminated sputum expelled during patients' coughing attacks. In rare instances, transmission to humans occurs from direct contact with the pelts of infected animals.

In addition to carrying plague, fleas serve as vectors for the **murine** or **endemic typhus** organism *Rickettsia typhi* (Fig. 17–20), transmitted by contaminated flea feces being rubbed into the bite wound. Fleas acquire the rickettsia during feeding from a wide variety of infected animals, including humans, rats, and mice. *Xenopsylla cheopis* is the principal vector for this rickettsia, which causes a mild disease found throughout much of the temperate region of the world.

*Pasteurella tularensis,* the tularemia-causing organism, and *Salmonella enteritidis,* the salmonellosis-causing bacte-

**Figure 17–20**
**Scanning electron micrograph**
**of the causative agent of**
**epidemic typhus,** *Rickettsia*
*prowazecki.*

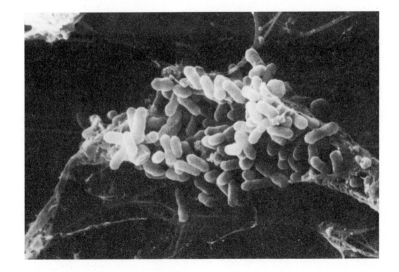

rium, are also transmitted to humans by fleas, and these insects also serve as intermediate hosts for two tapeworms that infect humans: *Dipylidium caninum* (see pp. 250–51) and *Hymenolepis nana* (see pp. 246–49).

## Lice

There are two orders of lice (Fig. 17–21): Mallophaga, the biting lice, and Anoplura, the sucking lice. Mouthparts of the biting louse are of the chewing type but are greatly reduced in size and number and are difficult to analyze without intensive study. Mouthparts of the sucking louse consist of an eversible set of five stylets through which it can suck host blood.

Among the mallophagans, one, *Trichodectes latus,* merits some concern as a transmitter of a potential human pathogen. *T. latus* can serve as an intermediate host for the dog tapeworm *Dipylidium caninum,* an occasional parasite of humans (see pp. 250–51).

Of the anoplurans, *Pediculus humanus,* the body louse—an ectoparasite of several animals, including humans—is also the major vector for three important human diseases: **relapsing fever, louse-borne** or **epidemic typhus,** and **trench fever.** A second anopluran species of medical importance is *Phthirus pubis,* the crab louse, which has been induced to transmit typhus-producing rickettsiae to laboratory animals. However, the body louse is the chief vehicle for transmision of the disease in nature.

**Figure 17–21**
**Lice.**
(a) *Pediculus humanus*.
(b) *Phthirus pubis*.
(c) *Trichodectes canis* of dogs.

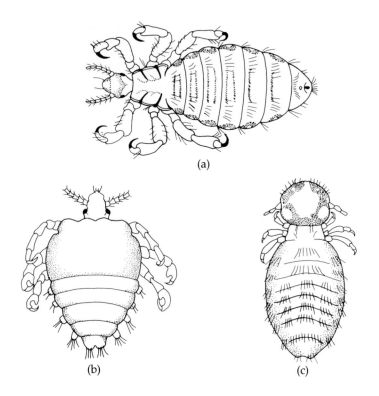

(a)

(b)                    (c)

Lice live in intimate contact with their human hosts. Because they are wingless and sluggish in movement, new infestations usually occur only through direct physical contact between humans. Low standards of personal hygiene, especially when exacerbated by warfare or disaster, create a favorable climate for louse infestation and, therefore, the spread of louse-borne diseases.

Relapsing fever is a cosmopolitan disease caused by the spirochete *Borrelia recurrentis*. The body louse ingests the spirochete while feeding upon an infected host. *B. recurrentis* lives and reproduces in the hemocoel of the louse, where it apparently can survive for the life of the vector with no adverse effect upon the insect. Since the spirochete has no available egress from the louse, transmission occurs when the louse's body is crushed and its contaminated body fluids enter the human host through mucus membranes or breaks in the skin. Louse-borne relapsing fever, an exclusively human disease, is characterized by intermittent high fever and rash and has a mortality rate of under 10%. The symptoms resemble those of typhus; consequently, the two were not recognized as distinct diseases until 1840.

Louse-borne, or epidemic, typhus is an ancient disease, once much dreaded; it is now limited to Asia, North Africa, and Central and South America. Caused by the rickettsia *Rickettsia prowazeki*, the last great typhus epidemic occurred in Europe immediately after World War I, with an estimated death toll of more than 3 million people. Unlike the spirochete responsible for relapsing fever, the typhus organism is transmitted from the feces of the louse. When ingested by the louse in a blood meal from an infected human, rickettsiae invade the epithelial cells of the insect's stomach, where they multiply. The cells eventually burst, releasing large numbers of the infective organism into the digestive tract, whence they exit with feces. Damage to the louse's intestinal tract is so extensive that ingested blood diffuses into the hemocoel in such quantities that the insect turns red and usually dies. The contaminated feces quickly dries into a fine powder that remains infective for several months. Rickettsiae are inhaled by human hosts, penetrate the mucus membranes of the eyes, or are rubbed into breaks in the skin along with contaminated louse feces. The disease is characterized by high fever accompanied by headache, nausea, delirium, and stupor, usually followed by the appearance of a dull, mottled rash on the body. Untreated victims either recover spontaneously or die in about two weeks, with a higher mortality rate among elderly victims than among children. Those who survive the disease may harbor infective organisms for many years.

Similar to but milder than typhus, trench fever is caused by a rickettsia, *Rochalimaea quintana*, and transmitted by contaminated louse feces. Unlike *R. prowazeki*, *R. quintana* is an extracellular pathogen in humans, causing typhuslike symptoms that culminate in a rash that disappears within 24 hours. The disease is debilitating but rarely fatal and, except for a few isolated outbreaks, rarely occurs today. However, it was one of the most common diseases during World Wars I and II.

# THE ACARINES

Ticks are the major acarine vectors of human disease-producing organisms, with mites playing a far lesser role. The acarine life cycle is similar to that of a number of other blood-feeding arthropods. Females lay clusters of eggs, from which hexapod larvae emerge in 1–4 weeks. The larvae and all subsequent stages are blood-feeders. Larvae metamorphose through four or five 8-legged nymphal stages, the final molt culminating in the adult stage. In some tick species, such as *Ixodes dammini*, the life cycle may extend over a period of up to 2 years.

## Ticks

These acarines (Fig. 17-22) are classified into two groups: soft ticks and hard ticks. One distinguishing characteristic is the relationship of the mouthparts to the rest of the body; in soft ticks, the mouthparts are completely concealed by the soft body, while in hard ticks they project from the body. Hard ticks also possess hard, shiny shields that in the male, cover the back completely but, in the female, do so only partially.

The two tick groups are also ecologically distinct. Soft ticks hide in cracks and crevices of houses, animal burrows, and similar areas during daylight hours, emerging at night to feed on host blood and to lay eggs. Hard ticks, on the other hand, spend most of their lives on host animals, and they spend the major portion of it gorging on blood. Female hard ticks produce far more eggs than their soft-bodied counterparts and usually die following oviposition. Some species of hard ticks spend their entire lives on one host; other species utilize two, some even three hosts. In multihost species, the ticks drop off the host animals indiscriminately, thereby infesting large areas of land.

*Ornithodoros* spp., soft-bodied ticks, transmit to humans several species of the spirochete genera *Spirocheta* and *Borrelia*. These cause **tick-borne relapsing fever,** a disease often endemic in the populations of tropical and subtropical regions of the world. Because of this endemicity, visitors, such as campers and hunters, are apt to suffer more acutely than natives, whose symptoms tend to be mild.

Like most tick-borne diseases, relapsing fever is zoonotic, being transmitted from wild rodents and other small mammals to humans. Spirochetes, ingested by a tick during a blood meal, gradually spread throughout the body of the arthropod, with those invading the salivary glands most likely to be transmitted to a vertebrate host during subsequent feeding.

Symptoms of the disease are similar to those of the louse-borne variety. The primary attack, characterized by se-

**Figure 17–22**
**Ticks.**
(a) *Dermacentor andersoni* (hard tick) (male left, female right).
(b) *Ornithodoros moubata* (soft tick) (dorsal aspect left, ventral aspect right).

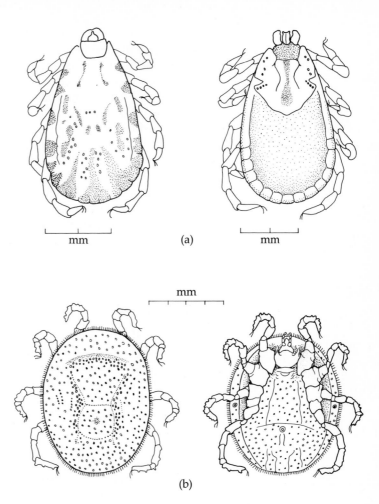

vere headache and high fever, lasts a few days and, if left untreated, is usually followed by several relapses occurring at short intervals. The patient usually recovers after 3 to 6 relapses, although in the African variety there may be as many as 11 relapses.

A group of closely related rickettsial diseases are transmitted by hard ticks. For example, **Rocky Mountain spotted fever,** caused by *Rickettsia rickettsi*, is indigenous to North America, and **tick-borne typhus,** caused by *Rickettsia conorii*, is found throughout the world. While Rocky Mountain spotted fever is considered a dangerous disease if left untreated, most tick-borne rickettsial diseases are not particularly serious. They are usually zoonotic, with humans rarely being sources of the organisms.

*Dermacentor andersoni* is the principal vector for *R. rickettsi* in the Rocky Mountain states, and *D. variabilis*, the American dog tick, in the central and eastern states. Several species of *Rhipicephalus* serve as vectors for *R. conorii* in Africa and the Mediterranean area. The rickettsiae, acquired when the tick feeds on an infected vertebrate, spread throughout the body of the arthropod, causing no apparent harm. The microorganisms penetrate both the egg cells in the ovaries and the cells of the salivary glands, allowing transmission of the rickettsiae to progeny as well as to other animals. Numerous wild animals serve as reservoirs for *R. rickettsi*, while *R. conorii* is harbored only by canines.

Symptoms of Rocky Mountain spotted fever are high fever accompanied by chills and headache and, at times, a typhus-like stupor. These are followed, after 4 to 5 days, by the appearance of a rash over the entire body. The disease, sometimes fatal to older patients, is far more pernicious than tick-borne typhus, which is rarely fatal.

Another hard tick, *Ixodes dammini*, the deer tick, is the principal vector for the spirochete *Borrelia burgdorferi*, the causative agent of **Lyme disease** in the United States. Recently, in the southeastern United States, *I. scapularis* has also been reported to harbor the spirochete. Lyme disease is currently considered the most frequently diagnosed tick-transmitted disease of humans in the United States and, possibly, the world.

First reported in 1975 in Lyme, Connecticut, Lyme disease has now been reported in Europe, Australia, the USSR, China, Japan, and Africa. The disease, which produces symptoms similar to rheumatoid arthritis, begins as a rash at the site where the tick takes a blood meal. Fatigue, fever, chills, and headache may also occur during this stage, which may last up to 30 days. Neurological complications with muscular pains may then become evident. A small percentage of patients (5%) may also show transitory cardiac malfunctions lasting from 3 days to 6 weeks. Several months after the appearance of the rash, rheumatoid arthritis affecting the knees and other large joints becomes evident. These symptoms persist indefinitely unless treated. Treatment with any of several broad-spectrum antibiotics has proven effective.

While ticks are second only to mosquitoes as vectors for viruses, the assortment of diseases ascribed to such arboviruses is confined mainly to Europe and Asia. Among such diseases are several types of encephalitis, with mortality rates varying from virtually 0% to as high as 25–30%, depending upon the type of virus. Almost all are zoonotic, with small mammals and birds serving as sylvatic reservoirs and hard ticks serving as the usual vectors.

## Mites

The larvae of harvest mites and allied forms (Fig. 17–23), like those of hard ticks, often remain on hosts for long periods of time, dropping off at random. They, too, infest entire, large areas frequented by their hosts and are not limited to nests, dens, and other abodes.

Mites are responsible for the transmission of *Rickettsia tsutsugamushi*, the causative agent for **scrub typhus,** also known as "mite disease" or tsutsugamushi fever. Scrub typhus occurs over large areas of Asia, including Japan and the southern USSR. Humans become infected from the bite of larval chigger mites of the genus *Leptotrombidium.* The larval mites that serve as vectors acquire the rickettsiae from natural reservoir hosts such as voles, rats, and other small mammals. The rickettsiae are then harbored in the mites' salivary glands and transmitted to human hosts. The infected mite carries the rickettsial population throughout its entire development from nymph to adult; and, even though the adult mite is free-living and feeds on insect eggs and minute arthropods, it passes the rickettsiae on, via the egg, to the next generation.

The pathology of the disease varies, ranging from mild to grave. Symptoms usually appear after an incubation period of 4–10 days following the bite of an infected larval mite. An ulcer commonly forms at the site of the bite, and symptoms such as high fever and headache are common.

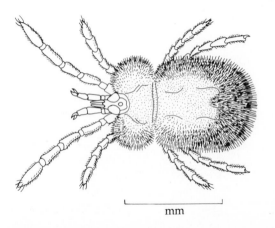

**Figure 17–23**
*Trombicula,* a mite vector of scrub typhus.

mm

⎯⎯⎯⎯⎯⎯⎯⎯◇⎯⎯⎯⎯⎯⎯⎯⎯
# SELECTED READINGS

Busvine, J. R. 1979. Arthropods: Vectors of disease. In *Studies in Biology*, Edward Arnold Publishers, London.

Harwood, R. F., and James, M. T. 1979. *Entomology in Human and Animal Health*, 7th ed. Macmillan, New York.

Jonas, G. 1978. Africa: Taming of the tsetse. *RF Illustrated* 4, 1–4.

McDaniel, B. 1979. *How to Know the Ticks and Mites*. William C. Brown, Dubuque, IA.

Piesman, J. 1987. Emerging tick-borne diseases in temperate climates. *Parasitology Today* 3, 197–199.

Spielman, A. 1988. Lyme disease and human babesiosis: Evidence incriminating vector and reservoir hosts. In *The Biology of Parasitism* (Englund, P. T., and Sher, A., eds.), Pp. 147–65. Alan R. Liss, New York.

---

# CLASSIFICATION OF THE ARTHROPODA*

**PHYLUM ARTHROPODA**

**Subphylum Uniramia**

## CLASS INSECTA

### ORDER DIPTERA
With functional forewings and reduced, knoblike hindwings **(halteres)**; mouthparts variable (piercing-sucking or rasping-lapping) as is body form; with complete metamorphosis.

*Suborder Orthorrhapha*

#### SUPERFAMILY NEMATOCERA

*Family Simuliidae*
Bodies short and stout. Thorax much arched, giving hump-backed appearance; legs comparatively short; antennae 10- or 11-jointed, slightly longer than the head; ocelli absent; compound eyes on males large and contiguous, those on females widely separated; proboscis not elongate; palpi 4-jointed. (Genus mentioned in text: *Simulium*.)

*Family Psychodidae*
Bodies mothlike; antennae slender, clothed with whorls of hair, and long in males; wings with 9 to 11 long, parallel veins, with no cross-veins except at base. (Genera mentioned in text: *Phlebotomus, Lutzomyia*.)

*Family Ceratopogonidae*

*Family Culicidae*
Bodies slight; abdomen long and slender; wings narrow (Fig. 19.5); antennae with 15 segments, plumose in males; proboscis long and slender; wings with fringe of scalelike setae on margins, compound eyes large, occupying a large portion of surface of head; ocelli lacking. (Genera mentioned in text: *Aedes, Anopheles, Culex, Mansonia*.)

#### SUPERFAMILY BRACHYCERA

*Family Tabanidae*
Bodies comparatively large, 7–30 mm long; wings well developed with veins evenly distributed; eyes large and widely separated (dichoptic) in females, contiguous in males (holoptic), antennae usually short and three-jointed, third joint with 4–8 annuli. (Genera mentioned in text: *Chrysops, Tabanus*.)

*Family Rhagionidae*

*Suborder Cyclorrapha*

---

*Only those taxa that include parasitic species mentioned in this text are defined.

*SUPERFAMILY ASCHIZA (OR ASCHIZA GROUP)*

*Family Syrphidae*

*SUPERFAMILY SCHIZOPHORA (OR SCHIZOPHORA GROUP)*

*Family Muscidae*
Typical flies; hypopleural or pteropleural bristles present; basal abdominal bristles reduced; antennae plumose. (Genera mentioned in text: *Musca, Glossina.*)

*Family Calliphoridae*
Bodies, especially abdomens, are metallic green or blue, less frequently violet or copper colored; large flies; antennae are plumose; hypo- and pteropleural bristles present; posterior-most posthumeral bristle present and more ventral than pre-sutural bristle; second ventral abdominal sclerite lies with edges overlying or in contact with ventral edges of corresponding dorsal sclerites. (Genus mentioned in text: *Calliphora.*)

*Family Sarcophagidae*

*Family Gasterophilidae*

*Family Oestridae*

*Family Cuterebridae*

*Family Chloropidae*

*Family Nycteribiidae*

*Family Streblidae*

*Family Hippoboscidae*

*Family Conopidae*

*Family Phasiidae*

*Family Cordyluridae*

*Family Tachinidae*

*Family Braulidae*

## ORDER HEMIPTERA
Primarily ectoparasitic; bodies medium size; with piercing-sucking mouthparts forming a beak; antennae six- to ten-segmented; eyes compound and large; with two pairs of wings; **corium** (thickened portion) present at base of outer wing; thinner extremities of outer wing overlap on dorsum when insect is at rest; wing venation reduced; abdomen lacks cerci; holometabolous metamorphosis.

*Family Cimicidae*

*Family Reduviidae*
Beak short, three-jointed, attached to tip of head; distal end of beak rests on prosternum in groove when not in use; ocelli present in winged species (with few exceptions); antennae

four-jointed. (Genera mentioned in text: *Triatoma, Rhodnius, Panstrongylus.*)

*Family Polyctenidae*

## ORDER HYMENOPTERA

*Suborder Symphyta ( = Chalastogastra)*

*Family Oryssidae*

*Suborder Apocrita ( = Clistogastra)*

*SUPERFAMILY ICHNEUMONOIDEA*

*SUPERFAMILY CHALCIDOIDEA*

*SUPERFAMILY PROCTOTRUPOIDEA*

*SUPERFAMILY CYNIPOIDEA*

*SUPERFAMILY CHRYSIDOIDEA*

*SUPERFAMILY SCOLIOIDEA*

## ORDER COLEOPTERA
Few species endoparasitic in other insects; with two pairs of wings; forewings (elytra) veinless, hard, covering dorsal aspect of abdomen while in resting position, meeting along middorsal line; mouthparts of chewing type; antennae of 10 to 14 segments; compound eyes conspicuous; legs heavily sclerotized; holometabolous metamorphosis. (Genus mentioned in text: Family Tenebrionidae—*Tenebrio.*)

## ORDER STREPSIPTERA

*Family Mengeidae*

*Family Stylopidae*

*Family Elenchidae*

*Family Halictophagidae*

## ORDER SIPHONAPTERA
Adults small and wingless; ectoparasitic on birds and mammals; bodies laterally compressed; legs long, stout, and spinose; antennae short and clubbed, and fit in depressions alongside of head when not extended; mouthparts of piercing-sucking type; holometabolous metamorphosis.

*Family Ceratophyllidae*

*Family Pulicidae*
Three thoracic tergites together longer than first abdominal tergite; head evenly rounded along margin; no vertical suture from dorsal margin of head to bases of antennae; abdominal tergites with one row of setae. (Genera mentioned in text: *Pulex, Xenopsylla.*)

## ORDER MALLOPHAGA
Ectoparasitic on birds and mammals; bodies small to medium

size, usually dorsoventrally flattened and wingless; with chewing mouthparts; antennae short, three- to five-segmented; with reduced compound eyes and no ocelli; thorax small; legs stout and short; no cerci on abdomen; hemimetabolous metamorphosis.

*SUBORDER AMBLYCERA*

*Family Gyropidae*

*Family Menoponidae*

*Family Boopiidae*

*Family Ricinidae*

*Family Tungidae*

*Family Ischnopsyllidae*

*Family Hystrichopsyllidae*

*Family Macropsyllidae*

*SUBORDER ISCHNOCERA*
Antennae three- or five-segmented, filiform, not concealed; maxillary palpi absent, mandibles vertically orientated; parasitic on birds and mammals.

*Family Trichodectidae*
Antennae three-jointed; with one claw on tarsi; parasitic on mammals. (Genus mentioned in text: *Trichodectes*.)

*Family Philopteridae*

*SUBORDER RHYNCHOPHTHIRINA*

*ORDER ANOPURA*
Ectoparasites of mammals; bodies small to medium size, dorsoventrally flattened, and wingless; mouthparts modified as piercing-sucking organ that is retractile; antennae short, three- to five-segmented; some with legs terminating as hooked claws; thorax fused; abdomen of five to eight distinct segments; hemimetabolous metamorphosis.

*Family Echinophthiriidae*

*Family Pediculidae*
Parasites of primates, including humans; bodies fairly robust, not covered with dense spines; abdomen armed with pleural plates (paratergites) and with tergal and sternal plates in most species; with well-developed eyes, comprised of pigment granules and a lens; with legs approximately equal in length or with first pair slightly smaller. (Genera mentioned in text: *Pediculus, Phthirus*.)

*Family Haematopinidae*

*Family Haematopinoididae*

## Subphylum Chelicerata

### ORDER ACARINA

Highly specialized Arachnida with body divided into protero-soma and hysterosoma which are distinguishable as boundary between second and third pairs of legs; segments of mouth and its appendages situated on capitulum (gnathostoma), more or less sharply set off from rest of body; typically with four pairs of legs; usually six podomeres of legs but may vary from two to seven; positions of respiratory and genital openings variable.

#### Suborder Metastigmata (Ixodides)

Large parasitic acarines known as ticks; mouth with recurved teeth modified for piercing; a tracheal spiracle located behind third or fourth pair of coxae.

##### Family Ixodidae (Hard Ticks)

Body ovoid; scutum present in all stages; scutum of adult males extends to posterior margin of body; scutum of adult females, like that of larvae and nymphs, restricted to propo-dosomal zone; capitulum anterior and visible from dorsal view; festoons usually present; eyes, if present, situated dor-sally on sides of scutum; segments of pedipalps fused, not movable; porose areas present on base of capitulum in fe-males; stigmatal plates large, posterior to coxa IV; only fe-males distended when engorged with blood; with marked sexual dimorphism. (Genera mentioned in text: *Dermacentor, Ixodes, Rhipicephalus.*)

##### Family Argasidae (Soft Ticks)

Integument leathery in nymphal and adult stages, and wrin-kled, granulated, mammillated or having tubercles; scutum absent in all stages; capitulum either subterminal or protrud-ing from anterior margin of body in nymphs and adults, sub-terminal or terminal in larvae; capitulum lies in distinctly or indistinctly marked depression (camerostome) in all stages; pedipalps freely articulate in all stages; porose area absent in both sexes; eyes usually absent (if present, or supracoxal folds); stigmata near coxa III lack stigmal plates; both sexes distended when engorged with blood; sexual dimorphism slight. (Genus mentioned in text: *Ornithodoros.*)

#### Suborder Notostigmata

#### Suborder Tetrastigmata (Holothyroidea)

#### Suborder Mesostigmata

# GLOSSARY

**Acquired immunity**   a host's immune response to previous parasitic infection.

**Amastigote**   a form of hemoflagellate that develops intracellularly and is characterized by subspherical shape and the presence of a very short flagellum.

**Amphids**   small depressions or pits located anteriorly on the body surface of most nematodes and believed to be chemoreceptors.

**Anthrax**   a bacterial disease of humans, cattle, and sheep, transmitted by tabanid flies.

**Antibody**   a protein synthesized in response to an antigen or, in varying degrees, to molecules of similar structure; an antibody usually binds with a specific antigen.

**Antigen**   any substance, usually proteinaceous, capable, under appropriate conditions, of inducing the host to synthesize antibodies.

**Apical complex**   a combination of structures found in the apical region of sporozoites and merozoites of members of the phylum Apicomplexa.

**Apolysis**   the release of gravid, or egg-filled, proglottids from tapeworm strobila.

**Arbovirus**   a virus transmitted from one human to another by an arthropod.

**Autoinfection**   reinfection of a parasitic organism without its leaving the host.

**Axoneme**   a microtubular element usually extending the length of a flagellum or cilium.

**Axostyle**   a tube-shaped sheath of microtubules, observed in many flagellates, that usually extends from a basal body to the posterior end.

**B cell**   a specialized lymphocyte that produces humoral, or circulatory, antibodies.

**Basal body**   an organelle, morphologically identical to a centriole, from which the flagellum or cilium originates.

**Biological vector**   an arthropod used by a disease-producing organism for transmission and as a vehicle for reproduction and/or development.

**Blackwater fever**   massive lysis of vertebrate erythrocytes that, at times, accompanies falciparum malaria.

**Blepharaphast**   See *basal body*.

**Bothrium**   groove on the scolex of some tapeworms.

**Breakbone fever**   an arbovirus-caused disease. See *dengue*.

**Calabar swelling**   a transient, subcutaneous swelling caused by the nematode *Loa loa*.

**Capitulum** a small, anterior projection of acarines that bears the mouthparts.

**Cell-mediated reaction** the effect produced by specialized cells, e.g., T lymphocytes, mobilized to arrest and, in most cases, eventually destroy a parasite.

**Cellular reaction** See *cell-mediated reaction*.

**Cercocystis** a modified cysticercoid larva of *Hymenolepis nana* found in the intestinal villus of the definitive host.

**Cercomer** the posterior extension of procercoid and cysticercoid larvae, usually retaining the oncospheral hooks.

**Chagas' disease** a disease, also known as American trypanosomiasis, caused by *Trypanosoma cruzi*.

**Chigger** a mite of the family Trombiculidae.

**Chromatoidal bar** a structure considered by many to be deposits of nucleic acids in members of the genus *Entamoeba*.

**Cirrus** the penis or ejaculatory duct of a flatworm.

**Coenurus** a larval tapeworm of certain cyclophyllideans in which numerous scolices bud from an internal germinal epithelium.

**Commensalism** a symbiotic relationship in which neither the commensal nor the host is physiologically dependent upon the other.

**Conoid** a truncated cone of spirally arranged, fibrillar structures in the apical complex of certain members of the suborder Eimeriina, e.g., *Toxoplasma gondii*.

**Coracidium** an oncosphere surrounded by a ciliated embryophore.

**Corrion's disease** a severe, often fatal, bacterial infection found among inhabitants of parts of South America and transmitted by sandflies.

**Costa** a striated rod, associated with basal bodies of many flagellates, that courses along the base of an undulating membrane.

**Creeping eruption** the irritation and rash caused by hookworm larvae in an unnatural host.

**Cutaneous larval migrans** a condition caused by the migration of nematode larvae in the skin of an unnatural host. See *creeping eruption*.

**Cysticercoid** the tapeworm larva, featuring a cercomer and a fully developed scolex enclosed within a multilayered cyst wall, that develops from the oncosphere of some cyclophyllideans.

**Cysticercosis** infection with cysticercus larvae.

**Cysticercus** a tapeworm larva, developing from the oncosphere of some cyclophyllideans, that is characterized by a fully developed scolex invaginated into a fluid-filled vesicle, or bladder; also called "bladderworm".

**Cystogenous glands**   in some cercariae of digenetic trematodes, secretory cells that give rise to metacercarial cysts.

**Definitive host**   See *host, definitive.*

**Delayed hypersensitivity**   increased reactivity to a specific antigen, mediated by cells rather than antibodies, usually requiring up to 24 hours to reach maximum intensity. See T lymphocyte.

**Dengue**   a disease caused by a mosquito-transmitted virus; also known as "blackwater fever".

**Ectoparasite**   a parasite that lives on the exterior surface of the host.

**Ectopic site**   abnormal or unexpected site of infection.

**Edema**   fluid accumulation in intercellular spaces, resulting in localized swelling.

**Endoparasite**   a parasite that lives inside the host.

**Epidemiology**   the study of the occurrence of a particular disease, including ecological factors, transmission, prevalence, and incidence.

**Epimastigote**   a form of hemoflagellate, equipped with a short undulating membrane, in which the kinetoplast lies near, but anterior to, the nucleus.

**Espundia**   a disease caused by *Leishmania braziliensis*, also known as mucocutaneous leishmaniasis, uta, pian bois, and chiclero ulcer.

**Facultative parasite**   an organism that, given the opportunity, can assume a parasitic existence.

**Flame cell excretory system**   a protonephridial excretory system with a current-producing mechanism at the closed end.

**Gastrodermis**   the tissue lining the digestive tract, as found in digenetic trematodes.

**Genital atrium**   a circumscribed area in the body wall of flatworms into which male and female genital ducts open; also known as common genital pore.

**Germ cell cycle**   asexual reproduction in digenea during which progeny arise through differentiation of germinal cells passed from one generation to the next.

**Glycocalyx**   the carbohydrate-containing outer coat found on the free surface of most cells.

**Glycosome**   a membrane-bound, microbodylike organelle, peculiar to the hemoflagellates, that contains enzymes essential for glycolysis.

**Gonotyl**   the muscular sucker or specialized structure surrounding the genital pore of some digeneans.

**Ground itch**   a localized irritation and rash caused by penetrating larvae and the accompanying bacteria of hookworms of humans.

**Gynaecophoral canal**   the ventral fold or groove in male schistosomes in which female worms are held *in copula.*

**Halzoun**   the disease resulting from nasopharyngeal blockage due to the attachment of worms, such as pentastomids or young digenea, to buccal or pharyngeal membranes.

**Hemocoel**   the major body cavity of arthropods, typically containing blood or hemolymph.

**Hemozoin**   granules, seen in erythrocytes infected with *Plasmodium malariae,* that may represent residues from incomplete hemoglobin digestion.

**Heterogonic**   the term used to describe a life cycle in which free-living generations may alternate periodically with parasitic generations.

**Homogonic**   the term used to describe a lifestyle that is consistently either parasitic or free-living.

**Host, definitive**   the host in which a parasite attains sexual maturity.

**Host, intermediate**   the host in which a parasite undergoes developmental changes but does not yet reach sexual maturity.

**Host, paratenic**   the host in which a parasite resides without further development; a transfer host.

**Host, reservoir**   a host, usually nonhuman, in which a parasite lives and remains a source of infection but usually produces no symptoms.

**Host specificity**   the extent to which a parasite can exist in more than one host species.

**Humoral reaction**   the effect produced when specialized molecules of the circulatory system interact with a parasite, usually immobilizing or destroying it.

**Hydatid**   a larval tapeworm, of the cyclophyllidean genus *Echinococcus,* in which numerous scolices bud from secondary cysts.

**Hydrogenosome**   a membrane-bound organelle in the cytoplasm of some flagellates (e.g., Trichomonads) that is involved in carbohydrate metabolism, an end-product of which may be molecular hydrogen.

**Hypnozoite**   the dormant stage of *Plasmodium vivax* passed in hepatocytes of the human host.

**Hypobiosis**   a lag phase at some stage of development in the life cycle of a nematode.

**Hypodermis**   the tissue that secretes the nematode cuticle.

**Infraciliature**   in a ciliophoran, numerous basal bodies interconnected by fibrils.

**K-strategist**   an organism employing a survival strategy characterized by low reproductive capability, low mortality, long life span, and saturation of an environment.

**Kala-azar**   a disease, also known as visceral leishmaniasis and Dumdum fever, caused by *Leishmania donovani*.

**Kinetosome**   See *basal body*.

**Laurer's canal**   a canal, originating on the surface of the oviduct near the seminal receptacle in some digenetic trematodes, that may represent a vestigial vagina.

**Leishmaniasis**   a disease caused by members of the genus *Leishmania*.

**Lymphokine**   any of several chemical mediators, released by T cells, that react with other cells essential to the inflammatory process.

**Lysosomotropic agents**   a group of chemical compounds, such as chloroquine, that demonstrate an affinity for lysosomes.

**Macrogametocyte**   the cell that gives rise to a macrogamete.

**Malpighian tubules**   excretory organs of terrestrial insects and most acarines.

**Maurer's dots**   aggregates in cytoplasm of erythrocytes infected with *Plasmodium falciparum*.

**Mechanical vector**   a passive carrier of a disease-producing agent.

**Mehlis' gland**   a group of unicellular glands that empty into the ootype region of flatworms.

**Merozoite**   one of many cells resulting from schizogony.

**Metacercaria**   the larval stage between cercaria and adult in the life cycle of many digenetic trematodes.

**Metacyclic**   the term used to describe a form of parasite infective to its vertebrate host, e.g., metacyclic trypomastigote.

**Metacystic trophozoite**   a small trophozoite of *Entamoeba* spp. that emerges from the cyst in the intestine of the host.

**Metraterm**   the muscular, distal portion of the uterus of digenetic trematodes.

**Microfilaria**   the juvenile, first-stage larva of filarial nematodes.

**Microgametocyte**   the cell that gives rise to microgametes.

**Micronemes**   small, convoluted structures that lie parallel to rhoptries and appear to merge with them at the apices of sporozoites and merozoites.

**Microthrix** (plural, *microthrices*)   a specialized microvillus that projects from the outer, limiting membrane of the tapeworm tegument.

**Miracidium**   the ciliated larva that emerges from the egg of digenetic trematodes.

**Molecular mimicry**   production of or covering by hostlike molecules, especially on the body surface of a parasite.

**Mutualism**   a symbiotic relationship in which each partner is physiologically dependent on the other.

**Nagana**   a disease of domestic ruminants, caused by *Trypanosoma brucei brucei, T. congolense,* and *T. vivax.*

**Natural immunity**   the type of immunity conferred by the presence in an organism of certain naturally occurring proteins that exhibit structural properties of antibodies to specific antigens even in the absence of previous exposure to those antigens.

**Oncosphere**   the hexacanth embryo of a tapeworm.

**Oocyst**   a rounded cyst containing sporoblasts.

**Ookinete**   the motile, elongated zygote of many apicomplexans.

**Ootype**   a specialized region of the flatworm oviduct that is surrounded by Mehlis' gland.

**Open circulatory system**   the system, characteristic of arthropods and molluscs, in which blood flows slowly through large sinuses (hemocoel) back to a dorsal, tubular heart.

**Operculum**   a lidlike structure at one end of the eggshell of many digenetic trematodes and some cestodes.

**Oriental sore**   a disease, also known as cutaneous leishmaniasis, caused by *Leishmania tropica.*

**Parasitism**   a symbiotic relationship in which only one of the organisms, the parasite, is physiologically dependent upon the other, the host.

**Parasitophorus vacuole**   within a cell, a vacuole containing a parasite (e.g., amastigote).

**Paratenic host**   See *host, paratenic.*

**Parenchyma**   in flatworms, mesodermal tissue filling all available body spaces.

**Parthenogenesis**   development of an unfertilized egg to a new individual.

**Phasmids**   small, sensory pits, believed to be chemoreceptors, located posteriorly on the body surface of members of the nematode class Secernentea.

**Phoresis**   a form of commensalism in which one organism is mechanically carried by the other; the relationship is nonobligatory.

**Plasma cell**   an effector B cell that secretes into the circulation large numbers of antibodies of the same specificity as its cell surface receptors.

**Plerocercoid**   the larval form that develops from the procercoid, as in *Diphyllobothrium latum.*

**Polar rings**   electron-dense structures, circling the apical region, that constitute part of the apical complex of sporozoites and mero-zoites of apicomplexans such as *Plasmodium* spp.

**Polyembryony**   the formation of multiple embryos from a single zygote with no intervening gamete stage.

**Premunition**   a form of acquired immunity dependent upon reten-tion of the infective agent.

**Procercoid**   the larval form that develops from the coracidium.

**Proglottid**   one segment in a tapeworm strobila complete with a full complement of reproductive organs.

**Promastigote**   a hemoflagellate form bearing an anterior flagellum and a kinetoplast well anterior to the nucleus.

**Protoscolex**   the immature scolex found in coenurus and hydatid larvae.

**Pseudocyst**   a cluster of amastigotes of *Trypanosoma cruzi* in a mus-cle fiber.

**Parabasal body**   the Golgi complex of protozoans.

**Parabasal filament**   a fibril running from the cisternae of the Golgi complex to one or more basal bodies.

**R-strategist**   an organism employing a survival strategy character-ized by high reproductive rates, high mortality, and short life span.

**Receptor cell**   a functionally specialized lymphocyte that produces a specific antibody.

**Recrudescence**   a sudden increase in a previously persistent, low-level parasite population (e.g., *Plasmodium malariae*).

**Redia**   a larval form that arises asexually from within a sporocyst or a primary redia of a digenetic trematode.

**Renette**   a large, unicellular gland that empties to the exterior through a pore and serves as the basic component of the nematode excretory system.

**Reservoir host**   See *host, reservoir*.

**Resistance**   the ability of an organism to withstand infection.

**Retroinfection**   reinfection by nematode larvae (e.g., *Enterobius vermicularis*) that hatch on skin and re-enter the host's body.

**Rhoptry**   part of the apical complex of the sporozoites and mero-zoites of apicomplexans, composed of electron-dense bodies ex-tending posteriorly from the apex.

**Romaño's sign**   early symptoms of Chagas' disease, consisting of unilateral, periorbital edema and conjunctivitis.

**Rostellum**   the small, rounded projection, sometimes bearing hooks, on the apex of the scolex of some tapeworms.

**Schistosomule**   in a blood fluke, the juvenile stage that develops following cercarial penetration of the definitive host. Sometimes called a schistosomulum.

**Schizogony**   a form of asexual reproduction characterized by rapid organelle and nuclear divisions, followed by cytoplasmic divisions, and resulting in many simultaneous daughter cells.

**Schizont**   a multinucleated cell undergoing schizogony, prior to cytoplasmic division.

**Schüffner's dots**   fine granules distributed throughout erythrocytes infected with *Plasmodium vivax*.

**Scolex**   the holdfast organ of tapeworms.

**Scrub typhus**   rickettsial disease transmitted by chigger mites.

**Shell-yolk glands**   clusters of cells each of which synthesizes globules essential to eggshell formation in many flatworms.

**Sleeping sickness**   a disease caused by *Trypanosoma brucei rhodesiense* and *T. b. gambiense* in Africa; also, any one of many arboviruses transmitted by mosquitoes and causing encephalitis.

**Sparganosis**   infection with plerocercoid larvae.

**Sporoblasts**   in the oocyst of apicomplexans, cells that divide into sporozoites while still enclosed by the sporoblast membrane.

**Sporocyst**   the larval stage of a digenetic trematode into which the miracidium metamorphoses, usually in a mollusc.

**Sporogony**   multiple divisions of a zygote.

**Stichocytes**   a series of unicellular glands surrounding the capillarylike esophagus of many adenophorean nematodes, e.g., *Trichuris trichiura*.

**Strobila**   in tapeworms, a chain of segments formed by budding.

**Strobilization**   the formation of a strobila by a tapeworm.

**Sylvatic animal**   an animal that lives in the wild.

**Syngamy**   the union of gametes.

**T cell**   a specialized lymphocyte, processed through the thymus, that elicits cell-mediated reactions.

**Tachyzoite**   a form of merozoite in *Toxoplasma*, found in parasitophorous vacuoles of vertebrate hosts.

**Tegument**   the syncytium that covers the surface of trematodes and cestodes.

**Trophozoite**   the motile, feeding stage of protozoans.

**Trypomastigote**   a hemoflagellate form with an elongated undulating membrane and kinetoplast located posterior to the nucleus.

**Tularemia**   a bacterial disease of humans transmitted by tabanid flies and for which rabbits often serve as sylvatic reservoir hosts.

**Undulating membrane**   that portion of a plasma membrane or cytoplasm of a flagellate that is drawn away from the cell during the beating of a recurrent flagellum.

**Vagina**   in tapeworms, a tubular organ that joins the oviduct and carries sperm from the genital atrium to the oviduct.

**Variant antigenic types**   divergent surface antigens that arise as the result of the ability of trypomastigote populations circulating in the bloodstream to change the chemical composition of the glycocalyx.

**Vector**   any agent, most commonly an arthropod, that actively transmits a disease-producing organism.

**Vermicle**   the infective stage, analogous to sporozoite, of *Babesia* spp. from ticks.

**Visceral larval migrans**   migration of second-stage larvae of nematodes in the internal organs of unnatural hosts.

**Vitellaria**   See *shell-yolk gland.*

**Winterbottom's sign**   symptom of African sleeping sickness characterized by enlarged, sensitive cervical lymph nodes.

**Xenodiagnosis**   diagnostic technique in which researchers identify a disease by infecting a laboratory animal and assessing its symptoms.

**Yaws**   a fly-transmitted disease that is caused by the spirochete *Treponema.*

**Yellow fever**   a viral disease transmitted by the mosquito *Aedes aegypti.*

**Zoonosis**   a disease of animals that can be transmitted to humans.

# APPENDIX A

## DRUGS FOR PARASITIC INFECTIONS: PARTIAL LIST OF GENERIC AND BRAND NAMES

**Amphotericin B**    Fungizone (Squibb)

*"**Antimony dimercaptosuccinate**" (stibocaptate)    Astiban (Hoffman-LaRoche, Switzerland)

**Benzyl benzoate**    Scabanca (Anca Labs., Canada); others

***Bithionol**    Bithin (Tanabe Seiyaku, Japan)

**Chloroquine**    Aralen (Winthrop); others

**Cupric oleate**    Cuprex (Beecham Research Labs., England)

**Crotamiton**    Eurax (Ciba-Geigy, Switzerland); Crotan (Alcon Labs.)

***Dehydroemetine**    Hoffman-LaRoche, Switzerland

**Diethylcarbamazine citrate**    Hetrazan (Lederle Labs.)

**Diiodohydroxyquin (iodoquinol)**    Glenwood Labs.

***Diloxanide furoate**    Furamide (Clin-Comar-Byla, France)

**Furazolidone**    Furoxane (Norwich-Eaton)

***Ivermectin**    Merck & Co.

**Lindane (gamma benzene hexachloride)**    Kwell (Reed & Carnrick); others

**Mebendazole**    Vermox (Janssen, Belgium)

***Melarsoprol**    Arsobal (Specia, France)

***Metrifonate (trichlorfon)**    Bilarcil (Bayer, Germany)

**Metronidazole**    Flagyl (Searle)

***Niclosamide**    Yomesan (Bayer, Germany)

***Nifurtimox**    Lampit (Bayer, Germany)

***Niridazole**    Ambilhar (Ciba-Geigy, Switzerland)

**Oxamniquine**    Vansil (Pfizer)

**Paromomycin sulfate**    Humatin (Parke, Davis)

***Pentamidine isethionate**    Lomidine (Rhône-Poulenc, France)

**Piperazine citrate**    Antepar (Burroughs Wellcome); others

***Praziquantel**    Biltricide (Bayer, Germany)

**Primaquine diphosphate**    Primaquine (Winthrop)

**Pyrantel pamoate**    Antiminth (Roerig)

**Pyrethrins and piperonyl butoxide**

**Pyrimethamine**    Daraprim (Burroughs Wellcome)

**Pyrimethamine plus sulfadoxine**    Fansidar (Hoffman-LaRoche, Switzerland)

**Pyrvinium pamoate**   Povan (Parke, Davis)

**Quinacrine hydrochloride**   Atabrine dihydrochloride (Winthrop)

****Spiramycin**   Rovamycin (Rhodia Pharma GmbH, West Germany)

***Sodium stibogluconate (antimony sodium gluconate)**   Pentostam (Burroughs Wellcome)

***Suramin sodium**   Germanin (Bayer, Germany)

**Tetrachloroethylene**   Nema Worm Capsules, Vet (Parke, Davis)

**Thiabendazole**   Mintezol (Merck Sharpe & Dohme)

****Tinidazole**   Fasigyn (Pfizer)

**Trimethoprim–sulfamethoxazole**   Bactrim (Hoffman-LaRoche, Switzerland); Septra (Burroughs Wellcome)

****Tryparsamide**

---

*Available from the Parasitic Diseases Division, Centers for Disease Control, U.S. Public Health Service, Atlanta, GA.

**Not available in the United States.

***Available in the United States only on an investigational basis from manufacturers.

# APPENDIX B

# CURRENT CHEMOTHERAPEUTIC REGIMENS

## Amoebiasis (Entamoeba histolytica)

| Infection | | Drug | Adult Dose | Pediatric Dose |
|---|---|---|---|---|
| *Asymptomatic* | | | | |
| Drug of choice: | | Diiodohydroxyquin | 650 mg tid × 20d | 30–40 mg/kg/d in 3 doses × 20d |
| Alternative(s): | | Diloxanide furoate | 500 mg tid × 10d | 20 mg/kg/d in 3 doses × 10d |
| | | Paromomycin sulfate | 25–30 mg/kg/d in 3 doses × 7d | 25–30 mg/kg/d in 3 doses × 7d |
| *Mild to moderate intestinal disease* | | | | |
| Drug of choice: | | Metronidazole | 750 mg tid × 5–10d | 35–50 mg/kg/d in 3 doses × 10d |
| | | *plus* | | |
| | | Diiodohydroxyquin | 650 mg tid × 20d | 30–40 mg/kg/d in 3 doses × 20d |
| Alternative: | | Paromomycin sulfate | 25–30 mg/kg/d in 3 doses × 7d | 25–30 mg/kg/d in 3 doses × 7d |
| *Severe intestinal disease* | | | | |
| Drug of choice: | | Metronidazole | 750 mg tid × 5–10d | 35–50 mg/kg/d in 3 doses × 10d |
| | | *plus* | | |
| | | Diiodohydroxyquin | 650 mg tid × 20d | 30–40 mg/kg/d in 3 doses × 20d |
| Alternative(s): | | Dehydroemetine | 1–1.5 mg/kg/d IM (max 90 mg/d) for up to 5d | 1–1.5 mg/kg/d IM (max 90 mg/d) in 2 doses, up to 5d |
| | | *plus* | | |
| | | Diiodohydroxyquin | 650 mg tid × 20d | 30–40 mg/kg/d in 3 doses × 20d |
| | OR | Emetine | 1 mg/kg/d (max 60 mg/d) IM for up to 5d | 1 mg/kg/d (max 60 mg/d) IM for up to 5d |
| | | *plus* | | |
| | | Diiodohydroxyquin | 650 mg tid × 20d | 30–40 mg/kg/d in 3 doses × 20d |
| *Hepatic abscess* | | | | |
| Drug of choice: | | Metronidazole | 750 mg tid × 5–10d | 35–50 mg/kg/d in 3 doses × 10d |
| | | *plus* | | |
| | | Diiodohydroxyquin | 650 mg tid × 20d | 30–40 mg/kg/d in 3 doses × 20d |
| Alternative(s): | | Dehydroemetine *followed by* | 1–1.5 mg/kg/d (max 90 mg/d) IM for up to 5d | 1–1.5 mg/kg/d (max 90 mg/d) IM, in 2 doses, up to 5d |
| | | Chloroquine | 600-mg base (1 g) daily × 2d, then 300-mg base (500 mg)/d × 2–3wks | 10-mg base/kg/d (max 300 mg-base/d) × 2–3 wks |
| | | *plus* | | |
| | | Diiodohydroxyquin | 650 mg tid × 20d | 30–40 mg/kg/d in 3 doses × 20d |
| | OR | Emetine *followed by* | 1 mg/kg/d (max 60 mg/d) IM for up to 5d | 1 mg/kg/d in 2 doses IM (max 60 mg/d), up to 5d |
| | | Chloroquine | 600-mg base (1 g) daily × 2d, then 300-mg base (500 mg) daily × 2–3 wks | 10-mg base/kg/d (max 300 mg-base/d) × 2–3 wks |
| | | *plus* | | |
| | | Diiodohydroxyquin | 650 mg tid × 20d | 30–40 mg/kg/d in 3 doses × 20d |

**Amoebic Meningoencephalitis, Primary (*Naegleria* spp.; *Acanthamoeba* spp.)**
Drug of choice:    Amphotericin B — 1 mg/kg/d IV, uncertain duration | 1 mg/kg/d IV, uncertain duration

**Ancylostoma duodenale (hookworm)**
Drug of choice:    Mebendazole — 100 mg bid × 3d | 100 mg bid × 3d for children > 2 yrs
    OR   Pyrantel pamoate — Single dose of 11 mg/kg (max 1 g) | Single dose of 11 mg/kg (max 1 g)

**Anisakiasis (*Anisakis* spp.)**
Treatment of choice:   Surgical removal
Alternative:    Thiabendazole — 25 mg/kg bid × 3d | 25 mg/kg bid × 3d

**Ascaris lumbricoides (roundworm)**
Drug of choice:    Mebendazole — 100 mg bid × 3d | 100 mg bid × 3d for children > 2 yrs
    OR   Pyrantel pamoate — Single dose of 11 mg/kg (max 1 g) | Single dose of 11 mg/kg (max 1 g)
Alternative:    Piperazine citrate — 75 mg/kg (max 3.5 g/d × 2d) | 75 mg/kg (max 3.5 g/d × 2d)

**Babesia**
There are no completely satisfactory drugs available for the therapy of *Babesia* infections in humans. Chloroquine has been used and produces symptomatic improvement but does not reduce parasitemia. Pentamidine isethionate also has been used. Recently one patient was successfully treated with clindamycin and quinine.

**Balantidium coli**
Drug of choice:    Tetracycline — 500 mg qid × 10d | 10 mg/kg qid × 10d (max 2 g/d)
Alternative:    Diiodohydroxyquin — 650 mg tid × 20d | 40 mg/kg/d in 3 doses × 20d

**Brugia malayi. See Filariasis**

**Chagas' Disease. See Trypanosomiasis**

**Clonorchis sinensis. See Flukes**

**Cutaneous Larval Migrans (creeping eruption)**
Drug of choice:    Thiabendazole — Topically and/or 25 mg/kg bid (max 3 g/d) × 2–5d | Topically and/or 25 mg/kg bid (max 3 g/d) × 2–5d

**Dientamoeba fragilis**
Drug of choice:    Diiodohydroxyquin — 650 mg tid × 20d | 40–50 mg/kg/d in 3 doses × 20d
    OR   Tetracycline — 500 mg qid × 10d | 10 mg/kg qid × 10d (max 2 g/d)

**Diphyllobothrium latum. See Tapeworms**

| Infection | Drug | Adult Dose | Pediatric Dose |
|---|---|---|---|
| ***Dracunculus medinensis* (guinea worm)** | | | |
| Drug of choice: | Niridazole | 25 mg/kg (max 1.5 g/d × 15d | 12.5 mg/kg bid (max 1.5 g/d) × 15d |
| Alternative: | Metronidazole | 250 mg tid × 10d | 25 mg/kg/d (max 750 mg/d) in 3 doses × 10d |
| ***Echinococcus.* See Tapeworms** | | | |
| ***Entamoeba histolytica.* See Amoebiasis** | | | |
| ***Enterobius vermicularis* (pinworm)** | | | |
| Drug of choice: | Pyrantel pamoate | Single dose of 11 mg/kg (max 1 g); repeat after 2 wks | Single dose of 11 mg/kg (max 1 g); repeat after 2 wks |
| | OR   Mebendazole | Single dose of 100 mg; repeat after 2 wks | Single dose of 100 mg for children > 2 years; repeat after 2 wks |
| Alternative(s): | Piperazine citrate | 65 mg/kg (max 2.5 g)/d × 7d; repeat after 2 wks | 65 mg/kg (max 2.5 g)/d × 7d; repeat after 2 wks |
| | Pyrvinium pamoate | 5 mg/kg single dose (max 350 mg); repeat after 2 wks | 5 mg/kg single dose (max 350 mg); repeat after 2 wks |
| ***Fasciola hepatica.* See Flukes** | | | |
| **Filariasis** | | | |
| *Wuchereria bancrofti, Brugia malayi, Loa loa* | | | |
| Drug of choice: | Diethylcarbamazine citrate | Day 1: 50 mg<br>Day 2: 50 mg tid<br>Day 3: 100 mg tid<br>Days 4–21: 2 mg/kg tid | Day 1: 25–50 mg<br>Day 2: 25–50 mg tid<br>Day 3: 50–100 mg tid<br>Days 4–21: 2 mg/kg tid |
| *Tropical eosinophilia* | | | |
| Drug of choice: | Diethylcarbamazine citrate | 2 mg/kg tid × 7–10d | 2 mg/kg tid × 7–10d |
| *Onchocerca volvulus* | | | |
| Drug of choice: | Diethylcarbamazine citrate | 25 mg/d × 3d, then 50 mg/d × 5d, then 100 mg/d × 3d, then 150 mg/d × 12d | 0.5 mg/kg tid × 3d (max 25 mg/d), then 1.0 mg/kg tid × 3–4d (max 50 mg/d), then 1.5 mg/kg tid × 3–4d (max 100 mg/d), then 2.0 mg/kg tid × 2–3 wks (max 150 mg/d) |
| | *followed by*<br>Suramin sodium | 100–200 mg (test dose) IV, then 1 g IV at weekly intervals × 5 wks | 10–20 mg (test dose) IV, then 20 mg/kg IV at weekly intervals × 5 wks |

**Flukes, Hermaphroditic**

*Clonorchis sinensis (Chinese liver fluke)*

| | | | |
|---|---|---|---|
| Alternative: | Mebendazole | 1 g bid × 28d | |

| | | Dose 1 | Dose 2 |
|---|---|---|---|
| Drug of choice: | Praziquantel | 25 mg/kg tid × 1d | 25 mg/kg tid × 1d |

*Fasciola hepatica (sheep liver fluke)*

| | | | |
|---|---|---|---|
| Drug of choice: | Praziquantel | 25 mg/kg tid × 1d | 25 mg/kg tid × 1d |
| Alternative: | Bithionol | 30–50 mg/kg on alternate days × 10–15 doses | 30–50 mg/kg on alternate days × 10–15 doses |

*Fasciolopsis buski (intestinal fluke)*

| | | | |
|---|---|---|---|
| Drug of choice: | Praziquantel | 25 mg/kg tid × 1d | 25 mg/kg tid × 1d |
| Alternative: | Tetrachloroethylene | 0.1–0.12 ml/kg (max 5 ml) | 0.1 ml/kg (max 5 ml) |

*Heterophyes heterophyes (intestinal fluke)*

| | | | |
|---|---|---|---|
| Drug of choice: | Praziquantel | 25 mg/kg tid × 1d | 25 mg/kg tid × 1d |
| Alternative: | Tetrachloroethylene | 0.1–0.12 ml/kg (max 5 ml) | 0.1 ml/kg (max 5 ml) |

*Metagonimus yokogawai (intestinal fluke)*

| | | | |
|---|---|---|---|
| Drug of choice: | Praziquantel | 25 mg/kg tid × 1d | 25 mg/kg tid × 1d |
| OR | Tetrachloroethylene | 0.1–0.12 ml/kg (max 5 ml) | 0.1 ml/kg (max 5 ml) |

*Paragonimus westermani (lung fluke)*

| | | | |
|---|---|---|---|
| Drug of choice: | Praziquantel | 25 mg/kg tid × 1d | 25 mg/kg tid × 1d |
| Alternative: | Bithionol | 30–50 mg/kg on alternate days × 10–15 doses | 30–50 mg/kg on alternate days × 10–15 doses |

**Giardiasis (Giardia lamblia)**

| | | | |
|---|---|---|---|
| Drug of choice: | Quinacrine hydrochloride | 100 mg tid pc × 5d | 2 mg/kg tid pc × 5d (max 300 mg/d) |
| Alternative(s): | Metronidazole | 250 mg tid × 5d | 5 mg/kg pc × 5d (max 300 mg/d) |
| | Furazolidone | 100 mg qid × 7d | 1.25 mg/kg qid × 7d |

**Hookworm. See Ancylostoma; Necator**

**Hymenolepis nana. See Tapeworms**

**Kala-azar. See Leishmaniasis**

**Leishmaniasis**

*Leishmania braziliensis (American mucocutaneous leishmaniasis) and L. mexicana (American cutaneous leishmaniasis)*

| | | | |
|---|---|---|---|
| Drug of choice: | Sodium stibogluconate | Not certain; probably 600 mg IM or IV/d × 6–10d (may be repeated) | 10 mg/kg/d IM or IV (max 600 mg/d) × 6–10d |
| Alternative: | Amphotericin B | 0.25–1 mg/kg by slow infusion daily or every 2d for up to 8 wks | 0.25–1 mg/kg by slow infusion daily or every 2d for up to 8 wks |

| Infection | Drug | Adult Dose | Pediatric Dose |
|---|---|---|---|
| **Leishmaniasis (continued)** | | | |
| *L. donovani (kala-azar, visceral leishmaniasis)* | | | |
| Drug of choice: | Sodium stibogluconate | 600 mg/d IM or IV × 6–10d (may be repeated) | 10 mg/kg/d IM or IV (max 600 mg/d) × 6–10d |
| Alternative: | Pentamidine isethionate | 2–4 mg/kg/d IM for up to 15 doses | 2–4 mg/kg/d IM for up to 15 doses |
| *L. tropica (Oriental sore, cutaneous leishmaniasis)* | | | |
| Drug of choice: | Sodium stibogluconate | 600 mg/d IM or IV × 6–10d (may be repeated) | 10 mg/kg/d IM or IV (max 600 mg/d) × 6–10d |
| Alternative: | Topical treatment | | |
| **Malaria (Plasmodium falciparum, P. ovale, P. vivax, and P. malariae)** | | | |
| *Suppression or chemoprophylaxis of disease while in endemic area (all Plasmodium except chloroquine-resistant P. falciparum)* | | | |
| Drug of choice: | Chloroquine | 300-mg base (500 mg) once weekly beginning 1 wk before and continued for 6 wks after last exposure in endemic area | < 50 kg; 5-mg base/kg once weekly beginning 1 wk before and continued for 6 wks after last exposure in endemic area |
| *Prevention of attack after departure from areas where P. vivax and P. ovale are endemic* | | | |
| Drug of choice: | Primaquine diphosphate | 15-mg base (26.3 mg)/d × 14d (with last 2 wks of chloroquine prophylaxis) | 0.3-mg base/kg/d × 14d (with last 2 wks of chloroquine prophylaxis) |
| *Treatment of uncomplicated attack (all Plasmodium except chloroquine-resistant P. falciparum)* | | | |
| Drug of choice: | Chloroquine | 600-mg base (1 g), then 300-mg base (500 mg) in 6 hrs, then 300-mg base (500 mg)/d × 2d | 10-mg base/kg (max 600-mg base), then 5-mg base/kg 6 hrs later, then 5-mg base/kg/d × 2d |
| *Treatment of severe illness, parenteral dosage—only if dose cannot be administered (regardless of severity) (all Plasmodium except chloroquine-resistant P. falciparum)* | | | |
| Drug of choice: | Quinine dihydrochloride | 600 mg in 300-ml normal saline IV over at least 1 hr; repeat in 6–8 hrs if oral therapy still cannot be started (max 1800 mg/d) | 25 mg/kg/d; administer half of dose in 1-hr infusion, then other half 6–8 hrs later if oral therapy still cannot be started (max 1800 mg/d) |
| OR | Quinacrine hydrochloride | 200-mg base (250-mg) IM q6h | Not recommended |
| *Prevention of relapses ("radical" cure after "clinical" cure) (P. vivax and P. ovale only)* | | | |
| Drug of choice: | Primaquine diphosphate | 15-mg base (26.3 mg)/d × 14d or 45-mg base (79 mg)/wk × 8 wks | 0.3-mg base/kg/d × 14d |

| Drug | Adult dosage | Pediatric dosage |
|---|---|---|
| *P. falciparum (chloroquine-resistant), suppression of chemoprophylaxis* | | |
| Drug of choice: Pyrimethamine *plus* Sulfadoxine | 1 tablet (25 mg pyrimethamine, 500 mg sulfadoxine) once weekly from 1 d before until 6 wks after exposure | 6–11 mos, 1/8 tablet; 1–3 yrs, 1/4 tablet; 4–8 yrs, 1/2 tablet; 9–14 yrs, 3/4 tablet: once weekly from 1d before until 6 wks after exposure |
| *Treatment of uncomplicated attack (chloroquine-resistant P. falciparum)* | | |
| Drug of choice: Quinine sulfate | 650 mg tid × 3d | 25 mg/kg/d in 3 doses × 3d |
| *plus* Pyrimethamine | 25 mg bid × 3d | < 10 kg: 6.25 mg/d; 10–20 kg: 12.5 mg/d; 20–40 kg: 25 mg/d |
| *plus* Sulfadoxine | 500 mg qid × 5d | 100–200 mg/kg/d in 4 doses × 5d (max 2 g/d) |
| Alternative: Quinine sulfate | 650 mg tid × 3d | 25 mg/kg/d in 3 doses × 3d |
| *plus* Tetracycline | 250 mg qid × 7d | 5 mg/kg qid × 7d |
| *Treatment of severe illness, parenteral dosage (chloroquine-resistant P. falciparum)* | | |
| Drug of choice: Quinine dihydrochloride | 600 mg in 300-ml normal saline IV over at least 1 hr; repeat in 6–8 hrs if oral therapy still cannot be started (max 1800 mg/d) | 25 mg/kg/d; administer half of dose in 1-hr infusion, then other half 6–8 hrs later if oral therapy still cannot be started (max 1800 mg/d) |

**Naegleria spp. See Amoebic Meningoencephalitis, Primary**

| Drug | Adult dosage | Pediatric dosage |
|---|---|---|
| *Necator americanus (hookworm)* | | |
| Drug of choice: Mebendazole | 100 mg bid × 3d | 100 mg bid × 3d for children > 2 yrs |
| OR Pyrantel pamoate | Single dose of 11 mg/kg (max 1 g) | Single dose of 11 mg/kg (max 1 g) |
| Alternative: Thiabendazole | 25 mg/kg bid (max 3 (g/d) × 2d | 25 mg/kg bid (max 3 g/d) × 2d |

**Onchocerca volvulus. See Filariasis**

**Paragonimus westermani. See Flukes**

**Pinworm. See Enterobius vermicularus**

| Drug | Adult dosage | Pediatric dosage |
|---|---|---|
| *Pneumocystis carinii* | | |
| Drug of choice: Trimethoprim–sulfamethoxazole | 20 mg/kg/d, 100 mg/kg/d in 4 doses × 14d | 20 mg/kg/d, 100 mg/kg/d in 4 doses × 14d |
| Alternative: Pentamidine isethionate | 4 mg/kg/d IM × 12–14d | 4 mg/kg/d IM × 12–14d |

| Infection | Drug | Adult Dose | Pediatric Dose |
|---|---|---|---|
| **Roundworm. See Ascaris lumbricoides** | | | |
| **Schistosomiasis** | | | |
| *Schistosoma haematobium* | | | |
| Drug of choice: | Metrifonate | 10 mg/kg every other wk × 3 | 10 mg/kg every other wk × 3 |
| Alternative: | Praziquantel | 40 mg/kg once | 40 mg/kg once |
| *S. japonicum* | | | |
| Drug of choice: | Praziquantel | 30 mg/kg twice in 1d | 30 mg/kg twice in 1 d |
| Alternative: | Niridazole | 25 mg/kg/d PO (max 1.5 g) × 10d | 25 mg/kg/d PO (max 1.5 g) × 10d |
| *S. mansoni* | | | |
| Drug of choice: | Oxamniquine | 15 mg/kg once | 15 mg/kg once |
| Alternative: | Praziquantel | 40 mg/kg once | 40 mg/kg once |
| **Sleeping sickness. See Trypanosomiasis** | | | |
| **Strongyloides stercoralis** | | | |
| Drug of choice: | Thiabendazole | 25 mg/kg bid (max 3 g/d) × 2d | 25 mg/kg bid (max 3 g/d) × 2d |
| **Tapeworms—Adult or intestinal stage** | | | |
| *Diphyllobothrium latum (fish tapeworm), Taenia saginata (beef tapeworm), Taenia solium (pork tapeworm), Dipylidium caninum (dog tapeworm)* | | | |
| Drug of choice: | Niclosamide | Single dose of 4 tablets (2 g) chewed thoroughly | 11–34 kg: single dose of 2 tablets (1 g); > 34 kg: single dose of 3 tablets (1.5 g) |
| Alternative: | Paramomycin | 1 g q/5min × 4 doses | 11 mg/kg q/5min × 4 doses |
| *Hymenolepis nana (dwarf tapeworm)* | | | |
| Drug of choice: | Niclosamide | Single daily dose of 4 tablets (2 g) chewed thoroughly × 5d | 11–34 kg: single daily dose of 2 tablets (1 g) × 5d; > 34 kg: single daily dose of 3 tablets (1.5 g) × 5d |
| OR | Praziquantel | 15–20 mg/kg once | 15–20 mg/kg once |
| | Paromomycin | 45 mg/kg once/d × 5–7d | 45 mg/kg once/d × 5–7d |

**Tapeworms—Larval or tissue stage**

*Echinococcus granulosus (sheep, cattle, human, and deer hydatid cysts)*

*Treatment:* Surgical resection of cysts is the treatment of choice. When surgery is contraindicated, or cysts rupture spontaneously during surgery, mebendazole (experimental for this purpose in the United States) can be tried.

*Cysticercus cellulosae (T. solium)*

*Treatment:* Surgical resection is the treatment of choice. When surgery is contraindicated, especially in neurocysticercosis, praziquantel can be tried.

**Toxocariasis. See Visceral Larval Migrans**

**Toxoplasmosis (*Toxoplasma gondii*)**
Drug of choice:  Pyrimethamine — 25 mg/d × 3–4 wks
  *plus*
  Trisulfapyrimidines — 2–6 g/d × 3–4 wks
Alternative:  Spiramycin — 2–4 g/d × 3–4 wks

**Trichinellosis (*Trichinella spiralis*)**
Drug of choice:  Steroids for severe symptoms
  *plus*
  Thiabendazole — 25 mg/kg bid × 5d
Alternative:  Mebendazole — 200–400 mg tid × 3d, then 400–500 mg tid × 10d

**Trichomonas vaginalis**
Drug of choice:  Metronidazole — 250 mg tid × 7d

**Trichuris trichiura (whipworm)**
Drug of choice:  Mebendazole — 100 mg bid × 3d

**Trypanosomiasis**
*T. cruzi (South American trypanosomiasis, Chagas' disease)*
Drug of choice:  Nifurtimox — 5 mg/kg/d orally in 4 divided doses, increasing by 2 mg/kg/d every 2 wks until dose reaches 15–17 mg/kg/d

*Trypanosoma brucei gambiense; T. b. rhodesiense (African trypanosomiasis, sleeping sickness)*
Hemolymphatic stage
Drug of choice:  Suramin sodium — 100–200 mg (test dose) IV; then 1 g IV on days 1, 3, 7, 14, and 21
Alternative:  Pentamidine isethionate — 4 mg/kg/d IM × 10d
Late disease with CNS involvement
Drug of choice:  Melarsoprol — 2–3.6 mg/kg/d IV × 3 doses; after 1 wk 3.6 mg/kg/d IV × 3 doses; repeat again after 10–21d
Alternatives:  Tryparsamide — One injection of 30 mg/kg IV every 5 d to total of 12 injections; may be repeated after 1 mo.
  *plus*

| Infection | Drug | Adult Dose | Pediatric Dose |
|---|---|---|---|
| **Trypanosomiasis (continued)** | Suramin sodium | One injection of 10 mg/kg IV every 5 d to total of 12 injections; may be repeated after 1 mo. | Unknown |
| **Visceral Larval Migrans**<br>Drug of choice: | Thiabendazole | 25 mg/kg bid × 5d | 25 mg/kg bid × 5d |
| **Whipworm. See *Trichuris trichiura*** | | | |
| ***Wuchereria bancrofti*. See Filariasis** | | | |

# APPENDIX C

# ADVERSE EFFECTS OF ANTIPARASITIC DRUGS

**Bithionol** *(Bithin)*
*Frequent:* photosensitivity skin reactions; vomiting; diarrhea; abdominal pain; urticaria.

**Chloroquine** *(Aralen; others)*
*Occasional:* pruritus; vomiting; headache; confusion; depigmentation of hair; skin eruptions; corneal opacity; irreversible retinal injury (especially when total dosage exceeds 100 g); weight loss; partial alopecia; extraocular muscle palsies; exacerbation of psoriasis, eczema, and other exfoliative dermatoses; myalgias.
*Rare:* discoloration of nails and mucous membranes of mouth; nerve-type deafness; blood discrasias; photophobia.

**Crotamiton** *(Eurax; Crotan)*
*Occasional:* skin rash, conjunctivitis.

**Dehydroemetine** Similar to emetine hydrochloride, but possibly less severe.

**Diethylcarbamazine Citrate USP** *(Hetrazan)*
*Frequent:* severe allergic or febrile reactions due to the filarial infection; GI disturbances.
*Rare:* encephalopathy; loss of vision.

**Diiodohydroxyquin** *(Iodoquinol)*
*Occasional:* rash; acne; slight enlargement of the thyroid gland; nausea; diarrhea; cramps; anal pruritus.
*Rare:* optic atrophy and loss of vision after prolonged use in high dosage (for months).

**Diloxanide Furoate** *(Furamide)*
*Frequent:* flatulence.
*Occasional:* nausea; vomiting; diarrhea; urticaria; pruritis.

**Emetine Hydrochloride USP**
*Frequent:* cardiac arrhythmias; precordial pain; muscle weakness; cellulitis at site of injection.
*Occasional:* diarrhea; vomiting; peripheral neuropathy; heart failure.

**Furazolidone** *(Furoxone)*
*Frequent:* nausea; vomiting.
*Occasional:* allergic reactions, including pulmonary infiltration; headache; orthostatic hypotension; hypoglycemia; polyneuritis; MAO inhibitor interactions.
*Rare:* hemolytic anemia in G6PD deficiency in infants less than one month old.

**Lindane** *(Kwell; Gamene)*
*Occasional:* eczematous skin rash; conjunctivitis.
*Rare:* convulsions; aplastic anemia.

**Mebendazole** *(Vermox)*
*Occasional:* diarrhea; abdominal pain.
*Rare:* leukopenia.

**Melarsoprol** *(Mel B; Arsobal)*
*Frequent:* myocardial damage; albuminuria; hypertension; colic; Herxheimer-type reaction; encephalopathy; vomiting; peripheral neuropathy.
*Rare:* shock.

**Metrifonate**   *(Bilarcil)*
*Occasional:* nausea; vomiting; bronchospasm; weakness; diarrhea; abdominal pain.

**Metronidazole**   *(Flagyl)*
*Frequent:* nausea, especially with single high dose; headache; dry mouth; metallic taste.
*Occasional:* vomiting; diarrhea; insomnia; weakness; stomatitis; vertigo; paresthesia; rash; urethral burning; phlebitis at injection site.
*Rare:* ataxia; encephalopathy; pseudomembranous colitis; neutropenia.

**Niclosamide**   *(Yomesan)*
*Occasional:* nausea; abdominal pain.

**Nifurtimox**   *(Bayer 2502; Lampit)*
*Frequent:* anorexia; vomiting; weight loss; loss of memory; sleep disorders, tremor; paresthesia; weakness; polyneuritis.
*Rare:* convulsions.

**Niridazole**   *(Ambilhar)*
*Frequent:* immunosuppression; vomiting; cramps; dizziness; headache.
*Occasional:* diarrhea; slight ECG changes; rash; insomnia; paresthesia.
*Rare:* psychosis; hemolytic anemia in G6PD deficiency; convulsions.

**Oxamniquine**   *(Vansil)*
*Occasional:* headache; fever; dizziness; somnolence; nausea; diarrhea; rash; insomnia; hepatic enzyme changes; ECG changes.
*Rare:* convulsions.

**Paromomycin**   *(Sulfate Humatin)*
*Frequent:* GI disturbance.
*Rare:* eighth-nerve damage (mainly auditory); renal damage.

**Pentamidine Isethionate**   *(Lomidine)*
*Frequent:* hypotension; hypoglycemia; vomiting; blood discrasias; renal damage; pain at injection site.
*Occasional:* may aggravate diabetes; shock; liver damage.
*Rare:* Herxheimer-type reaction; acute pancreatitis.

**Piperazine Citrate USP**   *(Antepar; others)*
*Occasional:* dizziness; urticaria; GI disturbances.
*Rare:* exacerbation of epilepsy; visual disturbances; ataxia; hypotonia.

**Praziquantel**   *(Biltricide)*
*Frequent:* sedation; abdominal discomfort; fever; sweating; nausea; eosinophilia.
*Occasional:* headache; dizziness.

**Primaquine Diphosphate USP**
*Frequent:* hemolytic anemia in G6PD deficiency.
*Occasional:* neutropenia; GI disturbances; methemoglobinemia in G6PD deficiency.
*Rare:* CNS symptoms; hypertension; arrhythmias.

**Pyrantel Pamoate**   *(Antiminth)*
*Occasional:* GI disturbances; headache; dizziness; rash; fever.

**Pyrimethamine USP**   *(Daraprim)*
*Occasional:* blood dyscrasias; folic acid deficiency.
*Rare:* rash; vomiting; convulsions; shock.

**Pyrvinium Pamoate USP**   *(Povan)*
*Frequent:* turns stool red.
*Occasional:* vomiting; diarrhea.
*Rare:* photosensitivity skin reactions.

**Quinacrine Hydrochloride USP**   *(Atabrine)*
*Frequent:* dizziness; headache; vomiting; diarrhea; yellow staining of skin.
*Occasional:* toxic psychosis; insomnia; bizarre dreams; blood dyscrasias; urticaria; blue and black nail pigmentation; psoriasislike rash.
*Rare:* acute hepatic necrosis; convulsions; severe exfoliative dermatitis; ocular effects similar to those caused by chloroquine.

**Quinine Dihydrochloride and Quinine Sulfate**
*Frequent:* cinchonism (tinnitus, headache, nausea, abdominal pain, visual disturbance).
*Occasional:* hemolytic anemia; other blood dyscrasias; photosensitivity reactions.
*Rare:* blindness; sudden death if injected too rapidly.

**Spiramycin**   *(Rovamycin)*
*Occasional:* GI disturbance.
*Rare:* allergic reactions.

**Sodium Stibogluconate**   *(Pentostam)*
*Frequent:* muscle pain and joint stiffness; bradycardia.
*Occasional:* colic; diarrhea; rash; pruritus; myocardial damage.
*Rare:* liver damage; hemolytic anemia; renal damage; shock; sudden death.

**Suramin Sodium**   *(Germanin)*
*Frequent:* vomiting; pruritus; urticaria; paresthesia; hyperesthesia of hands and feet; photophobia; peripheral neuropathy.
*Occasional:* kidney damage; blood dyscrasias; shock; optic atrophy.

**Tetrachloroethylene**   *(Nema Worm Capsules, Vet)*
*Frequent:* epigastric burning; dizziness; headache.
*Occasional:* drowsiness; Antabuse-like effect with alcohol.
*Rare:* hepatic necrosis.

**Thiabendazole**   *(Mintezol)*
*Frequent:* nausea; vomiting; vertigo.
*Occasional:* leukopenia; crystalluria; rash; hallucinations; olfactory disturbance; Stevens–Johnson syndrome.
*Rare:* shock; tinnitus.

**Tryparsamide**
*Frequent:* nausea; vomiting.
*Occasional:* impaired vision; optic atrophy; fever; exfoliative dermatitis; allergic reactions; tinnitus.

# PHOTO AND ILLUSTRATION CREDITS

## CHAPTER 1

**Fig. 1–1** From Thomas Cheng, 1986, *General Parasitology*, 2nd ed. Adapted with permission of Academic Press. **Fig. 1–2** Adapted with permission of Bobbs-Merrill Co., an imprint of Macmillan Publishing Company, from *Symbiosis: Organisms Living Together* by Thomas C. Cheng. Copyright © 1986 by Macmillan Publishing Company.

## CHAPTER 2

**Fig. 2–2** © Don Fawcett/Photo Researchers, Inc.

## CHAPTER 3

**Fig. 3–2** Reproduced from I. R. Gibbons and A. V. Grimstone in *Journal of Biophysical/Biochemical Cytology*, by copyright permission of Rockefeller University Press. **Fig. 3–3** Swanson/Webster, *The Cell*, 5th ed., © 1985, p. 215. Reprinted by permission of Prentice-Hall, Inc., Engelwood Cliffs, NJ. **Fig. 3–4** Reproduced by permission from Cleveland P. Hickman, Jr., Larry S. Roberts, and Frances M. Hickman, 1988, *Integrated Principles of Zoology*, 8th ed., St. Louis: © 1988 Times Mirror/Mosby College Publishing; original artwork by William C. Ober, M.D. **Fig. 3–5** Photo courtesy, Dr. Keith Vickerman, University of Glasgow. **Fig. 3–6** Swanson/Webster, *The Cell*, 5th ed., © 1985, pp. 215, 216. Reprinted by permission of Prentice-Hall, Inc., Englewood Cliffs, NJ. **Fig. 3–7** From *Cells and Organelles*, 2nd ed., by Alex B. Novikoff and Eric Holtzman, copyright © 1970 by Holt, Rinehart and Winston, Inc., reprinted by permission of the publisher. **Fig. 3–9** © Don Fawcett/Photo Researchers, Inc. **Fig. 3–10** © Don Fawcett/Photo Researchers, Inc. **Fig. 3–11** Photos courtesy, Dr. M. Aikawa, Case Western Reserve University, School of Medicine, from M. Aikawa, P. K. Hepler, C. G. Huff, and H. Sprintz, 1966, *Journal of Cell Biology*, **28**:362, by copyright permission of Rockefeller University Press.

## CHAPTER 4

**Fig. 4–3** Armed Forces Institute of Pathology, Negative No. 74–2981. **Fig. 4–4** © Institut Pasteur/Phototake, NYC. **Fig. 4–9a,b,c** Adapted from *Introduction to Animal Parasitology*, 2nd ed., by J. D. Smyth, published by Halsted Press, a division of John Wiley & Sons, Inc., copyright © 1970 J. D. Smyth. All rights reserved. **Fig. 4–9d** Photo courtesy, Dr. Lawrence Ash, University of California, Los Angeles, School of Public Health. **Fig. 4–10a,b,c** Adapted from *Introduction to Animal Parasitology*, 2nd ed., by J. D. Smyth, published by Halsted Press, a division of John Wiley & Sons, Inc., copyright © 1970 by J. D. Smyth. All rights reserved. **Fig. 4–10d** © Phototake, NYC. **Fig. 4–11** From Thomas Cheng, 1986, *General Parasitology*, 2nd ed. Adapted with permission of Academic Press.

## CHAPTER 5

**Fig. 5–2a, b** Photos courtesy, Dennis E. Feeley, University of Nebraska Medical Center, Lincoln, and Stanley L. Erlandsen, University of Minnesota, School of Medicine, reprinted from W. J. Bemrick and S. L. Erlandsen, "Giardiasis: Is it really zoonosis?" *Parasitology Today*, 4(3):69–70. **Fig. 5–2c** Photo courtesy, Dr. Robert L. Owen, University of California, San Francisco, Veterans Administration Medical Center, reprinted from *Journal of Infectious Diseases*, 140:222–28, by P. C. Nemanic, R. L. Owen, D. P. Stevens, and J. C. Mueller, by permission of The University of Chicago Press, © 1979 The University of Chicago. **Fig. 5–7** Reprinted with permission from D. R. Pitelka, *Electron Microscope Structure of Protozoa*, copyright © 1963, Pergamon Press PLC.

## CHAPTER 6

**Fig. 6–1** Adapted from *Introduction to Animal Parasitology*, 2nd ed., by J. D. Smyth, published by Halsted Press, a division of John Wiley & Sons, Inc., copyright © 1976 by J. D. Smyth. All rights reserved. **Fig. 6–2** Adapted from *Introduction to Animal Parasitology*, 2nd ed., by J. D. Smyth, published by Halsted Press, a division of John Wiley & Sons, Inc., copyright © 1976 by J. D. Smyth. All rights reserved. **Fig. 6–3** From A. M. Fallis (ed.), 1971, *Ecology and Physiology of Parasites*, p. 75. Adapted by permission of the University of Toronto Press. **Fig. 6–4** Adapted by permission of Dr. Keith Vickerman, University of Glasgow. **Fig. 6–5** From Keith Vickerman, 1971, "Morphological and physiological considerations of extra-cellular blood protozoa," in A. M. Fallis (ed.), 1971, *Ecology and Physiology of Parasites*, Fig. 13, p. 75. Adapted by permission of the University of Toronto Press and the author. **Fig. 6–6** Adapted from *Introduction to Animal Parasitology*, 2nd ed., by J. D. Smyth, published by Halsted Press, a division of John Wiley & Sons, Inc., copyright © 1976 by J. D. Smyth. All rights reserved. **Fig. 6–7** © James Webb/Phototake, NYC. **Fig. 6–8** © Institut Pasteur/Phototake, NYC. **Fig. 6–9** Adapted from *Rockefeller Foundation Illustrated*, 4(1), April 1978, by permission of The Rockefeller Foundation. **Fig. 6–10** Adapted from *Rockefeller Foundation Illustrated*, 4(1), April 1978, by permission of The Rockefeller Foundation. **Fig. 6–11** From K. Vickerman and J. D. Barry, 1982, "African trypanosomiasis," in S. Conen and K. S. Warren (eds.), *Immunology of Parasitic Infections*, 2nd ed., p. 210, Oxford: Blackwell Scientific Publications. Adapted with permission from K. Vickerman. **Fig. 6–12** After E. J. A. Brumpt, 1910, *Precis de Parasitologie*. Adapted with permission of MASSON, Paris. **Fig. 6–13** Courtesy, Dr. Julius P. Kreier, Department of Microbiology, Ohio State University.

## CHAPTER 7

**Fig. 7–2** Photos courtesy, R. E. Sinden, DSc., Imperial College of Science and Technology, London, and L. H. Bannister, University of London, Guy's and St. Thomas's Hospitals, from *Tropical Disease Research: Seventh Programme Report*, UNDP/World Bank/WHO Special Programme for Research and Training in Tropical Diseases, Geneva, World Health Organization, 1985. Reproduced with permission of the World Health Organization. **Fig. 7–3** Photos courtesy, Dr. M. Aikawa, Case Western Reserve University, School of Medicine, from M. Aikawa et al., 1978, "Erythrocyte entry by malarial parasites: A moving juncture between erythrocyte and parasite," *Journal of Cell Biology*, 77:75. **Fig. 7–4** Photos courtesy, Dr. M. Aikawa, Case Western Reserve University, School of Medicine, from M. Aikawa et al., 1966, "Comparative feeding mechanisms of avian and primate malarial parasites," in Research in Malaria: An International Panel Workshop, Contribution #95, from Army Research Program on Malaria, *Military Medicine*, 131(9):969–83, Supplement September 1966. **Fig. 7–5** From "Epidemiological assessment of malaria and chloroquine resistance, 1986," *World Health Statistics Quarterly*,

1988, **41**(2):69–71. Adapted with permission of the World Health Organization.   **Fig. 7–6** Photo courtesy, Dr. M. Aikawa, Cast Western Reserve University, School of Medicine, from *Tropical Disease Research: Seventh Programme Report*, UNDP/World Bank/WHO Special Programme for Research and Training in Tropical Diseases, Geneva, World Health Organization, 1985. Reproduced with permission of the World Health Organization.   **Fig. 7–8** From E. Scholtyseck, 1979, *Fine Structure of Parasitic Protozoa: An Atlas of Micrographs, Drawings and Diagrams*, Springer-Verlag, New York. Adapted with permission of the publisher.   **Fig. 7–9** From Y. Matsumoto and Y. Yoshida, 1986, "Advances in *Pneumocystis* biology," *Parasitology Today*, **2**(5):137–42. Adapted by permission of Elsevier Science Publishers. Cambridge, UK.   **Fig. 7–10** Photo courtesy, Elsevier Science Publishers, from Y. Matsumoto and Y. Yoshida, 1986, "Advances in *Pneumocystis* biology," *Parasitology Today*, **2**(5):138. Reproduced with permission of the publisher.

**CHAPTER 8**

**Fig. 8–2** Courtesy, Dr. Burton J. Bogitsh.   **Fig. 8–4** Courtesy, Dr. Burton J. Bogitsh.   **Fig. 8–5** Courtesy, Dr. Burton J. Bogitsh.   **Fig. 8–6** From Thomas Cheng, 1986, *General Parasitology*, 2nd ed. Adapted with permission of Academic Press.   **Fig. 8–7** Courtesy, Dr. Burton J. Bogitsh.   **Fig. 8–8** From Asa C. Chandler and Clark P. Read, 1961, *Introduction to Parasitology*, 10th ed. Copyright © 1930, 1936, 1940, 1944, 1949 by Asa C. Chandler. Copyright © 1955, 1961 by John Wiley & Sons, Inc. All rights reserved.   **Fig. 8–9** From Thomas Cheng, 1986, *General Parasitology*, 2nd ed. Adapted with permission of Academic Press.   **Fig. 8–10** From Thomas Cheng, 1986, *General Parasitology*, 2nd ed. Adapted with permission of Academic Press.   **Fig. 8–12** Courtesy, Dr. Burton J. Bogitsh.   **Fig. 8–13** Courtesy, Dr. Burton J. Bogitsh.   **Fig. 8–14** From Thomas Cheng, 1986, *General Parasitology*, 2nd ed. Adapted with permission of Academic Press.   **Fig. 8–15a, b, c, e** © Phototake, NYC.   **Fig. 8–15d** © Camera M. D. Studios, 1989. All rights reserved.   **Fig. 8–15f** © John Durham/Science Photo Library/Photo Researchers, Inc.   **Fig. 8–17** D. L. Belding, *Textbook of Parasitology*, 3rd ed., copyright © 1965. Reprinted by permission of Appleton-Century-Crofts, Norwalk, CT.   **Fig. 8–20** Redrawn after T. C. Cheng and H. A. James, 1960,

*Transactions of the American Microscopical Society*. Adapted with permission of the American Microscopical Society.   **Fig. 8–22** From E. A. Meuleman et al., 1978, "Ultrastructural changes in the body wall of *Schistosoma mansoni* during the transformation of the mother sporocyst in the snail host, *Biophalaria pfeifferi*," *Parasitology Research*, **56**:227–42. Copyright © 1978, Springer-Verlag, New York. Adapted by permission of the publisher.   **Fig–24** D. L. Belding, *Textbook of Parasitology*, 3rd ed., copyright © 1965. Reprinted by permission of Appleton-Century-Crofts, Norwalk, CT.

**CHAPTER 9**

**Fig. 9–1a** Supplied by Carolina Biological Supply Company.   **Fig. 9–1b** Courtesy, Dr. Lawrence Ash, University of California, Los Angeles, School of Public Health.   **Fig. 9–2** Reprinted with permission of Macmillan Publishing Company from *Principles of Parasitology* by W. C. Marquardt and R. S. Demaree. Copyright © 1986 by William C. Marquardt and Richard S. Demaree.   **Fig. 9–3** From H. Yoshimura, 1965, "The life cycle of *Clonorchis sinensis*: A comment on the presentation in the Seventh Edition of Craig and Faust's *Clinical Parasitology*," *Journal of Parasitology*, **51**:961–66.   **Fig. 9–4** Supplied by Carolina Biological Supply Company.   **Fig. 9–5** Reprinted with permission of Macmillan Publishing Company from *Principles of Parasitology* by W. C. Marquardt and R. S. Demaree. Copyright © 1986 by William C. Marquardt and Richard S. Demaree.   **Fig. 9–7** Redrawn after Monnig, 1934, *Veterinary Helminthology and Entomology*, as adapted in Thomas Cheng, 1986, *General Parasitology*, 2nd ed. Adapted with permission of Academic Press.   **Fig. 9–8a** From Thomas Cheng, 1986, *General Parasitology*, 2nd ed. Adapted with permission of Academic Press.   **Fig. 9–8b** After R. T. Leiper, 1913, *Transactions of the Royal Society of Tropical Medicine & Hygiene*, London. Adapted by permission of the Royal Society of Tropical Medicine & Hygiene.   **Fig. 9–11a** © Bruce Iverson.   **Fig. 9–11b** From Thomas Cheng, 1986, *General Parasitology*, 2nd ed. Reproduced with permission of Academic Press.

**CHAPTER 10**

**Fig. 10–1** From *The Control of Schistosomiasis: Report of a WHO Expert Committee*, Geneva, World Health Organization, 1985, WHO Technical Report Series, No. 728, original maps drawn by Ch. Cheung.   **Fig. 10–4** © Bruce Iverson.   **Fig. 10–5** H. W. Brown

and F. A. Neva, *Basic Clinical Parasitology*, 5th ed., copyright © 1983. Reprinted by permission of Appleton-Century-Crofts, Norwalk, CT.   **Fig. 10–6** Courtesy, Dr. Burton J. Bogitsh.   **Fig. 10–7a** H. W. Brown and F. A. Neva, *Basic Clinical Parasitology*, 5th ed., copyright © 1983. Reprinted by permission of Appleton-Century-Crofts, Norwalk, CT.   **Fig. 10–7b** From Thomas Cheng, 1986, *General Parasitology*, 2nd ed. Adapted with permission of Academic Press.   **Fig. 10–8** H. W. Brown and F. A. Neva, *Basic Clinical Parasitology*, 5th ed., copyright © 1983. Reprinted by permission of Appleton-Century-Crofts, Norwalk, CT.   **Fig. 10–9** © Camera M. D. Studios, 1989. All rights reserved.

**CHAPTER 11**

**Fig. 11–2** © Bruce Iverson.   **Fig. 11–3** From E. Loser, 1965, "Die Eibildug bei Cestoden," *Zeitschrift fur Parasitenkunde*, **25**:556–80. Copyright © 1985, Springer-Verlag, Heidelberg. Adapted with permission of the publisher.   **Fig. 11–6** From Thomas Cheng, 1986, *General Parasitology*, 2nd ed. Adapted with permission of Academic Press.   **Fig. 11–11** From E. Loser, 1965, "Die Eibildug bei Cestoden," *Zeitschrift fur Parasitenkunde*, **25**:556–80. Copyright © 1985, Springer-Verlag, Heidelberg. Adapted with permission of the publisher.   **Fig. 11–13** © Bruce Iverson.

**CHAPTER 12**

**Fig. 12–4** H. W. Brown and F. A. Neva, *Basic Clinical Parasitology*, 5th ed., copyright © 1983. Reprinted by permission of Appleton-Century-Crofts, Norwalk, CT.   **Fig. 12–8** From Asa C. Chandler and Clark P. Read, 1961, *Introduction to Parasitology*, 10th ed. Copyright © 1930, 1936, 1940, 1944, 1949 by Asa C. Chandler. Copyright © 1955, 1961 by John Wiley & Sons, Inc. All rights reserved.

**CHAPTER 13**

**Fig. 13–1** Photo courtesy, Formosan Medical Association, Taiwan, Republic of China, from Wang and Cross, 1974, *Journal of the Formosan Medical Association*, **73**:173–77.   **Fig. 13–2** © Bruce Iverson.   **Fig. 13–3a** Photo by Dr. Warren Buss, provided courtesy of Dr. Gerald D. Schmidt, University of Northern Colorado, from Gerald D. Schmidt and Larry S. Roberts, 1985, *Foundations of Parasitology*, 3rd ed., St. Louis, copyright © 1985, Times Mirror/Mosby College Publishing. Reproduced with permission of the publisher.   **Fig. 13–3b** Photo courtesy, Dr. A. Flissner, Ciudad Universitaria,

Instituto de Investigaciones Biomedicas, from chapter by Dr. Genaro Horacio-Zenteno-Alanis in A. Flissner (ed.), 1982, *Cysticercosis: Present State of Knowledge and Perspectives.* Reproduced with permission of Academic Press. **Fig. 13–4** Adapted from Frank A. Brown (ed.), 1950, *Selected Invertebrate Types,* copyright © 1950 by John Wiley & Sons, Inc. All rights reserved. **Fig. 13–5** From D. P. McManus and J. D. Smyth, 1986, "Hydatidosis: Changing concepts in epidemiology and speciation," *Parasitology Today,* **2**(6):163–68. Adapted by permission of Elsevier Science Publishers, Cambridge, UK. **Fig. 13–6** Adapted from Frank A. Brown (ed.), 1950, *Selected Invertebrate Types,* copyright © 1950 by John Wiley & Sons, Inc. All rights reserved. **Fig. 13–7** From D. P. McManus and J. D. Smyth, 1986, "Hydatidosis: Changing concepts in epidemiology and speciation," *Parasitology Today,* **2**(6):163–68. Adapted by permission of Elsevier Science Publishers, Cambridge, UK. **Fig. 13–8** Photos by Dr. Calum McPherson, provided courtesy Dr. D. P. McManus, Imperial College of Science and Technology, London, from D. P. McManus and J. D. Smyth, 1986, "Hydatidosis: Changing concepts in epidemiology and speciation," *Parasitology Today,* **2**(6):163–68. Reproduced by permission of Elsevier Science Publishers, Cambridge, UK.

## CHAPTER 14

**Fig. 14–1** Reprinted with permission of Macmillan Publishing Company from *Introduction to Parasitology* by W. C. Marquardt and R. S. Demaree. Copyright © 1986 by William C. Marquardt and Richard S. Semaree. **Fig. 14–2** Photo courtesy, Dr. Don L. Lee, University of Leeds, UK, from Don L. Lee, 1977, *Comparative Biology of Skin,* Zoological Society of London Symposia, Vol. 39:150. **Fig. 14–3** From Thomas Cheng, 1986, *General Parasitology,* 2nd ed. Adapted with permission of Academic Press. **Fig. 14–4** From Thomas Cheng, 1986, *General Parasitology,* 2nd ed. Adapted with permission of Academic Press. **Fig. 14–6** Reproduced from *Journal of Cell Biology,* 1965, **26**:580, by copyright permission of Rockefeller University Press. **Fig. 14–7** Adapted from *Introduction to Animal Parasitology,* 2nd ed., by J. D. Smyth, published by Halsted Press, a division of John Wiley & Sons, Inc. Copyright © 1979 by J. D. Smyth. All rights reserved. **Fig. 14–8a, b** From H. D. Crofton, 1966, *Nematodes,* Hutchinson University Library, published by Unwin Hyman, Ltd.,

London. Adapted by permission of the publisher. **Fig. 14–8c** From Thomas Cheng, 1986, *General Parasitology,* 2nd ed. Adapted by permission of Academic Press. **Fig. 14–9** From F. G. W. Jones, 1959, *Plant Pathology: Problems and Progress 1908–1958,* © 1959 University of Wisconsin Press. Adapted with permission of the publisher. **Fig. 14–10** Adapted from *Introduction to Animal Parasitology,* 2nd ed., by J. D. Smyth, published by Halsted Press, a division of John Wiley & Sons, Inc. Copyright © 1979 by J. D. Smyth. All rights reserved. **Fig. 14–11a** After S. Vottenlogel, 1902, *Zoologische Jahrbeucher Abteilung Anat.* Adapted with permission of VEB Gustav Fisher Verlag, DDR. **Fig. 14–11b, c** After J. G. de Man, 1907, *Memoires de la Société Zoologique de France.* Adapted with permission of the Société Zoologique de France. **Fig. 14–13a, b, e** © Bruce Iverson. **Fig. 14–13c** © Martin Rotker/Phototake, NYC. **Fig. 14–13d** Courtesy, Dr. Lawrence Ash, University of California, Los Angeles, School of Public Health. **Fig. 14–13f** © James Webb/Phototake, NYC. **Fig. 14–14** From Don L. Lee, 1965, *The Physiology of Nematodes.* Adapted with permission of Oliver and Boyd, Publishers, London. **Fig. 14–11a** After S. Vottenlogel, 1902, *Zoologische Jahrbeucher Abteilung Anat.* Adapted with permission of VEB Gustav Fisher Verlag, DDR. **Fig. 14–11b, c** After J. G. de Man, 1907, *Memoires de la Société Zoologique de France.* Adapated with permission of the Société Zoologique de France. **Fig. 14–13a, b, e** © Bruce Iverson. **Fig. 14–13c** © Martin Rotker/Phototake, NYC. **Fig. 14–13d** Courtesy, Dr. Lawrence Ash, University of California, Los Angeles, School of Public Health. **Fig. 14–13f** © James Webb/Phototake, NYC. **Fig. 14–14** From Don L. Lee, 1965, *The Physiology of Nematodes.* Adapted with permission of Oliver and Boyd, Publishers, London. **Fig. 14–15** From Thomas Cheng, 1986, *General Parasitology,* 2nd ed. Adapted with permission of Academic Press.

## CHAPTER 15

**Fig. 15–1** H. W. Brown/F. A. Neva, *Basic Clinical Parasitology,* 5th ed., copyright © 1983. Reprinted by permission of Appleton-Century-Crofts, Norwalk, CT. **Fig. 15–2** H. W. Brown/F. A. Neva, *Basic Clinical Parasitology,* 5th ed., copyright © 1983. Reprinted by permission of Appleton-Century-Crofts, Norwalk, CT. **Fig. 15–3** Adapted from *Introduction to Parasitology,* 2nd ed., by J. D. Smyth, published by Halsted Press, a division of John Wiley & Sons, Inc. Copyright © 1976 by J. D. Smyth. All

rights reserved. **Fig. 15–5a** © Dickson Despommier/Photo Researchers, Inc. **Fig. 15–5b** From Thomas Cheng, 1986, *General Parasitology,* 2nd ed. Adapted with permission of Academic Press. **Fig. 15–5c** © Dickson Despommier/Photo Researchers, Inc. **Fig. 15–6** After E. W. Faust, 1949, *Human Helminthology: A Manual for Physicians, Sanitarians and Medical Zoologists.* Adapted with permission from Kimpton Medical Publications, London. **Fig. 15–10** © James Webb/Phototake, NYC. **Fig. 15–11** Adapted from *Introduction to Parasitology,* 2nd ed., by J. D. Smyth, published by Halsted Press, a division of John Wiley & Sons, Inc. Copyright © 1976 by J. D. Smyth. All rights reserved. **Fig. 15–12** H. W. Brown/F. A. Neva, *Basic Clinical Parasitology,* 5th ed., copyright © 1983. Reprinted by permission of Appleton-Century-Crofts, Norwalk, CT. **Fig. 15–13** Courtesy, Dr. Burton J. Bogitsh. **Fig. 15–14** © Camera M.D. Studios. All rights reserved. **Fig. 15–15** Reprinted with permission of Macmillan Publishing Company from *Invertebrate Zoology Laboratory Workbook,* 3rd. ed., by D. E. Beck and L. F. Braithwaite. Copyright © 1968 by Macmillan Publishing Company. **Fig. 15–16** Reprinted with permission of Macmillan Publishing Company from *Introduction to Parasitology* by W. C. Marquardt and R. S. Demaree. Copyright © 1986 by William C. Marquardt and Richard S. Demaree. **Fig. 15–17** © Phototake, NYC.

## CHAPTER 16

**Fig. 16–2** © Institut Pasteur/Phototake, NYC. **Fig. 16–3** Reprinted with permission of Macmillan Publishing Company from *Introduction to Parasitology* by W. C. Marquardt and R. S. Demaree. Copyright © 1986 by William C. Marquardt and Richard S. Demaree. **Fig. 16–4a** © Bruce Iverson. **Fig. 16–4b** Armed Forces Institute of Pathology, Negative No. 68–7638–3. **Fig. 16–5** Armed Forces Institute of Pathology, Negative No. 67–5368–1. **Fig. 16–6** © James Webb/Phototake, NYC. **Fig. 16–7** © Phototake, NYC.

## CHAPTER 17

**Fig. 17–1** (top) Courtesy, National Center for Communicable Diseases, U.S. Public Health Service, Atlanta, GA. **Fig. 17–1** (bottom) From Thomas Cheng, 1986, *General Parasitology,* 2nd ed. Adapted with permission of Academic Press. **Fig. 17–4b, d** From Thomas Cheng, 1986, *General Parasitology,* 2nd ed. Adapted with permission of

Academic Press.    **Fig. 17–4c** Adapted from C. L. Metcalf and W. P. Flint, 1962, *Destructive and Useful Insects*, with permission of McGraw-Hill, New York.    **Fig. 17–5** After R. E. Snodgrass, *Smithsonian Miscellaneous Collection 110*, Number 10, Fig. 2.7. Reprinted by permission of the Smithsonian Institution Press.    **Fig. 17–6** From Thomas Cheng, 1986, *General Parasitology*, 2nd ed. Adapted with permission of Academic Press.    **Fig. 17–7** From Thomas Cheng, 1986, *General Parasitology*, 2nd ed. Adapted with permission of Academic Press.    **Fig. 17–8** Courtesy, National Center for Communicable Diseases, U.S. Public Health Service, Atlanta, GA.    **Fig. 17–9** © 1986 L. West/Photo Researchers, Inc.    **Fig. 17–10a, d** From Thomas Cheng, 1986, *General Parasitology*, 2nd ed. Adapted with permission of Academic Press.    **Fig. 17–10b, c** From W. Byam and R. G. Archibald, 1921–23, *The Practice of Medicine in the Tropics*, Hodder & Stoughton, N. Pomfret, VT.    **Fig. 17–11a** Adapted from Robert Matheson, 1950, *Medical Entomology*, 2nd ed. Copyright © 1950 by Comstock Publishing Company, Inc. Used by permission of the publisher, Cornell University Press.    **Fig. 17–11b, c** From Thomas Cheng, 1986, *General Parasitology*, 2nd ed. Adapted with

permission of Academic Press.    **Fig. 17–12** Armed Forces Institute of Pathology, Negative No. 75–5783.    **Fig. 17–13a** Adapted from E. Francis, 1919, *Public Health Reports*, U.S. Department of Health and Human Services.    **Fig. 17–13b** From Thomas Cheng, 1986, *General Parasitology*, 2nd ed. Adapted with permission of Academic Press.    **Fig. 17–14** From Thomas Cheng, 1986, *General Parasitology*, 2nd ed. Adapted with permission of Academic Press.    **Fig. 17–14b** After E. A. Brumpt, 1910, *Precis de Parasitologie*, adapted with permission of MASSON, Paris.    **Fig. 17–15** Armed Forces Institute of Pathology, Negative No. 65–5015.    **Fig. 17–16** Courtesy, National Center for Communicable Diseases, U.S. Public Health Service, Atlanta, GA.    **Fig. 17–17** Adapted from G. T. Strickland, *Hunter's Tropical Medicine*, 6th ed., copyright © 1984 by Saunders College Publishing, a division of Holt, Rinehart and Winston, Inc., reproduced by permission of the publisher.    **Fig. 17–18** From A. W. Bacot and C. S. Martin, 1914, *Journal of Hygiene, Epidemiology, Microbiology and Immunology*. Adapted with permission of Karger Libri AG, Basel, Switzerland.    **Fig. 17–19** Armed Forces Institute of Pathology, Negative No. 219900–7B.    **Fig. 17–20** © Institut Pasteur/Phototake, NYC.    **Fig. 17–21a, b** From D. Keilin

and G. H. F. Nuttall, 1930, *Parasitology*. Adapted with permission of Cambridge University Press, Cambridge, UK.    **Fig. 17–21c** From Thomas Cheng, 1986, *General Parasitology*, 2nd ed. Adapted with permission of Academic Press.    **Fig. 17–22** From James R. Busvine, 1975, *Arthropod Vectors of Disease*, Studies in Biology, No. 55, Edward Arnold Publishers, London. Adapted with permission of the author.    **Fig. 17–23** From James R. Busvine, 1975, *Arthropod Vectors of Disease*, Studies in Biology, No. 55, Edward Arnold Publishers, London. Adapted with permission of the author.

## COLOR SECTION

**Page 1** © Lennart Nilsson.    **Page 2** © World Health Organization.    **Page 3** © World Health Organization.    **Page 4** © World Health Organization.    **Page 5** © World Health Organization.    **Page 6** (top) Courtesy, Dr. Burton J. Bogitsh.    **Page 6** (middle) Courtesy, Dr. Burton J. Bogitsh.    **Page 6** (bottom) Courtesy, Dr. Burton J. Bogitsh.    **Page 7** (top) © Bruce Iverson.    **Page 7** (bottom) © Eric V. Grave/Photo Researchers, Inc.    **Page 8** (top) Drawing by Cecile Duray-Bito.    **Page 8** (bottom left) © Lennart Nilsson.    **Page 8** (bottom right) © Alfred Pasieka/Bruce Coleman, Inc.

# INDEX

References to photographs and illustrations are printed in boldface type.